# New Frontiers in Nursing

# New Frontiers in Nursing

Edited by Byrant Hill

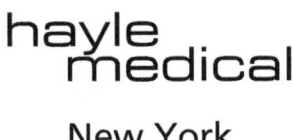

hayle
medical

New York

Hayle Medical,
750 Third Avenue, 9th Floor,
New York, NY 10017, USA


Visit us on the World Wide Web at:
www.haylemedical.com

ISBN: 978-1-63241-541-7

**Cataloging-in-Publication Data**

New frontiers in nursing / edited by Byrant Hill.
    p. cm.
Includes bibliographical references and index.
ISBN 978-1-63241-541-7
1. Nursing. 2. Nursing--Practice. I. Hill, Byrant.
RT42 .N49 2019
610.73--dc23

# Table of Contents

# Preface

Nursing is a health care profession that involves the promotion of health, prevention of illness and provision of care to disabled, sick and dying individuals. To achieve these objectives, nursing integrates principles of social science, technology, physical science and nursing theory. Nurses help in patient care by coordinating with other physicians, therapists, dieticians, etc. It also involves treating patients, taking records of their medical history, providing emotional support and follow-up-care. This book covers in detail some existing theories and modern approaches to nursing. Selected topics that redefine this profession have been presented in this book. For someone with an interest and eye for detail, this book covers the most significant topics in this field.

The researches compiled throughout the book are authentic and of high quality, combining several disciplines and from very diverse regions from around the world. Drawing on the contributions of many researchers from diverse countries, the book's objective is to provide the readers with the latest achievements in the area of research. This book will surely be a source of knowledge to all interested and researching the field.

In the end, I would like to express my deep sense of gratitude to all the authors for meeting the set deadlines in completing and submitting their research chapters. I would also like to thank the publisher for the support offered to us throughout the course of the book. Finally, I extend my sincere thanks to my family for being a constant source of inspiration and encouragement.

**Editor**

# Developing and Evaluating the Integration of Life and Social Sciences Teaching to First-Year Nursing Students

**John J Power***, **Johanna McMullan** and **Tony O'Connor**

*School of Nursing and Midwifery, Queen's University Belfast, Ireland*

**\*Corresponding author:** John J Power, School of Nursing and Midwifery, Queen's University Belfast, Ireland, E-mail: j.power@qub.ac.uk

## Abstract

**Title:** Evaluating the integrating of life and social sciences teaching to first-year nursing students.

**Objectives:** To evaluate an integrated teaching and learning approach to first-year nursing students, combining the life, social sciences and public health with a more integrated and clinical focused approach to teaching delivery

**Background:** Historically within the School of Nursing and Midwifery the life sciences and social sciences had been taught as separate modules with separate teaching teams. This had reflected in a somewhat dis-integrated approach to student learning and understanding without clear clinical focus on application. With focus upon student learning the teaching teams engaged with a stepped, incremental and progressive movement towards developing and delivering a more integrated structure of learning, combining the life sciences, social sciences and public health teaching and learning within the one extended first-year module. The focus was particularly on integrated understanding and clinical relevance. This paper discusses both the approach to developing the integrated model of teaching and the evaluation of that teaching.

**Results:** The module combining life, social science and Public health teaching was positively evaluated by the students. Evaluations are compared and contrasted from 2 nursing student groups of admissions.

- integrated learning
- clinical relevance
- combining life and social science teaching

## Introduction and Background

Before commencement of the academic year 2012/2013 the social sciences, public health and the biomedical sciences were taught and assessed as separate modules in the first year. This tended to reinforce the idea off separate disciplines and in the minds off certainly some of the younger students a failure to appreciate the interconnectedness (whole person) perspective on health; with separate modules taught and assessed in separate silos(a teacher centred, subject specific and specialized discipline). This became evident from earlier evaluations of the modules and impact of teaching and learning with some evidence of disproportionality in terms of delivery and impact on student nurse education.

Porter and Ryan in 1996 [1] discuss the need to 'break the boundaries' between nursing and sociology. Benbasset et al. in 2003 [2] in addressing some of the barriers to the teaching and learning of the behavioural and social sciences to medical students, suggest the importance of integrated courses and ideally begun early in the curriculum. Satterfield et al. in 2004 [3] also suggest the value of an early integration of the social and behavioural sciences within the medical curriculum to help address a more holistic approach to care and treatment. Borrell- Carrio et al. in 2004 [4] discuss the value of Engels earlier concept a bio - psychosocial model in promoting health and managing patients care. Cohen in 2015 [5] argues for the importance of holistic nursing and to better achieve this students' need

to be educated holistically; significantly to reduce or eliminate disciplinary division and fragmentation in health education.

Young and Paterson in 2007 [6] and Bruce in 2007 [7] suggest that historically there was perhaps a tendency towards an over structured curriculum and categorisation; the current focus would not necessarily negate 'fixed information' but with more of an emphasis on integration better reflecting the need to prepare students for social political and clinical situations that are complex moralistic and unpredictable' (p.423). In a significant and landmark work in nurse education, Wynne et al. in 1997 [8] discussed the position of the biological sciences within pre-registration nurse education as an 'incomplete holism' and the need for teachers to 'impart biological knowledge in a manner that can be readily applied by students to inform their clinical practice' (p.470). Connie and Rowles in 2012 [9] discuss the effective use of the student centred innovation and a more collective/integrated approach to the teaching of the sciences.

Jillings in 2007 [10] and Billings and Halstead in 2012 [11] discuss some of the barriers to student centred learning which include addressing traditional silos of knowledge and expertise in a teacher led approach, rather than focusing on the impact of student learning. The Nursing and Midwifery Council in 2010 [12] Standards for Preregistration Nursing and Midwifery Education focus the need for an integrated model of learning reflective of both the physical but also the psychosocial reality and living environment of patients and clients.

## Developing Health and Wellbeing

As a result of significant discussion and interdisciplinary negotiation, the life, social sciences public health/ health education were drawn together in the one module for the academic year 2012/13. The module seeks to provide the undergraduate students with an introduction in understanding of Life Sciences, psychology, sociology and public health and their contribution within the context of adult nursing, mental health, learning disability children's nursing and midwifery. The intention is to provide the student with a more integrated understanding and teaching to both building and sustaining health individually and to the health of the community within a social context.

The module runs in three phases across the student's first-year and teachers to nursing and midwifery students. They represent the fields of adult nursing, mental health nursing, learning disability, children's nursing and the midwifery students on the three year degree programme. Key weekly lectures are delivered in the social sciences and the Life Sciences (Hub) and developed within the structure of the tutorials and seminars (Spokes) [13,14] which is substantially matched against the topic areas delivered within the Nursing Values module for that particular phase and week. The Nursing Values module runs parallel to this module during the first year and addresses practical clinical application and nursing skills. It is then hoped that the student will not only achieve a more integrated perception of the physical and psychosocial needs of individuals and society but can more directly translate this to nursing care. The significant and predominant emphasis of the module in on health and health promotion (practical holism and the building and sustaining of homoeostasis) rather than the management of disease and disability. The tutorial or seminar topic is addressed in the week following the lecture in order that the student can better collect material and research the topic areas. Teaching is delivered by face to face lectures and by online e-learning resources including an e-virtual community reflecting aspects of social life within N. Ireland. Whilst subject specialists deliver the lectures, the tutorials and seminars are delivered by all lecturers, with the need at least initially to prepare themselves within their non-specialist areas and revise life sciences, social sciences or public health theory as appropriate-in order to ensure appropriate depth of knowledge and understanding reflected in teaching delivery. The development of both a more integrated model of teaching and learning, but also one with a more developed (and on-going development) focus on clinical work, was significantly helped by having colleagues who were also still engaged in practice (joint lecturing and clinical appointments)involved in the development planning and delivery of teaching to the integrated module.

## Phase 1

This provides a broad introduction to the subject areas and the initial grounding in theory. The subject areas include tissues, cells, homeostasis, and overview of the cardiovascular system, the renal system and fluid homeostasis and the immune system and immune resistance. In addition to a broad introduction to the disciplines of psychology and sociology the students are introduced to be theory of attitude development and approaches to attitude and behavioural change. They also explore power relationships particularly within the patient client situation and the characteristics off and approaches to care delivery contrasting compliant models of nursing care with more cooperative and empowering approaches to care. Mapping against (mirroring/reflecting in parallel) the physiology of the immune system the students are introduced to the psychology of stress, homeostasis and psychoneuroimmunology. The Assessment comprises a group project involving the development of and presentation to a health-promoting poster addressing both life and social sciences with a particular public health/health education focus. The group work provides an opportunity for the students in developing team working skills; research; research presentation and teaching delivery. The group work is summatively assessed.

## Phase II

The teaching programme focuses more within a case study delivery. By phase 2 of the students should have completed at least one substantial clinical placement. Within this phase the nervous system, respiratory system, musculoskeletal system and an introduction to pharmacology are addressed within the Life Sciences. Mapping against that and with an introduction to public health principles the particular example of smoking cessation is explored together with some of the theories and models of health related behaviour. Other examples include the exploration of power differentials within medicine and health consultation, addiction and substance misuse, patterns of disordered eating, inequalities in health and homelessness and the students are introduced to Health Care in the Community. The Assessment comprises a class test which consist of multiple choice questions single answer questions or true/false questions. This comprehensively addresses all subject areas from phase 1 and phase 2 of the module.

## Phase III

With at least two placements by then completed the students in this phase further develop the practical application of the life, social sciences and public health with particular focus on maintaining homeostasis in addition to exploring the biology of pain, the endocrine system and the physiology of human reproduction. This again is mirrored within the social sciences and reflecting the approach to death and dying and palliative care delivered within the Nursing Values module, the social science dimension of the module explores death and dying from a psycho-social perspective. In addition this phase of the module introduces the students by way of the key lecture to the historical experience of trauma and civil war within Northern Ireland 'the Troubles', from a health professional's perspective. This is then developed within tutorials which are substantially led by the victims of the Northern Ireland Troubles although overseen by the model teaching team. The Assessment at the end of this phase is in two parts. (1) A written short answer questions examination addressing both life and social science issues within phase III of the module. Questions are delivered in two related sections addressing (a) particular systems of the body (for example, the respiratory system), its description, structure and function and (b) the related and public health approaches to health maintenance and health promotion. (2) A 2000 word formal essay on a particular question which requires the students to address the life sciences, social sciences, public health and health education dimensions of the question within a clinical context. It also encourages the students to reflect theory against case study examples drawn from their practical experience to date. Again the focus is on health maintenance and health promotion.

## Evaluation of the Module and Learning Experience

The module and learning experience was evaluated in two phases. The first phase involved evaluation by first year adult nursing students from the student intake February 2014. The total student intake for that phase was 80 students all to the adult field (N=68). The second phase of evaluation involved adult nursing students from the student intake September 2014 (n=66).

## Data collection

The student's evaluation was investigated by means of a questionnaire and comprised of a number of multiple choice questions using a five point Likert type scale. There was no evident pre-existing scaled questionnaire for this form of evaluation. The questionnaire was therefore developed from an exploration of the literature, discussion with students and with lecturing colleagues. The questionnaire was reviewed and examined by several experienced teachers including fellow Lecturers, Information Technology experts and an Education Technologist who had all been briefed on the study. The questionnaire was fist piloted with any earlier cohort of students.

In order to facilitate larger groups, to ensure confidentiality, ease of collation of data and to keep the time needed to complete to a minimum the Personal Response System (PRS) was used to facilitate the data collection.

## Ethical considerations

Students were informed verbally at the start of the module review what the purpose of the evaluation was and that participation was entirely voluntarily and there would be no repercussions if they chose not to, nor personal benefit gained if they did and that responses would be completely anonymous.

## Results of Evaluation

**February 2014:** 77% of the students found the module stimulating and challenging (39% Good; 38% Very good). 62% of the students rated the module as Good and 26% as Excellent. By way of example and exploring particular aspects of the module, 785 of the students agreed or strongly agreed that the teaching on victims and survivors within the context of 'the troubles' was useful with 82% agreeing or strongly agreeing that the teaching would equip them for dealing with issues regarding victims and survivors that arise within nursing practice.

**Sept 2014:** 93% of the students suggested that the module's aims and objectives were well met (with 37% recording an excellent score against these criteria). Again some 93% of the students felt that the module was well or excellently organised. 90% of the students also found the module stimulating and challenging (47%=Good and 43% as Excellent) overall the module received ratings of 52% Good and 40% Excellent (92%). 7% rated the module as Acceptable and only 1% as Poor. The teaching to victims and survivors of the troubles again seems to have made the students more aware of its relevance to them as health care professionals.

**Examples of the questionnaire evaluations are contained in the Appendix (Figure 1,2):** As these were only first year students it was not considered entirely appropriate to enquire of the practical application of teaching and learning to their clinical experience as they had only by then engaged with three placements. However, informal discussion with the students, suggested significant acknowledgement of the practical application of theory to clinical experience.

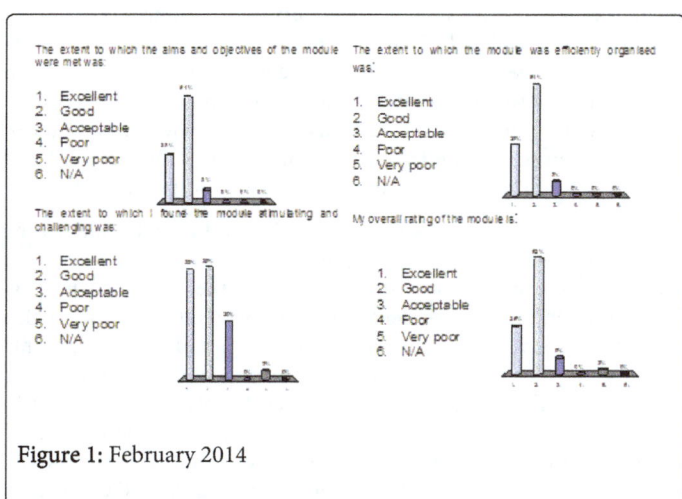

**Figure 1:** February 2014

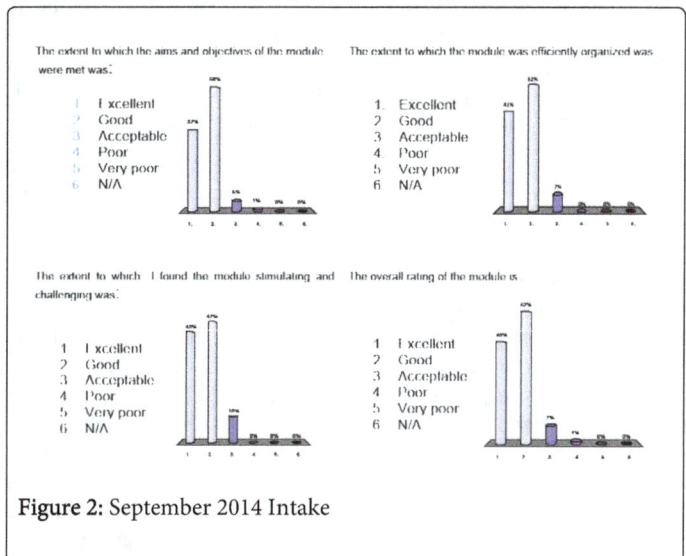

**Figure 2:** September 2014 Intake

## Limitations

This evaluation did not comprise a detailed and constituted study. Substantially to engage the students only a short questionnaire was used, and this could contribute to the limitations of the evaluation. This was a single centred study based in one Higher Education Institution in the United Kingdom. The results also need to be taken cautiously as they examine in some instances perceived effect, it is difficult to assess as yet actual positive effects.

## Discussion and Conclusions

This approach to audit and evaluation has helped to guide the development of the module and a more integrated approach to teaching and learning.

There were difficulties experienced both in developing and combining the life and social sciences and in developing a teaching module that could effect such combination in relation to practice. There was need for effort and goodwill on the part of the existing teaching teams in drawing together the life and social sciences with clear focus on what was in the best interests of facilitating learning to students. The focus was on what could best/better integrate the clinical learning experience for first year students [15]; Wynne et al. in 1997 [8]; Bruce in 2007 [7]. This has involved a stepped/incremental approach with detailed reflection on delivery and evaluation from September 2012 when this innovative combination of teaching for the school was first delivered. Whilst this did not amount to a detailed study of the impact and effect of teaching, this approach to audit and evaluation is of some teaching and potentially clinical value.

By 2014 both intakes of students would seem to have evaluated the module as effective and engaging and this was perhaps even more marked with larger number of students and the combined nursing fields and midwifery students in the September 2014 intake. Significantly, whilst 77% of the smaller group of adult field only students in the February 2014 intake evaluated the module as stimulating and challenging (good/excellent). This figure reflected in 88% for the later and larger September 2014 intake. Although overall ratings for the module for both groups were not dissimilar (88% February 2014 and 92% September 2014) some 26% of the February 2014 rated the module overall as excellent, but by way of significant contrast, some 40% of the September 2014 intake rated the module as excellent. It is not entirely clear why there is some degree of notable difference here but again after each module delivery and module evaluation, incremental changes in teaching delivery are made.

Traditionally within the school the life and social sciences had been taught as separate modules. This seemed to separate both the teaching teams and streams of teaching, but also the learning experience for the students [8,13]. Certainly in combining life and social sciences a number of the lecturers had to recover and develop their depth of knowledge and currency in respect of one or other field of science. However, student evaluations do suggest some degree of significant impact and efficacy in this combined approach- relative to earlier module evaluations, when the subject areas were taught as separate modules. Possibly of a particular relevance was the focus on health and the whole person and although phase 1 of the module was perhaps more grounded in theory phase 2 and phase 3 work was increasingly applied to clinical and case study examples drawn to help the students develop an integrated approach to life ,social sciences and practice. Currently module coordinators are involved with student representatives in remodelling aspects of the module teaching delivery for the coming academic year 2015/2016 together with service user and carer representatives to better reflect and facilitate learning and clinical care needs.

## References

1. Porter S, Ryan S (1996) Breaking the boundaries between nursing and sociology: a critical realist ethnography of the theory-practice gap. J Adv Nurs 24: 413-420.

2. Benbassat J, Baumal R, Borkan JM, Ber R (2003) Overcoming barriers to teaching the behavioral and social sciences to medical students. Acad Med 78: 372-380.

3. Satterfield JM, Mitteness LS, Tervalon M, Adler N (2004) Integrating the social and behavioral sciences in an undergraduate medical curriculum: The UCSF essential core. Acad Med 79: 6-15.

4. Borrell-Carrio F, Suchman AL, Epstein RM (2004) The Biopsychosocial Model 25 Years Later: Principles, Practice and Scientific Enquiry. Annals of Family Medicine, 2: 576-582.

5. Cohen R (2015) We Must Educate Nurses Holistically to Practice Holistically. American Holistic Nursing Association.

6. Young LE, Paterson BL (2007) (Eds) Teaching Nursing Developing a Student Centred Learning Environment: Lippincott Williams Wilkins, Philadelphia.

7. Bruce A (2007) in Young LE And Paterson BL (Eds) Teaching Nursing Developing a Student Centred Learning Environment: Lippincott Williams Wilkins, Philadelphia.

8. Wynne N, Brand S, Smith R (1997) Incomplete holism in pre-registration nurse education: The position of the biological sciences. J Adv Nurs 26: 470-474.

9. Connie J, Rowles D (2012) in Billings DM and Halstead JA ( 2012) (Eds.,) Teaching in nursing- a guide for faculty, St Louis: Elsevier Saunders.

10. Jillings C. Barriers to Student-Centred Teaching: Overcoming Institutional and Attitudinal Obstacles in Young LE and Paterson BL (2007) (Eds.,) Teaching Nursing Developing a Student Centred Learning Environment Philadelphia: Lippincott Williams Wilkins.

11. Billings DM, Halstead JA ( 2012) Teaching in nursing a guide for faculty (fourth edition) St Louis: Elsevier Saunders.

12. Nursing and Midwifery Council (2010) Standards for Education.

13. Crookes K, Crookes PA, Walsh K (2013) Meaningful and engaging teaching techniques for student nurses: A literature review. Nurse Educ Pract 13: 239-243.

14. Nielsen AE, Noone J, Voss H, Mathews LR (2013) Preparing nursing students for the future: an innovative approach to clinical education. Nurse Educ Pract 13: 301-309.

15. Benner P (1984). From novice to expert: Excellence and power in clinical nursing. Menlo Park, CA: Addison-Wesley.

# Job Satisfaction and Associated Factors among Nurses in East Gojjam Zone Public Hospitals Northwest Ethiopia, 2016

**Dessalegn Haile[1*], Tenaw Gualu[1], Haymanot Zeleke[1] and Berhanu Dessalegn[2]**

[1]Department of Nursing, College of Health Sciences, Debre Markos University, Debre Markos, Ethiopia

[2]Department of Nursing and Midwifery, College of Health Sciences, School of Allied Health Sciences, Addis Ababa University, Addis Ababa, Ethiopia

*Corresponding author: Dessalegn Haile, Department of Nursing, College of Health Sciences, Debre Markos University, Debre Markos, Ethiopia, E-mail: dessalegnhaile@gmail.com

## Abstract

**Background:** Job satisfaction represents one of the most complex areas facing today's managers when it comes to managing their employees. The low job satisfaction among nurses results negative outcome that affect both quality and cost of patient care. Dissatisfaction not only gives poor quality, but also less efficient care.

**Objective:** To assess the level of job satisfaction and associated factors among nurses in East Gojjam Zone Public hospitals northwest Ethiopia 2016.

**Method:** Institutional based Cross-sectional study design was employed. Sampling method was simple random sampling and data was collected from March 8 to 23, 2016. Source population of the study were all nurses who work at public hospitals in East Gojjam zone public hospitals and sample size was 181 nurses from the four hospitals. After nurses were proportionally allocated to size from the four hospitals. Data were collected through pretested self-administered structured questionnaire. Both descriptive and inferential statistics were used to present the data

**Results:** A total of 178 nurses were voluntarily agreed to participate in the study with a response rate of 98.3%. Overall average prevalence rate of job satisfaction of this study was 54.2%. The most highly satisfied subscale for study participants was nature of work and the most dissatisfied sub scale was promotion. There was a significance mean difference of job satisfaction between age groups, between sex of respondents and between nurses who had children and nurses who had no children.

**Conclusion:** The average job satisfaction of nurses was at moderate level.

**Keywords:** Job satisfaction; East Gojjam; Nurses

## Introduction

Job satisfaction refers to the attitude and feelings people have about their work. Positive and favorable attitudes towards the job indicate job satisfaction. Negative and unfavorable attitudes towards the job indicate job dissatisfaction [1].

The phenomenon of job satisfaction and dissatisfaction is the function of two needs systems of physiological and psychological. Physiological needs are called extrinsic or hygiene factors which includes: payment, supervision, fringe benefits, operating procedures, coworkers, and communication. Psychological needs are called intrinsic or motivator factors which includes: nature of work, promotion and contingent rewards. The motivation factors come from the nature of the job itself, not from external rewards or job conditions which can lead to satisfaction but their absence can lead only to lack of satisfaction and not dissatisfaction. The hygiene factors are related to the work environment which are external to employees and are controlled by another person rather than the person himself which can lead to dissatisfaction and at best they can produce only lack of dissatisfaction rather than satisfaction [2].

Job satisfaction causes a series of influences on various aspects of organizational life such as the influence of job satisfaction on employee performance, loyalty and absenteeism. For example satisfaction of workers leads to departmental and organizational level improvements, the higher the degree of job satisfaction the higher is the level of employee loyalty and vice versa and when satisfaction is high, absenteeism tends to be low; when satisfaction is low, absenteeism tends to be high [1].

The low job satisfaction among nurses results negative outcome that affect both quality and cost of patient care. Even though the cost of nurse job dissatisfaction has not been directly measured, the high cost of turnover rate has been well established. Moreover, poor patient outcomes increase the length of stay, increase resource utilization and increase the cost of treatment. Nurses who were not satisfied at work were also found to distance themselves from their patients and their nursing chores [3]. With this regard a descriptive cross-sectional study done in Ekiti State, Nigeria showed that majority (67.1%) of the nurses had low degree of job satisfaction while only few nurses (3.1%) reported high degree of satisfaction with job. A significant positive strong correlation was found between overall work environment and the general job satisfaction of the nurse [4]. Another study done among hospital nurses in Kampala, Uganda showed that only 17.4% nurses reported satisfaction with their job [5]. Furthermore study done in Public Hospitals in Ethiopia Tigray region, almost half of Nurses were dissatisfied with their job [6].

There are two approaches to the study of job satisfaction the global approach and the facet approach. The global approach treats job satisfaction as a single, overall feeling toward the job. The facet approach focus on job facets or different aspects of the job. The facet approach permits a more complete picture of job satisfaction. An individual typically has different levels of satisfaction with the various facets [2]. Therefore this study was done based on the facet approach.

The results of this study might be used to guide policy makers and nurse managers to develop a strategies to increase job satisfaction among nurses in hospital setting. Because when job satisfaction nurses improved, then nursing care of the patients might be increased and it might reduce costs for the healthcare organizations as well as individual patients.

## Methods

### Study design and sampling procedure

Institutional based cross-sectional study design was employed. The study was conducted in East Gojjam Zone Public Hospitals. In East Gojjam Zone there were 4 hospitals with a total of 284 nurses during this study. By simple random sampling 181 nurses were included in the study as the study participant.

### Measurement tool

A structured self-administered questionnaire was used to collect data from study participants. Job satisfaction of the nurses was assessed with job satisfaction survey (JSS). The JSS instrument is a 36 item, nine-facet scale with each 4 item of self-report instrument which provides an overall job satisfaction score after assessing nine facets .The sub scales are: pay, promotion, supervision, fringe benefits, contingent rewards, operating conditions, coworkers, nature of work and communication. The respondents agree or disagree on a 6-point likert-scale of: (1) very much disagreement, (2) disagree moderately, (3) disagree slightly, (4) agree slightly, (5) agree moderately, and (6) agree very much. Some items are worded positively while others are worded negatively. Therefore reverse scoring has been made before total summation of the score. The total satisfaction score of the 36 items ranging from 36-216. Therefore scores with a mean item response of 4 or more represents satisfaction, whereas mean responses of 3 or less represents dissatisfaction. Mean scores between 3 and 4 are ambivalence. These scores were then transformed to for 36-216 score. Score of 36-108,109-143 and 144-216 was considered as dissatisfied, ambivalent and satisfied respectively with their jobs. Reliability of the instrument was established with an overall Cronbach's alpha score of 0.91 [7].

### Ethical clearance

Ethical clearance and approval to conduct this research was obtained from research and ethical review board of department of nursing and midwifery, school of allied health science, college of Health science, Addis Ababa University. After thoroughly discussing, the ultimate purpose and method of the study, permission was sought from the study hospitals. The study participants were informed about the objective and expected outcomes of the study and written consent was provided for guaranteeing their choice of participation or refusal.

All the information was recorded anonymously and confidentiality was assured throughout the study.

## Data processing and analysis

The collected data were coded and entered into Epi data version 3.1. Then the cleaned data were exported to SPSS version 23.00. Recoding and reverse coding was done for negative statements. Data analysis was done using descriptive and inferential statistics. Statistical analyses were performed with the use of Independent-Samples T Test, One Way ANOVA and Pearson correlation.

## Results

### Socio demographic and work characteristics of respondents

A total of 181 eligible nurses were included in the study. Among this, about 178 nurses were voluntarily agreed to participate in this study, only 2 were not returned the questionnaires. This resulted in a response rate of 98.3%.

Out of 178 respondents, 102 (57.3%) were males. Moreover, the age of the participants included in this study ranged between 21 and 54 years with mean age of 28.77 (SD=±5.816) years. In addition 90 (50.6%) were married and 65 (36.5%) had children.

Half percent of the participants were nurses with less than or equal to 4 years of work experience. Nearly all participants (93.3%) reported working eight hours standard shift on a typical day. Most of the participants had been working in inpatient departments. From all participants only 28 (15.7%) participants had extra responsibility on the wards/units (Table 1).

| Variables | Category | Frequency | Percentage |
|---|---|---|---|
| Sex | Male | 102 | 57.3 |
| | Female | 76 | 42.7 |
| Age | <25 years | 50 | 28.1 |
| | 26-30 years | 92 | 51.7 |
| | >30 years | 36 | 20.2 |
| Marital status | Single | 88 | 49.4 |
| | Married | 90 | 50.6 |
| Level of education | Diploma | 81 | 45.5 |
| | Bachelor | 97 | 54.5 |
| Work experience | <5 years | 89 | 50 |
| | 5-10 years | 69 | 38.8 |
| | >10 years | 20 | 11.2 |
| Work unit | Inpatient department | 132 | 74.2 |
| | Outpatient department | 46 | 25.8 |
| Extra responsibility | Yes | 28 | 15.7 |
| | No | 150 | 84.3 |

| Working hours/day | 8 h | 166 | 93.3 |
|---|---|---|---|
| | >8 h | 12 | 6.7 |

**Table 1:** Socio demographic and work characteristics of nurses in East Gojjam Zone public hospitals, Ethiopia, June, 2016 (n=178).

## Job satisfaction among nurses

From the descriptive analysis of JSS, respondents reported low satisfaction for payment, promotion, fringe benefits, contingent rewards and operating conditions subscales. The most dissatisfied sub scale was promotion. Study participants were reported moderate satisfaction for supervision. However study participants were highly satisfied for relationship with co-workers, nature of work and communication. The most highly satisfied subscale for study participants was nature of work. In general the mean satisfaction level for all nurses 54.5 %( Table 2).Therefor the average job satisfaction of nurses in east Gojjam zone public hospital was at a moderate level of satisfaction.

| Subscales | Average mean of satisfaction | SD | Average satisfaction (%) |
|---|---|---|---|
| Payment | 2.51 | 1.12 | 41.8 |
| Promotion | 2.18 | 1.24 | 36.3 |
| Supervision | 3.78 | 1.38 | 63.0 |
| Fringe Benefits | 2.40 | 1.10 | 40.0 |
| Contingent Rewards | 2.63 | 1.29 | 43.8 |
| Operating Conditions | 2.83 | 0.76 | 47.2 |
| Relationship with Co-workers | 4.52 | 1.02 | 75.3 |
| Nature of Work | 4.54 | 1.38 | 75.7 |
| Communication | 4.03 | 1.62 | 67.2 |

| Overall average | 3.27 | 0.60 | 54.5 |
|---|---|---|---|

**Table 2:** Subscales with overall average mean, SD and satisfaction level of nurses at East Gojjam Zone public Hospitals, 2016.

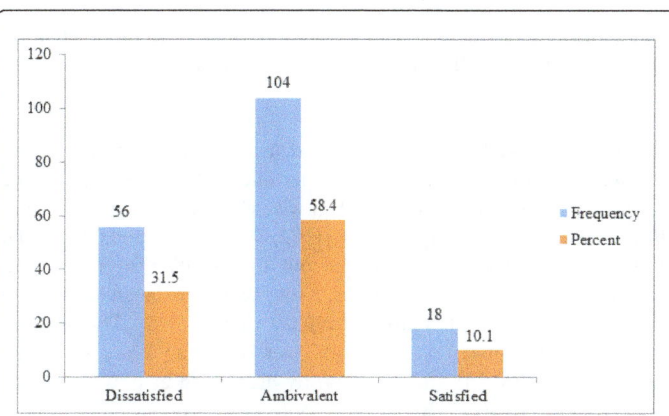

**Figure 1:** Level of job satisfaction among nurses in East Gojjam Zone public hospitals, 2016.

According to Spector JSS, score of 36-108,109-143 and 144-216 was considered as dissatisfied, ambivalent and satisfied respectively with their jobs. Accordingly majority of respondents 104 (58.4%) were ambivalent, 56 (31.5%) were dissatisfied and 18 (10.1%) of participants were satisfied (Figure 1).

## Factors associated with job satisfaction

From the independent sample t-test there was significantly difference mean score of job satisfaction between males and females of respondents. In the same way, there was a significantly difference mean score of job satisfaction between nurses who had children and had no children at $p<0.05$ (Table 3).

| Variables | | Job satisfaction | Mean difference | t | 95% C.I | |
|---|---|---|---|---|---|---|
| | | Mean (SD) | | | Lower | Upper |
| *Sex | Male | 3.18 (0.64) | -0.2 | -2.196 | -0.37 | -0.02 |
| | Female | 3.38 (0.52) | | | | |
| Marital status | Single | 3.20 (0.56) | -0.14 | -1.566 | -0.32 | 0.04 |
| | Married | 3.34 (0.63) | | | | |
| *Having child | Yes | 3.39 (0.51) | 0.2 | 2.195 | 0.02 | 0.38 |
| | No | 3.19 (0.63) | | | | |
| Level of education | Diploma | 3.28 (0.55) | 0.03 | 0.314 | -0.15 | 0.21 |
| | Bachelor | 3.25 (0.63) | | | | |
| Extra responsibility | Yes | 3.42 (0.50) | 0.18 | 1.52 | -0.06 | 0.43 |
| | No | 3.24 (0.61) | | | | |
| Working hours/day | 8 h | 3.26 (0.60) | -0.03 | -0.163 | -0.38 | 0.32 |

| | >8 h | 3.29 (0.54) | | | | |
|---|---|---|---|---|---|---|
| Wok unit Inpatient department | | 3.29 (0.59) | 0.09 | 0.844 | -0.12 | 0.29 |
| Outpatient department | | 3.20 (0.62) | | | | |

**Table 3:** Independent t-test with selected demographic variables of nurses at East Gojjam Zone public hospitals, 2016, *Significant at p –value < 0.05, C.I=Confidence Interval, SD=Standard Deviation.

One way ANOVA was performed to see the relation of job satisfaction with age and work experience. But only age of the respondents was significant at P<0.05 where at least one group means differs from others group means [F (2,175)=3.476, p=0.033]. Then turkey post-hoc testing was carried out to identify the group mean difference in the specific age groups. Accordingly the mean satisfaction level of greater than 30 years old nurses (mean=3.45, SD=0.49) was higher than the mean satisfaction level of 26-30 years of nurses (mean=3.16, SD=0.56) and significantly associated at p=0.036 with a mean difference -0.29 and 95% confidence interval of -0.56 to -0.2.However there was no statistically significant mean difference between less than or equal 25 years nurses and 26-30 years of nurses or between less than or equal 25 years nurses and greater than 30 years old nurses (Table 4).

| Variables | | Job satisfaction | ANOVA, p value |
|---|---|---|---|
| | | Mean (SD) | |
| | <25 years | 3.33 (0.69) | |
| Age* | 26-30 years | 3.16 (0.56) | F=3.476, p=0.033 |
| | >30 years | 3.45 (0.49) | |
| | <5 years | 3.25 (0.63) | |
| Work experience | 6-10 years | 3.23 (0.56) | F=1.592, p=0.206 |
| | >10 years | 3.49 (0.58) | |

**Table 4:** One way ANOVA between age groups and work experience of nurses at East Gojjam Zone public hospitals, Ethiopia 2016.

The Pearson correlation coefficient (r) was tested to examine the relationships between overall job satisfaction score and nine job satisfaction dimension. Overall job satisfaction was significantly and positively correlated with each dimension. Strong correlation was seen between Promotion and total job satisfaction with correlation coefficient (r=0.625) at p=0.01.All other dimensions were moderately correlated with total job satisfaction score (Table 5).

| S. No. | 1 | 2 | 3 | 4 | 5 | 6 | 7 | 8 | 9 | 10 |
|---|---|---|---|---|---|---|---|---|---|---|
| 1 | 1 | | | | | | | | | |
| 2 | 0.488** | 1 | | | | | | | | |
| 3 | 0.625** | 0.538** | 1 | | | | | | | |
| 4 | 0.462** | -0.123 | 0.12 | 1 | | | | | | |
| 5 | 0.575** | 0.340** | 0.485** | 0.126 | 1 | | | | | |
| 6 | 0.543** | 0.375** | 0.319** | 0.025 | .320** | 1 | | | | |
| 7 | 0.300** | 0.172* | 0.257** | -0.091 | 0.073 | 0.279** | 1 | | | |
| 8 | 0.328** | 0.081 | 0.014 | 0.076 | -0.005 | 0.061 | -0.03 | 1 | | |
| 9 | 0.406** | 0.049 | 0.023 | 0.104 | 0.037 | 0.012 | -0.076 | 0.180* | 1 | |
| 10 | 0.592** | -0.086 | 0.101 | 0.473** | 0.197** | 0.083 | 0.098 | 0.143 | 0.243** | 1 |

**Table 5:** Pearson correlations between general job satisfaction of nurses and dimensions of job satisfaction in East Gojjam Zone public hospitals June, 2016, **Correlation is significant at the 0.01 level (2-tailed), *Correlation is significant at the 0.05 level (2-tailed), 1: Overall job satisfaction, 2: Payment, 3: Promotion, 4: Supervision, 5: Fringe benefits, 6: Contingent rewards, 7: Operating conditions, 8: Co-workers, 9: Nature of work, 10: Communication.

## Discussion

This cross-sectional study revealed that the overall average prevalence rate of job satisfaction of this study was at moderate level (54.2%) which was slightly consistent compared with study done in turkey with mean satisfaction level of nurses (58%) [8], in Slovenian hospitals job satisfaction of nurses was at a medium level [9], in Jordan with mean satisfaction level of nurses (57%) [10] and study done in Jordanian and Saudi nurses [11] with mean satisfaction of nurses was moderate level. The possible explanation for slight difference could be due socio economic and organizational difference. And when it was compared with study done Sidama zone public health facilities, south Ethiopia with overall job satisfaction of nurses (52.5%) [12], the current study is slightly high. This minimal difference could be due to study time and the tool used difference.

In this study age of the respondents was significantly associated with job satisfaction. The mean satisfaction level of greater than 30 years old nurses (mean=3.45) was higher than the mean satisfaction level of 26-30 years of nurses (mean=3.16) and significantly associated at p=0.036. Even though the means plot didn't show increasing job satisfaction with increasing age group, older nurses showed more satisfied. This finding was consistent with study in Tigray region [6], where Nurses with older age were more satisfied than nurses with younger age group. This might be older nurse had no other option of jobs so that they were forced to like and satisfied with their current job. However this finding was inconsistent with study in Uganda [5] where younger nurses were more satisfied than older nurses.

The average mean scores for job satisfaction for males was 3.18, SD=0.64 and for females 3.38, SD=0.52). Thus, female's ratings of job satisfaction were significantly higher than male nurses at (t=-2.196, p=0.03).This was consistent with a study in Turkey [8], where female nurses slightly more satisfied than male nurses. The possible explanation might be nursing still perceived to be a job for females rather than males. However this finding contradicted when compared with study in Uganda [5], where no significance difference was seen between female and male.

Nurses who had children, ratings of job satisfaction (mean=3.40, SD=0.51) were significantly higher than nurses had no children (mean=3.20, SD=0.63) at (t=2.2, p=0.03).Having child might be increase personal responsibility which intern dues to the person to like his or her job.

Level of nursing education was not statistically significant in job satisfaction levels. This finding was contradicted with the finding in Uganda [5], where enrolled nurses were more satisfied than registered nurses and in Slovenian hospitals Nurses with a higher education were more satisfied with the job than with lower education [9]. The possible explanation might be in this study area, there was no clear cut job description based on level of nursing education. But this study was consistent with study done in India [3], where no significant association was found between satisfaction and educational level. There was a positive significant correlation between subscales of JSS with total job satisfaction. This was consistent with a study in Cross River State Nigeria and Turkey [8,13], where positive and significant correlation was seen.

Respondents were dissatisfied for payment, promotion, fringe benefit, contingent rewards, and operating conditions. However they were highly satisfied for relationship with co-workers, nature of work and communication and this result was consistent with study done in Jordan and Turkey [8,10]. But this result was inconsistent related with communication with study done in Saudi Arabia [14], where respondents lowest level of satisfaction regarding the communication inside the organization. From the nine sub scales nature of work was got the highest mean satisfaction score and this result was congruent with study in Saudi Arabia and Philippines [15,16]. This might be, even though average satisfaction level of nurse was moderate level still study participants like their profession.

## Conclusion

Averagely, nurses were neither satisfied nor dissatisfied with their jobs, i.e., moderate level of satisfaction. The sub scales in which, nurses indicated satisfaction were nature of work, relationship with co-workers and communication. However the sources of dissatisfaction were promotion, fringe benefits, payment, contingent rewards and operating conditions. Individual factors like age, sex and nurses who had child were significantly associated with total job satisfaction score. All the sub scale were positively and significantly correlation with overall job satisfaction among nurses.

## Recommendation

Based on the findings of the study the following were recommended:

- The Amhara Regional Health Bureau should give great concern on nurses' job satisfaction by reviewing financial and non-financial benefit packages to increase job satisfaction among nurses in hospital setting.

- The study hospital manager should balance the benefit package and internal promotion to increase job satisfaction. The hospital managers should give emphasis for conducive environment for work, appropriate rewards and recognition for achievements among nurses.

- More studies should be conducted on a larger scale especially in a nationwide to identify factors that enhance job satisfaction for the hospital based nurses.

## Acknowledgement

We are grateful to Addis Ababa University and Debre Markos University for funding this study and other supports. We would also like to express our deepest gratitude to study participants.

## References

1. Aziri B (2011) Job satisfaction: A literature review. Mana Res Prac 3: 77-86.

2. Spector PE (1999) Industrial and organizational psychology: Research and practice (2nd eds.) John Wiley and sons Inc., New York.

3. Gulavani A, Shinde M (2014) Occupational stress and job satisfaction among nurses. Int J Scie Res 3: 733-740.

4. Ayamolowo SJ (2013) Job satisfaction and work environment of primary health care Nurses in Ekiti State, Nigeria: An exploratory study.

5. Rose N, Kathleen B, Erica PEHM (2011) Occupational stress, job satisfaction and job performance among hospital nurses in Kampala, Uganda. J Nurs Man 19: 760-768.

6. Medhin G, Berhe H (2012) Job satisfaction of nurses and associated factors in public hospitals in Tigray Region, Northern Ethiopia. Greener J Med Sci 4: 22-37.

7. Spector PE (2011) Job satisfaction survey, JSS Page.

8. Masum AKM, Azad MAK, Hoque KE, Beh L, Wanke P, et al. (2016) Job satisfaction and intention to quit: An empirical analysis of nurses in Turkey. Peer J 4: e1896.

9. Lorber M, Skela Savič B (2012) Job satisfaction of nurses and identifying factors of job satisfaction in Slovenian Hospitals. Croat Med J 53: 263-270.

10. Raddaha AHA, Alasad J, Albikawi ZF, Batarseh KS, Realat EA et al. (2012) Jordanian nurses @TM job satisfaction and intention to quit. Leadership in Health Service 25: 216-231.

11.   Aburuz ME (2014) A comparative study about the impact of stress on job satisfaction between Jordanian and Saudi nurses. Eur Sci J 10: 162-172.

12.   Asegid A, Belachew T, Yimam E (2014) Factors influencing job satisfaction and anticipated turnover among nurses in Sidama Zone Public Health Facilities, South Ethiopia. Nurs Res Pract 26.

13.   Edoho SP, Bamidele E, Neji OI, Frank AE (2015) Job satisfaction among Nurses in Public Hospitals in Calabar, Cross River State Nigeria. Am J Nurs 4: 231-237.

14.   Kamal SM, Al-Dhshan MI, Abu-Salameh KA, Abuadas FH, Hassan MM (2012) The effect of nurses' perceived job related stressors on job satisfaction in Taif Governmental Hospitals in Kingdom of Saudi Arabia. J Am Sci 8: 119-125.

15.   Rosales RA, Labrague, LJ, Rosales GL (2013) Nurses ' Job satisfaction and Burnout: Is there a connection? Int J Adv Nurs Stud 2: 1-10.

16.   Saleh AM, Saleh MM, AbuRuz, ME (2013) The impact of stress on job satisfaction for nurses in King Fahad Specialist Hospital-Dammam-KSA. JAS 9: 371-377.

# 3

# Knowledge and Attitude Regarding Pubertal Changes among Pre-Adolescent Boys: An Interventional Study in Rural Area in India

Poonam Sheoran*, Manisha Rani, Yogesh Kumar and Navjyot Singh

*M.M. Institute of Nursing, Mullana, Ambala, India*

*Corresponding author: Poonam Sheoran, Principal, M.M. Institute of Nursing, Mullana, Ambala, India, E-mail: principalmmin@mmumullana.org

## Abstract

**Purpose:** During puberty growth is rapid and confusing, especially compared to the relatively earlier period of childhood. The purpose of this study was to compare the knowledge and attitude regarding pubertal changes among pre–adolescent boys before and after the pubertal preparedness programme (PPP) in experimental and comparison/control group or control group.

**Methods:** A Quasi experimental (non-equivalent comparison/control group pre-test post-test) design was adopted with 100 pre-adolescent boys (50 in each experimental and comparison/control/control group) of age 12-14 years, selected by purposive sampling from two different rural government schools of Ambala District. The Knowledge and attitude of both groups were assessed using structured knowledge questionnaire (KR-20=0.77) and 5 point likert scale (Cronbach's alpha=0.76), respectively. On the same day of pre-test, pubertal Preparedness Programme (PPP) was administered only to the experimental group and on 12th day Frequently Asked Questions (FAQs) reinforcement session was held only for experimental group. After 28 days, post-test was taken to both groups.

**Results:** The computed t value of pre-test scores of knowledge and attitude of pre-adolescent boys were 1.96 vs. 1.75 respectively in experimental and comparison/control/control group which was found to be non-significant at 0.05 level of significance which shows that both group didn't differ significantly in their knowledge and attitude before the administration of PPP intervention. Findings of unpaired 't' value of post-test knowledge and attitude scores of pre-adolescent boys were 14.25 vs. 10.98 respectively in experimental and comparison/control/control group were found significant at 0.05 level of significance. Thus, knowledge and attitude of pre-adolescent boys were improved with PPP and FAQs session.

**Conclusion:** PPP and FAQs (frequently asked questions) reinforcement session are effective in enhancing knowledge and developing favorable attitude among pre-adolescent boys.

**Keywords:** Preadolescence; Pubertal preparedness programme; Pubertal changes; Sex education

## Introduction

Adolescence is a period of transition between childhood and adulthood – a time of rapid physical, cognitive, social and emotional maturation as the boy prepares for manhood. The precise boundaries of adolescence are difficult to define, but this period is customarily viewed as beginning with the gradual appearance of secondary sexual characteristics at about 11 or 12 years of age and ending with cessation of body growth at 18 to 20 years. Adolescence which literally means, "to grow into maturity". It involves three distinct sub phases: early adolescence (pre adolescence) (age 11 to 14 years), middle adolescence (ages 15 to 17 years), and late adolescence (ages 18 to 20 years) [1]. Adolescents – defined by the United Nations as those between the ages of 10 and 19 – number 1.2 billion in 2010, forming 18 percent of world population [2]. Adolescent population in India has increased from 85 million in 1961 to 253 million in 2011 (in five decades) [3] and in Haryana, percentage of adolescent's population is approx. 21% [4].

The most dramatic changes related to adolescence are the physical changes that occur as a part of pubertal process [5]. Puberty includes maturational, hormonal and growth process that occurs when the reproductive organs begin to function and the secondary sex characteristics develop [1]. During puberty, growth is disorganized confusing and rapid, compared to the relatively stable earlier period of childhood. When pubescent children are not informed of the changes that take place at puberty, it is traumatic to undergo these changes and may develop unfavourable attitudes towards these changes [6].

Studies have shown that there are still many misconceptions and misbelieves regarding issues related to sexuality in adolescence, which should be tackled comprehensively by imparting formal puberty and sex education at proper age [5]. Another study shows that twenty eight percentages do not like the changes due to puberty, in their body. Twenty three percentages were worried about shape and size of their penis and 60% accept that they feel mood swings sometimes [7]. Various studies concluded that reproductive health is ignored and queries go unanswered [8]. Adolescent possess some knowledge about reproductive health but still effective educational intervention is required to encourage more sensible and healthy behaviour and results of a study shows health education sessions are very effective in increasing knowledge [7-9].

With this background, the study was aimed to assess and compare the knowledge and attitude of pre-adolescent boys in experimental and comparison/control group before and after the pubertal preparedness programme in rural areas.

## Methods

### Study design

This quantitative study was based on quasi experimental, non-equivalent comparison/control groups. Pre-test and post-test are design to test and compare two groups of participants at two specified time points: one group with and the other without PPP and an evaluation of both 28 days later.

### Design and settings

The study was conducted in two government rural schools of Mullana and Barara village of Ambala District Haryana, India selected by convenience sampling and randomized. Data was collected between December and January 2015 after obtaining clearance from the "institutional ethical committee" of MM University.

### Setting and sample

The study participants selected by purposive sampling technique comprised of 100 pre-adolescent boys (50 in each experimental and comparison/control/control group) of 12-14 years age group studying in 8th and 9th class from two rural government schools (selected by convenience sampling) of Mullana and Barara village of Ambala District Haryana, and randomized to experimental and comparison/control groups.

### Ethical consideration

Ethical approval was taken from the MM University institutional ethical committee (IEC) (under the project number 375). Written informed consent was obtained from the parents (legal guardian) and assent was obtained from all participants before starting the study.

### Measurements/instruments

Knowledge and attitude was assessed using a structured knowledge questionnaire and 5 point likert scale. Both tools were validated by 7 experts in the various nursing fields. Reliability of tools was checked. The reliability coefficient of structured knowledge questionnaire for boys was found 0.77 by Kudar Richardson-20 formula and for attitude scale it was found 0.76 for boys by Cronbach's alpha. Structured knowledge questionnaire containing 36 multiple choice questions was used with Areas like reproductive organs, concept of puberty, secondary sexual characteristics, nocturnal emission of semen and emotional changes. A five point likert scale ranging strongly agree to strongly disagree containing 33 statements was used, out of which 17 were positive statements and 16 were negative. The maximum score was 165 and minimum score was 33.

### Data collection/procedure

After obtaining the formal approval from the principals of Government rural schools of Mullana and Barara village of Ambala district, Haryana, India, the group could be studied. All the groups were given an initial pre-test to assess the knowledge and attitude regarding pubertal changes.

The experimental was given the pubertal preparedness programme (PPP) using audio visual aids. After that on 12th day a reinforcement session using FAQs (frequently asked questions) session was held to develop favourable attitude among pre-adolescent boys and post-test was conducted after 28 days of PPP (pubertal preparedness programme).

For comparison/control/control group, on first day pre-test and after 28 days post test was conducted to assess the knowledge and attitude regarding pubertal changes without giving any intervention.

### Intervention

Pubertal preparedness programme (PPP) is a presentation of 45-50 min duration and was structured to enhancing knowledge and to develop favourable attitude regarding pubertal changes.

The content outline included Introduction to the male reproductive system, a discussion of the various stages of the pubertal period, physical changes – secondary sexual characteristics, Nocturnal emission (wet dreams) and various emotional changes that occur during puberty.

Lecture cum discussion method was adopted for teaching.

### Data analysis

Data were entered into Microsoft Excel 2007 and analyzed using SPSS 17.0. Categorical data are presented as mean (Standard Deviation) or median based on the distribution of data. Statistical analysis was performed by using t test for continuous variables and chi square for categorical variables. A p value of 0.05 or less was considered significant.

### Results

Base line characteristics: Frequency, percentage distribution and chi square was computed to describe the sample characteristics of the sample and characteristics similarities of the sample in both experimental and comparison/control/control group. The baseline sample characteristics of the participants showed that in experimental group vs. comparison/control/control group more than half boys 54% vs. 60%, respectively were of 9th grade class and the remaining, 46% vs. 40% respectively, were of 8th grade class y. Among these 52% vs. 62%, respectively were aged 14. Most of boys 72% vs. 64%, respectively were Hindu. In the experimental group less than half of boys' fathers (30%) were illiterate and mothers 38% had education up to primary and 32% were illiterate and in comparison/control group 36% father and 34% mothers had education up to secondary. Majority of boys' father (72%) in experimental group and 46% in comparison/control group were labourer and mothers of majority of boys in experimental group, 74% vs. 82%, in comparison/control group were home maker. 98% of the boys in experimental group and 100% in comparison/control group had knowledge regarding puberty and for them source of information were parents and books.

Findings of the further study show that, for 27% of pre-adolescent boys, source of information regarding puberty was friends followed by internet (19.14%). Friends were major source of information regarding pubertal changes.

The computed chi square value for the sample characteristics of experimental and comparison/control groups' boys were found to be non-significant at 0.05 level of significance, revealing that boys in both groups had equal knowledge before the administration of pubertal preparedness programme.

Mean, mean percentage, median and standard deviation of pre- and post-test knowledge and attitude score of pre-adolescent boys in experimental and comparison/control group were calculated and presented in Table 1.

| Group | | Range of Score | | Mean | | | | Median | | Standard Deviation | |
|---|---|---|---|---|---|---|---|---|---|---|---|
| | | Pre-test | Post-test | Pre-test | % | Post-test | % | Pre-test | Post-test | Pre-test | Post-test |
| knowledge | (E) | 8-22 | 13-30 | 15.46 | 42.94 | 22.56 | 62.66 | 16 | 22 | 3.63 | 3.64 |
| | (C) | 6-22 | 7-20 | 13.98 | 38.83 | 12.84 | 35.66 | 14 | 12.5 | 3.9 | 3.15 |
| Attitude | (E) | 75-106 | 101-135 | 93.44 | 56.63 | 112.74 | 68.32 | 94 | 112 | 6.51 | 7.97 |
| | (C) | 72-111 | 74-106 | 91 | 55.15 | 94.94 | 57.33 | 91.5 | 96 | 7.39 | 8.23 |

**Table 1:** Range of score, mean, mean percentage, median and standard deviation of pre-test and post-test knowledge and attitude score of pre-adolescent boys regarding pubertal changes in experimental and comparison/control group, knowledge max score:-36, minimum score:-0, attitude max score:-165, minimum score:-33.

't' Value of pre- and post-test knowledge and attitude score of pre-adolescent boys in experimental and comparison/control group: The computed 't' value of pre-test knowledge and attitude scores of pre-adolescent boys 1.96 vs. 1.75, respectively was found to be statistically non-significant being more than 0.05 level of significance thus suggesting that both group (experimental and comparison/control) do not differ in their knowledge and attitude significantly before the administration of intervention. On the other hand, post-test findings

of unpaired 't' value of knowledge and attitude score of pre-adolescent boys, 14.25 vs. 10.98, respectively, in experimental and comparison/control group were found significant at 0.05 level of significance, Thus knowledge and attitude of pre-adolescent boys were improved with PPP and FAQs session.

In order to determine the significance between pre-test and post-test, area wise 't' value was computed and presented in Tables 2 and 3.

| Group | Area | Pre-test Mean | Post-test Mean | Mean $_D$ | SD $_D$ | SE $_{MD}$ | t value |
|---|---|---|---|---|---|---|---|
| Experimental group (n=50) | Reproductive organs | 2.36 | 3.82 | 1.46 | 1.89 | 0.26 | 5.44* |
| | Concept of puberty | 3.24 | 4.82 | 1.58 | 2.02 | 0.28 | 5.53* |
| | Secondary sexual characteristics | 3.38 | 4.76 | 1.38 | 1.96 | 0.27 | 4.96* |
| | Nocturnal emission of semen | 3.68 | 5.84 | 2.16 | 2.28 | 0.32 | 6.67* |
| | Emotional changes | 2.8 | 3.32 | 0.52 | 1.54 | 0.21 | 2.19* |
| Comparison group (n=50) | Reproductive organs | 2.34 | 2.36 | 0.02 | 2.05 | 0.29 | 0.06 [NS] |
| | Concept of puberty | 2.68 | 2.38 | 0.3 | 1.71 | 0.24 | 1.24 [NS] |
| | Secondary sexual characteristics | 3.3 | 2.88 | 0.42 | 2.43 | 0.34 | 1.22 [NS] |
| | Nocturnal emission of semen | 3.62 | 3.28 | 0.34 | 2.2 | 0.31 | 1.09 [NS] |
| | Emotional changes | 2.04 | 1.94 | 0.1 | 1.58 | 0.22 | 0.45 [NS] |

**Table 2:** Area wise mean, mean difference, standard deviation of difference standard error of mean difference and 't' value of pre-test and post-test knowledge score of pre-adolescent boys in experimental and comparison/control group, N=100, 't' (49)=1.68 (p ≤ 0.05), * significant, NS: Non-Significant.

| Group | Areas | Pre-test Mean | Post-test Mean | Mean Deviation | SD $_D$ | SE $_{MD}$ | t value |
|---|---|---|---|---|---|---|---|

| | | | | | | | |
|---|---|---|---|---|---|---|---|
| Experimental group (n=50) | Concept of puberty | 46.46 | 54.78 | 8.32 | 5.77 | 0.81 | 10.18* |
| | Secondary sexual characteristics | 10.5 | 14.82 | 4.32 | 5.92 | 0.83 | 5.15* |
| | Nocturnal emission of semen | 14.2 | 17.82 | 3.62 | 2.68 | 0.38 | 9.53* |
| | Emotional changes | 22.28 | 25.32 | 3.04 | 5.17 | 0.73 | 4.15* |
| Comparison group (n=50) | Concept of puberty | 44.88 | 47.88 | 3 | 7.29 | 1.03 | 2.91* |
| | Secondary sexual characteristics | 10.22 | 9.4 | 0.82 | 3.1 | 0.43 | 1.87 NS |
| | Nocturnal emission of semen | 13.78 | 15.08 | 1.36 | 3.7 | 0.52 | 2.59* |
| | Emotional changes | 22.18 | 22.58 | 0.4 | 4.37 | 0.62 | 0.65NS |

**Table 3:** Area wise mean, mean difference, standard deviation of difference standard error of mean difference and 't' value of pre-test and post-test attitude score of pre-adolescent boys in experimental and comparison/control group, N=100, 't' (49)=1.98 (p ≤ 0.05), * significant, NS- Non Significant

The computed 't' value for knowledge scores in the experimental group after PPP was found to be statistically significant at 0.05 level of significance in all areas that covered reproductive organs, concept of puberty, secondary sexual characteristics, nocturnal emission of semen and emotional changes but in comparison/control group, computed 't' values for all areas were found to be statistically non-significant at 0.05 level of significance (Table 2).

The computed 't' value for attitude scores in experimental group was found to be statistically significant at 0.05 level of significance in all areas that covered concept of puberty, secondary sexual characteristics, nocturnal emission of semen and emotional changes. However in comparison/control group computed 't' value for all areas was found to be statistically non-significant at 0.05 level of significance except area of nocturnal emission of semen (2.59), this increase in area could be because of sensitization of pre-test or some of them might had experienced nocturnal emission of semen in mean time (Table 3).

The finding of the present study revealed that 40.5% boys were aware about concepts of puberty, 39.33% boys have knowledge about reproductive organs and their functions, 42.3% boys were aware about secondary sexual characteristics and 46.7% boys were aware about emotional changes.

Findings regarding correlation: A significant, low, positive correlation was found between mean post-test knowledge and attitude scores of pre-adolescent boys regarding pubertal changes as evidenced by computed 'r' value of (0.28) as shown in Figure 1.

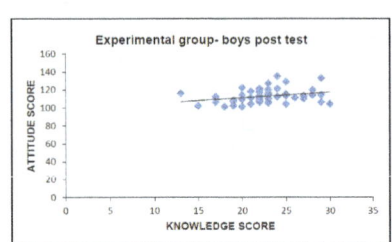

**Figure 1:** Scatter Plot Showing the correlation between knowledge and attitude scores obtained by pre-Adolescent boys in experimental group post test.

ANOVA/t values showing the association of the level of post knowledge and attitude scores of pre-adolescent boys with sample characteristics: The findings of ANOVA/t values showing the association of level of post knowledge and attitude scores of pre-adolescent boys with source of information (0.00) and (0.02), respectively were found to be significant at 0.05 level of significance. This denotes the association of source of information with the obtained knowledge and attitude scores.

## Discussion

The finding of the present study revealed that 40.5% boys were aware about concepts of puberty, 39.33% boys have knowledge about reproductive organs and their functions, 42.3% boys were aware about secondary sexual characteristics and 46.7% boys were aware about emotional changes. The study finding were consistent with finding of a cross sectional study conducted in block Beri, District Jhajjar (Haryana) regarding assessment of self-awareness of rural adolescent students regarding adolescent changes. Findings shows that 50% boys were aware about physical changes in their bodies during puberty, 30.6% boys have knowledge about sexual development changes and total 23% were aware about emotional changes during puberty [10].

The PPP was effective in enhancing the knowledge and attitude of pre-adolescent boys. In the presents study, mean post-test knowledge and attitude scores of pre-adolescents, in experimental group 24.33 vs. 94.21, respectively was higher than the mean pre-test knowledge and attitude scores 14.83 vs. 117.88 respectively. Similar findings were reported in an interventional study conducted in 2014 to assess knowledge and attitude regarding growing up changes among adolescents in Pune, findings showed that both knowledge and attitude scores improved significantly after intervention pre-test knowledge and attitude mean was 9.82 and 109.86 and post-test knowledge and attitude mean was 14.11 and 130.59, respectively [11]. These findings was also found inconsistent with a study held in Tanzania in 2011, shows that the boys' mean score in the knowledge pre-test was 6.4 and 7.0 in post-test, which increased significantly (t=4.5, p=0.000) but in attitude pre-test and post-test increase was not observed, mean (30.8) (t=0.00, p=0.973) was same in both in both [12].

Findings of present study further shows that, for 27% of pre-adolescent boys source of information regarding puberty was friends followed by 23.8% was elder siblings. 22% gain information from books and television followed by internet (19.14%). Almost similar findings were reported in a study conducted in Varanasi in 2014. The survey found that 10 percent boys discuss their problems with their parents. Teenagers are understandably more comfortable discussing their problems and personal experiences with their friends. It has been found that 51 percent boys discuss their problems with their friends [13]. Similarly in findings of study conducted in Tehran, Iran, shows that, Adolescents' preferred sources of in- formation about puberty were parents (17%), peers for 20% or teachers (21%). 12% of adolescents said that books and magazines were their preferred source of information on puberty [14].

## Conclusion

Pre-adolescent boys, who were exposed to PPP, had significantly higher knowledge and favorable attitude than pre-adolescent boys who were not exposed to pubertal preparedness programme. Pre-test knowledge and attitude scores were equal and deficient.

Therefore the study concluded that structured pubertal preparedness programme and a FAQs (frequently asked questions) reinforcement session was effective in terms of enhancing knowledge and developing favorable attitude of pre-adolescent boys regarding pubertal changes after 28 days.

It is recommended that these kinds of programmes need to be enforced in curriculum. As this was a study over 28 days with the FAQs possibly enhancing the scores, school need to give these programmes and repeat frequently.

## Strength

Pubertal preparedness programme and FAQs session were effective in enhancing knowledge and developing favourable attitude among pre-adolescent boys of rural areas.

## Limitations

- Sample taken for the study was only from 2 rural schools because of time constraints. This limits the generalization of the study.
- Study subjects were not selected by randomization.
- The study was limited only to rural pre-adolescent boys studying in government schools.
- In the present study the pubertal preparedness programme was administered only once to the pre-adolescent boys.

## Recommendation for the further studies

- A study can be replicated on a large sample of pre-adolescent boys in selected areas of Haryana for wider generalization of the findings.
- Same study can be conducted on school dropout pre adolescents.
- A study can be carried out using other teaching strategies like information booklet, SIM, etc.
- A study can be undertaken to assess the impact of child to child teaching on knowledge and attitude of pre-adolescent boys regarding pubertal changes.

- Comparative study can be conducted to assess the effectiveness of structured teaching programme and peer group teaching programme regarding pubertal changes.
- A qualitative study can be undertaken to assess the experience of pre-adolescent boys regarding pubertal changes.
- Comparative study can be conducted to assess knowledge, attitude and practice regarding reproductive health among Urban and Rural pre adolescents.
- A study can be conducted to assess parent's perception and attitude toward education regarding pubertal changes.
- A study can be conducted to assess teacher's perception and attitude toward special education camps/classes regarding pubertal changes at school level.
- A longitudinal study can be conducted to assess level of coping among pre adolescents regarding pubertal changes.

## References

1. Marilyn JH, Wilson David (2013) Wong's essentials of pediatric nursing. Elsevier publication, pp: 477-478.
2. Progress for Children (2012) A report card on adolescents by United Nations Children's Fund (UNICEF) [Internet] Division of Communication, New York, USA.
3. Size, Growth and Composition of Adolescent and Youth Population in India (2014) Dr. Kumar Sanjay National Programme Officer, UNFPA India, New Delhi.
4. Release of social and cultural tables – age data highlights census of India (2011) Dr. C Chandramouli Registrar General and Census Commissioner, India Ministry of Home Affairs August 2013.
5. Singh BP, Singh G, Singh KK (2014) Pubertal changes in teenagers of Varanasi - The spiritual city of India. Ind J Youth Adol Health 1: 39-43.
6. Sharma N (1998) A study of social and psychological problems related to puberty among high school students. J Inst Med 19: 1-5.
7. Upadhyay Dhungel K, Dhungel BA, Das PKL, Karki BMS (2012) Perception and knowledge regarding reproductive health among adolescent males of Lalitpur. Asian J Medical Science 3: 27-31.
8. Devidas T, Chandra Srkhar K, Kembhavi RS (2011) Perception of adolescent boys regarding pubertal changes (physical, emotional and psychological) from urban slum area of Mumbai. Indian J Public Health Res and Development 2: 42-46.
9. Moodi M, Zamanipour N, Sharifirad GR, Shahnazi H (2013) Evaluating puberty health program effect on knowledge increase among female intermediate and high school students in Birjand. Iran J Edu Health Promot 1: 223-236.
10. Jain RB, Kumar A, Khanna P (2013) Brief communication assessment of self-awareness among rural adolescents⊠: A cross-sectional study. Indian J Endocrinol Metab 17: 367-372.
11. Deshmukh Vaishali R, Kulkarni Aditi A, Apte Sarang S (2014) knowledge and attitude about growing up changes: An intervention study. Pediatric on call journal 54: 65-70.
12. Madeni F, Horiuchi S, Iida M (2011) Evaluation of a reproductive health awareness program for adolescence in urban Tanzania-A quasi-experimental pre-test post-test research study. Reproductive Health 8: 21.
13. Singh BP (2014) Pubertal changes in teenagers of Varanasi - The spiritual city of India. Ind J Youth Adol Health 1: 39-43.
14. Mohammadi MR, Mohammad K (2006) Reproductive knowledge, attitudes and behavior among adolescent males in Tehran, Iran. International Family Planning Perspectives 32: 35-44.

# 4

# Knowledge and Attitude Regarding Care of Elderly among Nursing Students: An Indian Perspective

**Sukhpal Kaur***, Anoop Kumar K.P, Baljeet Kaur, Bhawana Rani, Sandhya Ghai and Monaliza Singla

*National Institute of Nursing Education, Post Graduate Institute of Medical Education and Research, Chandigarh, India*

*****Corresponding author:** Dr Sukhpal Kaur, National Institute of Nursing Education, Post Graduate Institute of Medical Education and Research, Chandigarh, India; E-mail: sukhpal.trehan@yahoo.in, drsukhpalkaur@gmail.com

**Abstract:**

There is proportionate increase in the health problems along with increase in elderly population in India. Nurses need to be well equipped with knowledge and should also have a positive attitude regarding elderly care. The current cross sectional study was undertaken with an objective to assess the knowledge and attitude of nursing students regarding care of elderly. Using purposive sampling technique, 267 undergraduate nursing students were enrolled in the study. A pre validated self-administered questionnaire was used to assess the knowledge and attitude of nursing students regarding elderly care. The knowledge questionnaire consisted of 28 multiple choice questions with one right answer. Total score was further categorized as poor, average and good as per the score obtained by the subjects. The attitude was assessed on a Likert five-point scale, ranged from 'strongly agree' with 5 score to 'strongly disagree' with 1 score. It consisted of 16 items. The total score was further categorized as unfavorable, neutral and favorable attitude as per the scores obtained. Majority (95.5%) of the subjects were females. Mean age (yrs) ± SD was 22.61 ± 3.31 with the range of 19-48 yrs. More than half (53.9) were from urban locality. Only 29.2% were staying with the grandparents. Mean knowledge score ± S.D. was 22.10 ± 2.91, with the range of 9-27. Around two third (76.4) were in the good category of knowledge score. Mean attitude score ± S.D. was 60.38 ± 8.95 with the range of 22-78. 64.6% were in the positive category of attitude. Knowledge and attitude were positively correlated.

**Keywords:** Knowledge; Attitude; Nursing students; Elderly care

## Introduction

The percentage of elderly population is continuously increasing globally due to decline in overall death rate, decline in fertility and sustained improvement in survival. Worldwide, there are estimated 605 million people aged 60 years and above [1,2]. One out of every ten persons is 60 years or above. By 2050, this number is expected to be one out of five of 60 years or older and by 2150, one out of three persons will be 60 years or older [3]. As the age advances, there is decline in physical functions of the elderly. It leads to a loss of independence and the person become susceptible to both the acute and chronic health problems. In general, most organ systems demonstrate an age-related decline of about 0.5% per year [4]. As the people become aged, the patterns of diseases that they suffer and die from also changes. Different studies show varied results in the morbidity pattern [5-10]. The various risk factors for reduced physical function in elderly people, as identified in longitudinal studies, relate to comorbidities, physical and psychosocial health, environmental conditions, social circumstances, nutrition, and lifestyle [11,12].

Many more people thus need some kind of help for the problems caused by the diseases towards the end of life. Thus, the increased life expectancy rather has an element of morbidity and disability linked with it. Older people's continuing care needs are met in a variety of settings, including their own home, supported housing, residential care, a nursing home or hospital. Under the influence of modernization, the size and structure of families have undergone dramatic changes especially in India. Nuclear families are replacing the joint families. Families have become smaller, more dispersed and varied. This has affected the family care and support available to the aged persons to a certain extent.

So, the current demographic and health utilization trends strongly indicate a rapidly increasing demand for nurses who are well qualified to care for older adults. There is a growing need for motivated nurses to provide care for older people. Nurses have a pivotal role as providers of care to the older people and are in a unique position to influence the quality of care. Various functions of nurses that can contribute to the optimum health and overall wellbeing of the older people include supportive, restorative, educative, life-enhancing and managerial [13]. Cultivation of positive attitudes towards older adults and specialized knowledge about aging and the health care needs of older adults are of utmost priorities for nurses. It has been suggested that attitudes can influence an individual's behavior and that people with a positive attitude towards anyone will have more positive thoughts about them [14].

Because of these demographic changes, it is expected that nearly all nursing students will predominately have to work with older people after completing their primary education. Thus it is essential that nursing students are adequately prepared for taking care of this growing population [15]. Several studies investigating the nursing students' knowledge and attitudes toward care of older people and their willingness to work with them have been conducted in various countries. The majority of these studies have concluded that most nursing students have little knowledge and interest in working with older people [15-17]. But, there is scarcity of data regarding the topic under study in India. So, the current study was undertaken with the objective to assess the knowledge and attitude of nursing students regarding the care of elderly.

## Materials and Methods

This was a cross sectional study carried out at National Institute of Nursing Education, PGIMER, Chandigarh, India. The institution runs both the postgraduate and the undergraduate nursing programs. Using purposive sampling technique, 267 undergraduate nursing students willing to participate were enrolled in the study. A pre validated self-administered questionnaire was used to obtain the data. The questionnaires were developed by the researchers after extensive literature review. The content validity was established by circulating the tool among the experts. Information was obtained regarding socio demographic data of the study subjects, their knowledge (28 multiple choice questions with one right answer) and attitude regarding care of elderly. The attitude was assessed on a Likert five-point scale, ranging from 'strongly agree' to 'strongly disagree'. All items were scored from 1 to 5, where 5 stand for 'strongly agree' and 1 for 'strongly disagree. It consisted of 16 items. The total score was further categorized as unfavorable, neutral and favorable attitude as per the scores obtained. Total Knowledge score was also categorized as poor, average and good as per the score obtained by the subjects i.e. 9-14, 15-20, and 21-27 respectively. An informed consent was obtained from each subject. They were assured that the collected data would be used only for the research purposes, and that their decision to withdraw or refuse to participate will not have any impact on their studies.

The protocol was approved by ethics review committee of National Institute of Nursing Education. Data was collected as per the availability of the class. The routine of academic program was not disturbed. It took around 20-30 minutes by study subjects to fill the questionnaire. SPSS version 16 was used to analyze the data. Both descriptive (mean, S.D., range) and inferential statistics (Pearson Correlation test) was used. Probabilities of $p<0.05$ were assumed as statistically significant.

## Results

### Demographic profile of the subjects

The mean age of study subjects was 22.61 ± 3.31 with range of 19-48 years. Majority were females (95.55%), belonged to Hindu religion (63.3%) and were residing in urban localities (53.9%). 46.3% of study subjects had per capita income in between Rs 500-5000/month (Table 1)

| Variables | | n (%) |
|---|---|---|
| Age (yrs) | | |
| 19-23 | | 206(77.1) |
| 24-30 | Mean ± SD:22.61 ± 3.31Range: 19-48 | 053(19.8) |
| 31-36 | | 005(01.9) |
| ≥ 37 | | 003(01.2) |
| Gender | | |
| Male | | 012(04.5) |
| Female | | 255(95.5) |
| Religion | | 169(63.3) |
| Hindu | | 078(29.2) |
| Sikh | | 001(00.4) |
| Muslim | | 019(07.1) |
| Christian | | |
| Habitat | | |
| Urban | | 143(53.9) |
| Rural | | 124(46.1) |
| Per capita income (Rs) | | |
| 500-5000 | | 123(46.3) |
| 5100-10000 | Mean ± S.D: 7662.09 ± 499.3 Range: 500-30000 | 100(37.4) |
| 10100-20000 | | 041(15.4) |
| Above 20000 | | 003(01.1) |

Table 1: Demographic profile of the subjects (N=267).

| Items | n (%) |
|---|---|
| The client is helped to develop positive self concept and improved feeling of control by encouraging positive comments about self and give positive feedback about his/her accomplishment. | 260 (97.4) |
| The trauma in elderly can be prevented by keeping the bed in low position and side rail up as well as adequate lighting. | 259 (97.0) |
| Average caloric requirement in elderly is 1800 calories. | 256 (95.9) |
| The fear and anxiety related to inability to perform usual roles and to live independently can be reduced by maintaining a calm, unhurried, confident manner while interacting with client. | 254 (95.1) |
| Increase the physical mobility/activity tolerance in elderly by keeping supplies and personal articles within reach and use energy saving techniques. | 251 (94.0) |
| The urinary continence in elderly can be regained by performing perineal exercises and fixing a toileting schedule. | 249 (93.3) |
| Client can be made adjusted to changes in the family role and structure by encouraging verbalization of feelings about changes in the client and effect of these on family structure. | 249 (93.3) |
| The elderly people avoid to go to the doctor because of the fear of diagnosis of an unknown illness. | 246 (92.1) |
| Sound sleep can be encouraged in elderly by restricting visitors during rest period and provide care in groups. | 246 (92.1) |

| | |
|---|---|
| Dehydration can be prevented in elderly by assessing skin turgor, mucous membrane and urine output. | 246 (92.1) |
| Bed sores in elderly is prevented by keeping the skin clean and dry and the bed linens wrinkle free &dry. | 244 (91.4) |
| Nursing concentration directed to at health promotion in elderly are primarily focused on providing a sense of control over health problem. | 238 (89.1) |
| Memorizing capabilities of elderly person is affected due to structural changes in brain. | 233 (87.3) |
| The care can be provided to the elderly with altered sensory perception by reducing environmental noise and speak louder and slowly with a non verbal cues when appropriate. | 224 (83.9) |
| The constipation in elderly can be prevented by maintaining proper position, privacy and adequate ventilation, encourage to relax while attempts to defecate. | 222 (83.2) |
| The anatomical areas most often affected by the development of pressure sores in elderly are iliac crest, and ischial tuberosities. | 220 (82.4) |
| Balance and risk for falls are assessed in elderly by Get-up and go test instrument. | 198 (74.2) |
| The anxiety related to the unfamiliar environment of hospital can be reduced by orienting the client to the hospital environment and explain all the diagnostic procedure to the client and the relative. | 190 (72.3) |
| When checking the blood pressure of an elderly, the nurse needs to know that systolic blood pressure tends to rise with aging because of loss of elasticity of arteries. | 188 (70.4) |
| The urinary retention in elderly can be prevented by avoiding suppression of urge to urinate, provide privacy, assume normal position, run water and pour water over perineum. | 182 (68.2) |
| The advice can be given to diminish the pain and discomfort due to degenerative changes in joint cartilage is to go for mild exercises & gentle circular motion and avoid weight bearing exercise. | 174 (65.2) |
| The nurse is working with older clients in a long term care facility. The activities performed by the nurse fosters reminiscence among these clients is 'Having story telling hours'. | 170 (63.7) |
| Adequate nutrition can be maintained in elderly by assisting client to choose foods/fluids to provide nutritional needs as well as his/her preferences. | 151 (56.6) |
| Among the given theories, one theory explains the psychosocial development aspect 'integrity versus despair' is Erickson's theory. | 125 (46.8) |
| Person is considered elderly above the age of 65years. | 121 (45.3) |
| Orientation, memory, attention, language, recall are tested in elderly by the use of Folstien mini- mental status instrument. | 099 (39.1) |
| We age because of wear and tear of important organs by continuous functioning. | 092 (34.5) |
| The adequate respiratory function can be maintained in elderly by instructing the client deep breathing exercises. | 048 (18.0) |

Table 2 a: Knowledge regarding care of elderly among the nursing students (correct response).

| Categorization of knowledge score | | n% |
|---|---|---|
| Poor (9-14) | Mean ± S.D:22.10 ± 2.91 Range: 09-27 | 001 (00.4) |
| Average (15-20) | | 062 (23.2) |
| Good (21-27) | | 204 (76.4) |

Table 2b: Mean score and categorization of knowledge score regarding care of elderly (Maximum attainable score: 28).

### Knowledge regarding care of elderly

Table 2a shows the correct responses given by the subjects regarding care of elderly for the various questions in descending order. For majority of the questions, more than 80% of the subjects gave the correct answer. Mean knowledge score was 22.10 ± 2.91 with the range of 09-27. Most of the subjects (76.4%) had good knowledge regarding care of elderly. 23.2% of subjects had average knowledge. Only 0.4% of subjects had poor knowledge regarding care of elderly (Table 2b).

| Items | Strongly disagree | Disagree | Neither agree nor disagree | Agree | Strongly agree |
|---|---|---|---|---|---|
| In India, there is an urgent need to understand the health and disease profile of elderly and their care by nurses. | 15 (5.6) | 2 (0.7) | 8 (3.0) | 120 (44.9) | 122 (45.7) |
| Health needs of elderly are different from other age group population. | 15 (5.6) | 9 (3.4) | 8 (3.0) | 131 (49.1) | 104 (39) |

| | | | | | |
|---|---|---|---|---|---|
| Elderly are more prone to fall ill. | 14 (5.2) | 3 (1.1) | 32 (12) | 136 (50.9) | 82 (30.7) |
| Elderly are the burden on the family and the society. | 186 (69.7) | 37 (13.9) | 21 (7.9) | 8 (3.0) | 15 (5.6) |
| Elderly are abused/neglected. | 28 (10.5) | 27 (10.1) | 63 (23.6) | 125 (46.8) | 24 (9.0) |
| Alcoholism and drug is a problem among elderly. | 30 (11.2) | 79 (29.6) | 107 (40.1) | 41 (15.4) | 10 (3.7) |
| We need to focus on social support to elderly. | 7 (2.6) | 9 (3.4) | 17 (6.4) | 141 (52.8) | 93 (34.8) |
| There is the need to establish more special geriatric clinic. | 12 (4.5) | 5 (1.9) | 8 (3) | 112 (43.8) | 125 (46.8) |
| There is a need to promote elderly health by routine health check-ups, organizing health camps and health education | 11 (4.1) | 4 (1.5) | 2 (0.7) | 106 (39.7) | 144 (53.9) |
| There is a need for mobile clinics to reach the elderly population staying in rural/remote areas. | 12 (4.5) | 7 (2.6) | 17 (6.4) | 99 (37.1) | 132 (49.4) |
| Elderly who are unable to perform activities of daily living should be provided care, love, sympathy and assistance in the performance of the activities by the family members. | 11 (4.1) | 6 (2.2) | 11 (4.1) | 83 (31.1) | 156 (58.4) |
| It is more interesting to work in an elderly people ward rather working in other wards. | 8 (3.0) | 21 (7.9) | 115 (43.1) | 102 (38.2) | 21 (7.9) |
| Many elderly tends to behave like a child. | 10 (3.7) | 27 (10.1) | 77 (28.8) | 120 (44.9) | 33 (12.4) |
| Many elderly bore by narrating their past experiences. | 27 (10.1) | 96 (36) | 94 (35.2) | 47 (17.6) | 3 (1.1) |
| It is difficult to understand and convenience to elderly. | 10 (3.7) | 97 (36.3) | 76 (28.5) | 76 (28.5) | 8 (3.0) |
| Elderly may be cheerful and may have a good sense of humour. | 6 (2.2) | 30 (11.2) | 71 (26.6) | 132 (49.4) | 28 (10.5) |

**Table 3a:** Attitude regarding care of elderly among nursing students.

| Categorization of attitude | | n (%) |
|---|---|---|
| Negative (22-40) | Mean ± SD: 60.38 ± 8.95 | 014 (05.3) |
| Neutral (41-59) | Range: 22-78 | 078 (30.1) |
| Positive (60-78) | | 175 (64.6) |

**Table 3b:** Mean score and categorization of attitude score regarding care of elderly (Maximum attainable score: 80)

## Attitude regarding care of elderly among the nursing students (Table 3 a and 3 b)

Table 3a shows attitude of the nursing students regarding care of elderly in details. Most of the subjects (64.6%) had positive attitude regarding care of elderly. 30.1% subjects had neutral attitude. Only 5.3% had negative attitude regarding care of elderly. Mean attitude score was 60.38 ± 8.95 with the range of 22-78 (Table 3b).

## Correlation between knowledge and attitude

There was a significant correlation between knowledge and attitude regarding care of elderly (r=0.1). As knowledge increases the attitude became more positive (Table 4).

| | | Attitude | Knowledge |
|---|---|---|---|
| **Attitude** | Pearson Correlation | 1 | .155* |
| | Sig. (2-tailed) | | 0.011 |
| | N | 267 | 267 |
| **knowledge** | Pearson Correlation | .155* | 1 |
| | Sig. (2-tailed) | 0.011 | |

| | N | 267 | 267 |
|---|---|---|---|

**Table 4:** Correlation between knowledge and attitude

Correlation is significant at the 0.05 level (2-tailed).

## Discussion

There is tremendous rise in the elderly population worldwide. Since nursing students are the future care providers for the aged population, understanding their attitude and knowledge towards elderly is vital. The current study was conducted to elucidate the attitude and knowledge of nursing students regarding care of elderly.

Geriatric nursing as speciality is still in an infancy stage in India. Even there is no separate subject on elderly care in the undergraduate and post graduate nursing curricula. The topic of geriatric care is incorporated and taught to the students along with other nursing subjects such as medical surgical nursing and advanced nursing practice. The hospital where these nursing students go for nursing practice, there are no separate units/wards for the older people. The elderly people are admitted and being provided care along with other adult patients in the wards. Even then, the students in the current study demonstrated fairly good level of knowledge and attitude towards care of elderly people. However, in other studies, the mean knowledge score regarding aging has been reported to be 11.13 (46.37%) and 14 (56%) among the nursing students [18,19]. Lack of knowledge and interest in the issue of older people care has also been reported by Deltsidou A et al[20]. Duggan S et al has recommended to evaluate and revise the contents of the courses to ensure that the knowledge, skills and attitudes required to work with older people are accorded appropriate value and attention [21].

There was a significant correlation between knowledge and attitude regarding care of elderly in the current study. As knowledge increases the attitude became more positive. This could be explained by the fact that majority of the participants in the present study were female and females especially in the Indian situations are the one who take for each and every member of the family and have also been shown to be more positive attitudes toward older people than males. As the number (male vs females) in the current study was not comparable, so statistically no comparison was made. Another thing is that the culture of joint family is still prevailing in India, and this increases the bond amongst the family members. It has been documented that attitudes influence an individual's behavior and people with a positive attitude towards anyone have more positive thoughts about them [14]. Attitude towards the older people is considered as an important factor in providing them care. The positive attitude among nursing students toward older people has also been documented by other studies [22,23]. In the current study around 60% of the subjects strongly agreed that elderly are not the burden on the family and the society. They were of the opinion that there is a need to promote elderly health by routine health check-ups, organizing health camps and health education. Elderly who are unable to perform activities of daily living should be provided care, love, sympathy and assistance in the performance of the activities by the family members.

However, Oyetunde et al have reported that nurses have a negative attitude towards the care of the elderly even though they displayed a fairly good knowledge of geriatric care. It has been suggested that effective care of the elderly requires special training, provision of geriatric ward, adequate staffing to reduce stress and improve quality care. There is need for continuing education on quality care to improve nursing practice in the care of the elderly [24]. If students are provided with the relevant education, they can deliver quality care and develop positive attitudes in caring for older people in their professional practice [25,26].

The limitation of this study is that it is confined to the population of nursing students at one institute only. Therefore, these findings cannot be viewed as a good representation of all nursing students.

## Conclusion

In light of the above findings, it is concluded that nursing students have good knowledge and positive attitude regarding care of elderly. Because of the demographic transition, it is suggested that consideration should be given to the inclusion of more structured gerontology courses in the basic nursing curriculum. This study could be replicated to larger sample and in different settings to generalize the findings. This study may help the nursing educator to plan for increasing interest of nursing students by encouraging discussion related to the elderly, present their problems and emphasize the positive aspects of aging.

## Competing Interests

The authors declare that they have no competing interests.

## Acknowledgement

The authors would like to thank all nursing students who participated in this study.

## References

1. Anil JP, Joy B, Malini K, Kavita V, Perushottam P (2006) Morbidity pattern among the elderly population in the rural area of Tamil Nadu, India. Turkey Journal of Medical Sciences 36: 45-50.

2. Abdulraheem JP, Abdulrahman AC (2008) Morbidity pattern among the elderly population in a Nigerian tertiary health care institution: analysis of a retrospective study. Nigerian Medical Practitioner 54: 32-38.

3. Troisi J (2004) "Ageing in Africa: Older persons as a resource". International Conference on "Rapid Ageing and the changing role of the elderly in African households", Union for African Population Studies UAPS/UEPA (Senegal), South Africa.

4. Sehl ME, Yates FE. Kinetics of human aging: I (2001) Rates of senescence between ages 30 and 70 years in healthy people. J Gerontol Biol Sci 56A:B198-B208.

5. Purty AJ, Bazroy J, Kar M, Vasudevan K, Veliath A (2006) Morbidity Pattern among the elderly population in the rural area of Tamil Nadu, India. Turk J Med Sci 36: 45-50.

6. Joshi K, Kumar R, Avasthi A (2003) Morbidity profile and its relationship with disability and psychological distress among elderly people in Northern India. Int J Epidemiol 32: 978-87.

7. Singh MM, Murthy GV, Venkatraman R, Rao SP, Nayar S (1997) A study of ocular morbidity among elderly population in a rural area of central India. Indian J Ophthalmol 45: 61-5.

8. Dey AB, Soneja S, Nagarkar KM, Jhingan HP (2001) Evaluation of the health and functional Status of older Indians as a prelude to the development of a health programme. Natl Med J India 14:135-8.

9. Ahluwalia N (2004) Aging, nutrition and Immune function. J Nutr Health Aging 8: 2-6.

10. Singh P, Umesh K, Dey AB (2004) Prevalence of overweight and obesity among elderly patients attending a geriatric clinic in a tertiary care hospital in Delhi, India. Indian J Med Sci 58: 162-3.

11. Stuck AE, Walthert JM, Nikolaus T, Büla CJ, Hohmann C (1999) Risk factors for functional status decline in community-living elderly people: a systematic literature review. Soc Sci Med 48: 445-69.

12. Ayis S, Gooberman-Hill R, Bowling A, Ebrahim S (2006) Predicting catastrophic decline in mobility among older people. Age Ageing 35: 382-87.

13. Royal College of Nursing. Nursing Assessment and Older People 2004: A Royal College of Nursing Toolkit. Published by the royal College of Nursing. 20 Cavendish Square. London. WIG ORN.

14. Fishbein M, Ajzen I (1975) Belief, attitude, intention, and behavior: An introduction to theory and research.

15. Hweidi IM, Al-Obeisat SM (2006) Jordanian nursing students' attitudes toward the elderly. Nurse Educ Today 26: 23-30.

16. Shen J, Xiao LD (2011) Factors affecting nursing students' intention to work with older people in China. Nurse Educ Today 32: 219-223

17. Celik SS, Kapucu S, Tuna Z, Akkus Y (2010) Views and attitudes of nursing students towards ageing and older patients. Australian Journal of Advanced Nursing 27: 24.

18. Alsenany S (2009) Student nurses attitudes and knowledge towards the care of older people in Saudi Arabia.

19. Palmore E (1988) The Facts on Aging Quiz: A Handbook of Uses and Result: New York: Springer Inc.

20. Deltsidou A, Gesouli- Voltyraki E, Mastrogiannis D, Mantzorou M, Noula M (2010) Nurse teachers' and student nurses' attitudes towards caring the older people in a province of Greece. Health Science Journal 4: 245-57.

21. Duggan S, Mitchell EA, Moore KD (2013) 'With a bit of tweaking…we could be great'. An exploratory study of the perceptions of students on working with older people in a preregistration BSc (Hons) Nursing course. Int J Older People Nurs 8: 207-15

22. Howeidi I, Al-hassan M (2005) Jordanian nurses attitudes toward older patients in Acute Care Settings. International Nursing Review 52: 225-232.

23. McKinaly, Cowan (2003) Student nurses attitudes towards working with older patients. Journal of Advanced Nursing 43: 298-309.

24. Oyetunde MO, Ojo OO, Ojewale LY (2013) Nurses' attitude towards the care of the elderly: Implications for gerontological nursing training. Journal of Nursing Education and Practice 3: 150-58.

25. Baumbusch J, Dahlke S, Phinney A (2012) Nursing students' knowledge and beliefs about care of older adults in a shifting context of nursing education. J Adv Nurs 68: 2550-2558.

26. Koh LC (2012) Student attitudes and educational support in caring for older people--a review of literature. Nurse Educ Pract 12:16-20.

# 5

# Knowledge, Attitude and Practice of Infection Prevention Measures among Health Care Workers in Wolaitta Sodo Otona Teaching and Referral Hospital

**Hussen SH[1]\*, Estifanos WM[2], Melese ES[3] and Moga FE[2]**

[1]*Department of Reproductive Health, Arba Minch University, Arba Minch, Ethiopia*

[2]*Department of Nursing, Arba Minch University, Arba Minch, Ethiopia*

[3]*Department of Statistics, Arba Minch University, Arba Minch, Ethiopia*

\*Corresponding author: Hussen SH, Department of Reproductive Health, Arba Minch University, Arba Minch, Ethiopia, E-mail: sultanhussn@gmail.com

## Abstract

**Background:** Infection prevention is a systematic effort or process of placing barrier between susceptible host and the microorganisms. It also refers to all policies, procedures and activities which aim to prevent or minimize the risk of transmission of infectious disease at health care facility. As far as we know there is no similar study has been done on Wolaitta Sodo teaching and referral hospital, so this study is aim to assess Knowledge, Attitude and Practice on infection prevention and control measures among health professionals.

**Objectives:** The main objective of this study is to assess knowledge, attitude and practice of infection prevention measures among health care workers in Wolaitta Sodo teaching and referral hospital, SNNPR, Ethiopia, in March 2017.

**Methods:** The study was conducted at Wolaitta Sodo teaching and referral hospital, South East Ethiopia and Cross-sectional study design was conducted. From the total of 282 respondents, two hundred seventy one were responded to the study. Self-administered questionnaire were used to collect data. Data were entered in to SPSS version 20 for analysis. Both bivariable and multivariable variable logistic regression were done and for variables which had P-value less than 0.25 in bivariable analysis were inserted in to multivariable logistic regression. Then the variables with p-value of less than 0.05 were considered as predictors of the outcome variable. Data were checked for consistency and completeness. Letter of support was obtained from department of nursing and verbal consent was obtained from the institution and all participants.

**Results:** From the total 282 health care workers (HCWs), 271 HCWs were responded with response rate of 95.7%. Among the respondents 253 (93.4%) have good attitude towards infection prevention and 18 (6.6%) of the respondents have negative attitude towards infection Prevention. 269 (99.3%) of HCWs have good knowledge towards infection prevention and 2 (0.7%) have poor knowledge and 164 (60.5%) of HCWs have good practice towards infection prevention and the remaining 107 (39.5%) of health care workers had poor practice. According to this study sex, working in different departments and receiving formal training has significant association with infection prevention practice but educational status, work experience and job title has no significant association with infection prevention practice.

**Conclusion:** Majority of health care workers' knowledge and attitude toward infection prevention in Wolaitta Sodo Otona teaching and referral hospital were good and safe enough, but practice of health care workers towards infection control were not sufficient enough. Wolaitta Zone health bureau should monitor and supervise health care workers towards infection prevention practice and control measures with the routine services through preparing and introducing health care workers infection prevention guidelines, protocol, rules, regulation and opportunities to promote the desired team sprit at all health facility levels are recommended.

**Keywords:** Knowledge; Attitude; Practice; Infection prevention measure; Wolaita Sodo

## Introduction

Infection prevention is a systematic effort or process of placing barrier between susceptible host and the microorganisms [1]. Infection control also refers to all policies, procedures and activities which aim to prevent or minimize the risk of transmission of infectious disease at health care facility [2]. Reports indicate that standard precautions are effective in preventing both occupational exposure incident and associated infections [3].

Health care-associated infection is "An infection occurring in a patient during the process of care in a hospital or other healthcare facility which was not present or incubating at the time of admission." This includes infections acquired in the hospital but appearing after discharge, and also occupational infections among staff of the facility [4].

The endemic burden of health care-associated infection is also significantly higher in low- and middle-income than in high-income countries, in particular in patients admitted to intensive care units and in neonates [5].

Despite the availability of low-cost interventions for infection prevention and control, the compliance with standard infection control practices remains very low, particularly in low-income and middle income countries [6].

According to the fact sheet of World Health Organization (WHO) there are several factors which can cause health care-associated infections. Among this Prolonged and inappropriate use of devices and antibiotics, high-risk and sophisticated procedures, immune-suppression and other severe underlying patient conditions and insufficient application of standard precautions are some of factors which present regardless of the resources available [5].

To improve the control and prevention of infections in countries with limited resources, a multi-facet approach is needed that is based on improved healthcare structures, increased knowledge, effective guidelines, behavioral changes, attitude adjustment, better and efficient use of existing resources, as well as international cooperation [7].

Even though, some studies have focused on knowledge of and compliance with standard precautions, hand washing, knowledge and practice of infection control among hospital staff regardless of focusing in attitude. The information that has been generated on health care workers in Wolaitta Sodo Otona teaching and referral hospital about infection prevention measure is limited. Therefore, this study aimed to assess the knowledge, attitude and practice of infection prevention among all health care workers in Wolaitta Sodo Otona teaching and referral hospital.

## Materials and Methods

### Study setting

This institutional based cross study was conducted from March 1st to March 15th, 2017 in Wolaitta Sodo Otona hospital, which is one of the teaching and referral hospitals in SNNPR, located in Wolaitta Zone, Ethiopia with distance of 378 km South from Addis Ababa and 125 km distance from regional city Hawassa. Wolaittigna is spoken as a first language by 96.82% of the inhabitants. In Wolaitta Sodo town there are one governmental referral and one private hospital, three health centers, seven health posts and thirty private clinics. In Otona hospital there are 282 health care workers in total among them 52 were doctors, 113 were nurses of all type, 21 were laboratory workers and 96 were others such as pharmacy, technologists, radiologists and the likes.

### Sample size and sampling procedure

In this study the sample size was calculated by using single population proportion formula based on the following assumption: Based on the finding from previous study, 76.3 % of health care workers has good practice in the study in west Ethiopia in Mizan Aman hospital on infection prevention [8], expecting 5% margin of error (d) and confidence level of 95%, the total of 280 individuals were calculated as sample size. Since the calculated sample size and the HCWs in the hospital are similar in numbers, all HCWs were included in this study.

### Data collection

Data were collected from study participants using self-administered questionnaire. After reviewing of the relevant literature, the data collection tools were developed, as appropriate to address the study objectives. Five percent of total sample respondents were interviewed during the pre-test in another health institution. After this, the questionnaires were edited accordingly, and after adapting the final version of the questionnaire, the questionnaire was distributed for each participant in the form of hard copy.

### Data processing and analysis

The completeness and consistency of the data were checked, coded and double entered into Epi-Data 3.1. The data were exported to Statistical Package for the Social Sciences (SPSS) version 20 (IBM Corporation, Armonk, NY, USA) statistical soft-wares for further analysis. The analysis and modeling were conducted in several steps.

First, simple descriptive statistics such as a frequency distribution and percentages were performed to describe the characteristics of the study participant. At the second step, a bi-variable logistic model analysis was performed for each independent factor and outcome of interest to identify independent predictors. Upon the completion of the bivariable analysis, variables with a P-value<0.25 were selected for the multivariable analysis to control for confounding and interaction effect. Once the variables were identified, multivariable analysis was performed by enter method.

To decide whether or not a variable is significant, the P-value associated with each parameter was estimated using the P-value<0.05 as a cut-off point. The crude and adjusted odd ratios together with their corresponding 95% confidence intervals were computed and interpreted accordingly.

### Ethical consideration

A letter of clearance was obtained from Arba Minch University, College of Medicine and Health Science. After the letter has received we have disseminated it to Wolaitta zone health bureau, the study area health institution and other concerned bodies. A letter of approval was found from Wolaitta zone health bureau. Data was collected after explaining the rights and responsibilities of giving information and the purpose of the study to respondents and ascertain their confidentiality by explaining that no data were disclosed as an individual rather disseminated at community and health institution level in general. Finally informed consent was obtained from respondents, telling that they have the right not to answers the questions.

## Results and Discussion

### Socio demographic characteristics

A total of 282 HCWs with response rate of (95.7%) were found to complete and included in analysis. Among 271 respondents 156 (57.6%) were males and 115 (42.4%) were females. From the study participants, 39 (14.4%) of HCWs were less than 25 years old and 68 (25.1%) were in age group of 25-29 years and 5 (1.8%) were range in age group of above >44 years. Concerning the professional categories of respondents 111 (41%) were nurses, 50 (18.5%) were physicians and 99 (36.5%) were other health professionals. One hundred five (38.7%) of the respondents were professional with service year of less than five years and 113 (41.7.7%) between 5-10 years (Table 1).

| Variables | Classification | Frequency (%) |
|---|---|---|
| Age in years | <25 | 39 (14.4%) |
| | 25-29 | 68 (25.1%) |
| | 30-34 | 83 (30.6%) |
| | 35-39 | 56 (20.7%) |
| | 40-44 | 20 (7.4%) |
| | >44 | 5 (1.8%) |
| Sex of respondent | Male | 156 (57.6%) |
| | Female | 131 (48.3%) |
| Department | Medical | 41 (15.1%) |
| | Surgical | 55 (20.3%) |
| | Obs/gyni | 40 (14.8%) |
| | Pediatrics | 40 (14.8%) |
| | Others | 95 (35.1%) |
| Professions of respondents | Physician | 50 (18.5%) |
| | Nurses | 111 (41%) |
| | Others | 99 (36.5%) |
| Educational status of respondents | Diploma | 124 (45.8%) |
| | Bsc | 85 (31.4%) |
| | Others | 62 (22.9%) |
| Service years | <5 | 105 (38.7%) |
| | 05-Oct | 113 (41.7%) |
| | >10 | 53 (19.6%) |
| Marital status | Unmarried | 82 (30.2%) |
| | Married | 181 (66.8%) |
| | Others | 8 (9.2%) |

**Table 1:** Socio-demographic characteristics of HCW's, Wolaitta Sodo teaching and referral hospital, 2017.

## Knowledge on infection prevention measures

All of the respondents (271) knew the safety precautions for disposal of needles, syringes and the risk of nosocomial infections and 267 (98.5%) of the respondents were aware of for recommended guidelines for hand hygiene with alcohol based formulations. Among the respondents 264 (97.4%) were received training in hand hygiene and standard precautions.

From the respondents 250 (92.3%) know the impact of HCAIs in clinical outcome and 255 (94.1%) of the respondents knew the effectiveness of hand washing in preventing health care related infections. From the respondents 209 (77.1%) knew when to perform hand washing and 265 (97.8%) knew the transmission mode of nosocomial infections and also 269 (99.3%) of the respondents knew as infections can be transmitted through contact with blood and body fluids.

Among the respondents 252 (93%) knew the effectiveness of standard precautions and 149 (55%) not knew when to use glove. Two hundred two (74.5%) of the respondents knew the objective of standard precautions and 246 (90.8) knew the mechanism of bacteria and virus spread and 265 (97.8%) of knew what to do in the room with TB patients.

In general 269 (99.3%) of HCWs have good knowledge towards infection prevention and control measures and 2 (0.7%) have poor knowledge (Figure 1 and Table 2).

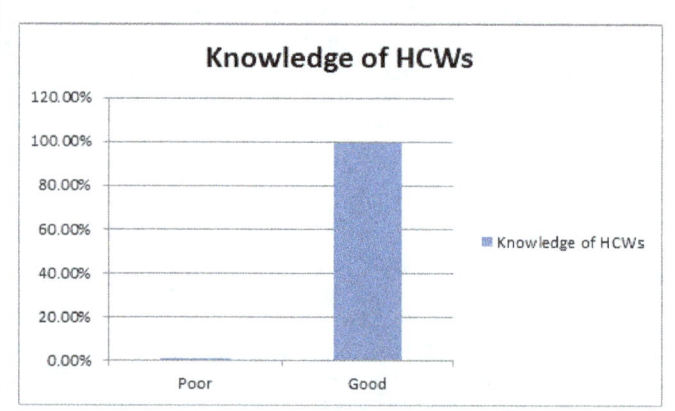

**Figure 1:** Knowledge on infection prevention measures of HCWs, Wolaitta Sodo Otona teaching and referral hospital, 2017.

| No. | Variables | Frequency (%) |
|---|---|---|
| | | Yes |
| 1 | Know about safety precautions for disposal of needles syringes and any wastes precautions for disposal of needles syringes and any wastes | 271 (100%) |
| 2 | Aware of recommended guide lines for hand hygiene | 267 (98.5%) |
| 3 | Is there infection control team? | 264 (97.4%) |
| 4 | Did you receive training in hand hygiene and standard precautions? | 264 (97.4%) |
| 5 | Is there a system for reporting accidental exposure to blood and body fluids? | 264 (97.4%) |
| 6 | Do you know the impact of HCAIs in clinical outcomes? | 250 (92.3%) |

| 7 | Do you know the effectiveness of hand washing in preventing HCAIs? | 255 (94.1%) |
|---|---|---|
| 8 | Do you know when to perform hand washing? | 209 (77.1%) |
| 9 | Do you know nosocomial infections can be transmitted through medical equipment's? | 265 (97.8%) |
| 10 | Do you know nosocomial infections can be transmitted through blood and body fluid contamination? | 269 (99.3%) |
| 11 | Do you know when to use standard precautions? | 252 (93%) |
| 12 | Do you think glove is effective substitute for hand washing? | 149 (55%) |
| 13 | Do you know the objective of standard precautions? | 202 (74.5%) |
| 14 | Do you know by what mechanism bacteria and virus spread through can? | 246 (90.8%) |
| 15 | Do you know what to do in room with TB patients to prevent the spread? | 265 (97.8%) |

**Table 2:** knowledge on infection prevention measures of HCWs, Wolaitta Sodo Otona teaching and referral hospital, 2017.

## Attitude on infection prevention and control measures

Out of 271 study participants 251 (92.6%) of HCWs had positive attitude (agree and strongly agree) towards that every patient should be asked for detail if they have any signs and symptoms of infection and 20 (7.4%) had negative (disagree, neutral and strongly disagree). From the total respondents 239 (88.2%) had positive attitude (agree and strongly agree) that every patient should be voluntarily counselled and tested for HIV/AIDs to know their status and 32 (11.8%) disagree, neutral, strongly disagree to advice every patient about VCT.

Among 271 study participants 251 (92.6%) tell coughing patients to follow cough hygiene procedures such as using masks, covering mouth while coughing and sneezing and 20 (7.4%)had negative attitude (disagree, neutral, and strongly disagree). From the total participants 262 (96.7%) had positive (agree and strongly agree) that opening windows and doors of the ward is important to make the ward ventilated and 9 (3.3%) of the respondents had negative (disagree, neutral and strongly disagree) to open windows and doors (Table 3).

| No. | Variable | Category | | | | |
|---|---|---|---|---|---|---|
| | | Strongly disagree | Disagree | Neutral | Agree | Strongly agree |
| | | Freq. (%) | Freq.(%) | Freq. (%) | Freq. (%) | Freq. (%) |
| 1 | I feel comfortable asking every patient if they have any symptoms of infection | 1 (0.4) | 12(4.4%) | 7 (2.6%) | 102 (37.6%) | 149 (55%) |
| 2 | Advising every patient to accept VCT | 4 (1.5%) | 9 (3.3%) | 19 (7%) | 134 (49.9%) | 105 (38.7%) |
| 3 | Feeling comfortable to tell coughing patients to follow cough hygiene procedures | 1 (0.4%) | 12(4.8%) | 6 (2.2%) | 152 (56.1%) | 99 (36.5%) |
| 4 | Ventilating the ward by opening windows and doors | 1 (0.4) | 3 (1.1%) | 5 (1.8%) | 127 (46.9%) | 135 (49.8%) |
| 5 | Using PPE | 0 (0%) | 6 (2.2%) | 4 (1.5%) | 128 (47.2%) | 133 (49.1%) |
| 6 | Washing hands before and after contact with patients | 2 (0.7%) | 9 (3.3%) | 5 (1.8%) | 107 (39.5%) | 148 (54.06%) |
| 7 | Do you believe PPE protect HCWs from infection | 0 (0%) | 4 (1.1%) | 10 (3.7%) | 136 (50.2%) | 121 (44.6%) |
| 8 | Do you agree that in the absence of universal precaution hospital facilities can be the source of infection | 1 (0.4%) | 4 (1.1%) | 11 (4.1%) | 148 (54.6%) | 107 (39.5%) |
| | | | | | | |
| 9 | Do you believe needles should be recapped after use | 24 (8.9%) | 27(10%) | 11 (4.1%) | 121 (44.6%) | 88 (32.5%) |
| 10 | Do you believe that nosocomial infection can pose serious outcome | 1 (0.4%) | 10(3.7%) | 17 (6.3%) | 130 (48%) | 113 (41.7%) |
| 11 | Do you agree that recapping is the cause for needle prick injury | 5 (1.8%) | 47(17.3%) | 29(10.7%) | 109 (40.2%) | 81 (29.9%) |

| 12 | Do you believe separating active TB patients from other patients is an effective strategy for trans. of TB | 3 (11%) | 9 (3.3%) | 8 (3%) | 102 (37.6%) | 149 (55%) |

**Table 3:** Attitude of HCWS on infection prevention measures in WSTRH in 2017.

## Practice towards infection prevention measures

Among the respondents 22 (8.1%) follows recommended guide lines for use of alcohol based solutions and other antiseptics after lifting and moving a patient and 121 (44.6%) recaps needle after use. From the total respondents 261 (96.3%) discard used needles and other wastes in to their container and 47 (17.3%) of the participants of the study removes rings and bracelets and watches before beginning hand hygiene and also 261 (96.3%) dispose sharps separately from other wastes. In general 164 (60.5%) of HCWs have good practice towards infection prevention and control measures and the remaining 107 (39.5%) of health care workers have poor practice (Table 4).

| No. | Variables | Frequency (%) |
|-----|-----------|---------------|
|     |           | Yes |
| 1 | Do you follow recommended guide lines for use of alcohol and other antiseptics after lifting and moving patient? | 22 (8.1%) |
| 2 | Do you recap used needle? | 121 (44.6%) |
| 3 | Do you discard wastes immediately in to their container? | 261 (96.3%) |
| 4 | Do you remove rings and bracelets before beginning hand hygiene? | 47 (17.3%) 17.3 |
| 5 | Do you have written guideline for those who are exposed to HIV, HBV, HCV and etc.? | 267 (98.5%) |
| 6 | Do you have written guide line on waste disposal? | 270 (99.6%) |
| 7 | If yes do all staffs apply the guide line? | 125 (46.1%) 99.6 |
| 8 | Do you have isolation criteria for those who are admitted with highly contagious diseases? | 261 (96.3%) |
| 9 | Do you discard sharp materials separately from other wastes? | 261 (96.3%) |

**Table 4:** Practice of HCWs on infection prevention in WSTRH in 2017.

## Factors associated with practice on infection prevention measure in WSTRH

According to this study sex and working in different department has significant association with infection prevention practice but educational status, work experience and job title has no significant association with infection prevention practice (Table 5).

| Variable | Category | P-value | COR (95% CI) | P-value | AOR (95% CI) |
|----------|----------|---------|--------------|---------|--------------|
| Sex | Male | 0.016 | 1.833 (1.118-3.007) | 0.005 | 0.379 (0.193-0.743) |
|  | Female (R) |  | 1 |  |  |
| Department | Medical (R) |  | 1 |  |  |
|  | Surgical | 0 | 11.054 (4.391-27.829) | 0 | 0.076 (0.028-0.206) |
|  | Oby/gyn | 0 | 7.353 (3.439-15.723) | 0 | 0.127 (0.054-0.03) |
|  | Pediatrics | 0.001 | 3.739 (1.748-8.232) | 0.001 | 0.17 (0.06-0.48) |
|  | Other | 0 | 12.897 (4.881-34.073) | 0 | 0.073 (0.026-0.203) |
| Educational status | Diploma (R) |  | 1 |  |  |
|  | B.Sc. | 0.001 | 0.289 (0.138-0.607) | 0.114 | 1.933 (0.851-4.532) |
|  | Other | 0 | 0.211 (0.097-0.459) | 0.307 | 1.654 (0.63-4.344) |
| Receiving formal training | Yes |  | 1 |  |  |

| | No | 0.037 | 0.103 (0.012-0.87) | 0.037 | 9.683 (1.49-81.605 |
|---|---|---|---|---|---|

**Table 5:** Bivariable and multivariable analysis of factors affecting infection prevention practice among HCWs in Wolaitta Sodo, Otona teaching and referral hospital in 2017.

From this study male health care workers were 62% less likely to practice infection prevention when compared with female health care workers (AOR=0.379 (0.193-0.743)). Health care workers who work in surgical ward were 92% less likely to practice infection prevention when compared with HCWs in medical ward (AOR=0.076 (0.028-0.206)) and HCWs in Obs/gyn were 87% less likely to practice infection prevention (AOR=0.127 (0.054-0.03)) also HCWs in pediatrics ward were 87% less practice infection prevention (AOR=0.17 (0.06-0.48)) and the remaining health care workers from other departments were 92% less likely to practice infection prevention (AOR=0.073 (0.026-0.203)). According to this study health care workers not received training on infection prevention were nearly 10 times more likely to practice infection prevention.

## Discussion

This study revealed that 99.3% of health care workers had good knowledge and 0.7% of them had poor knowledge. This study finding is high when compared with finding from Health institutions from Baghdad city which revealed that 69% of health care workers had poor knowledge and 31% had good knowledge [9], teaching hospital of Zabol which revealed that 43% of the participants had poor knowledge and the remaining 57% had good knowledge [10].

This study finding is also higher when compared with finding from Palestine hospital which revealed 53.9% of the study participants had good knowledge [11]. This study finding is almost similar with finding from Dessie referral hospital which revealed 95.19% had good knowledge and 4.81 of the health care workers had poor knowledge [12] and also higher than finding from Amhara regional state referral hospital which showed >50% of the study participants had poor knowledge on infection prevention and control [12] and Bahir-dar city health institutions which revealed 84.5% of health care workers had good knowledge [13].This discrepancy may be due to the difference in setting, in sample size and having of training, characteristics of the study participants and difference in health related policies and guide lines.

This study showed that 93.4% of health care workers had good attitude and 6.6% of health care workers had poor attitude towards infection prevention. This finding is higher when compared with finding from teaching hospital of Zabol which revealed 33% of HCWs had good attitude [10]. And also higher from the study result conducted from health institutions from Bahir-dar city which revealed 55.6% of health care workers had good attitude [13].This difference may be due to variation in setting of the study and it also may be due to difference in awareness of health care workers.

This study showed that 60.5% of health care workers had good practice and 39.5% of health care workers had poor practice on infection prevention and control measures. The finding from this study is higher when compared with finding from Zabol teaching hospital which showed 34% of the study participants had good practice [10]. This study finding is also higher than finding from Amhara regional state referral hospital which revealed that >50% of the study participants had poor practice on infection prevention and control

[12].This variation is may be due to difference in sample size, difference in participant's characteristics and due training and infection prevention guideline availability.

This study finding is almost similar with finding from health institutions of Bahir-dar city which showed 54.2% of study participants had good practice towards infection prevention and control measures [13].

This study finding is lower when compared with finding from Dessie referral hospital which revealed 87.5% of the study participants had good practice [13]. Also this study finding is lower when compared with finding from Palestine hospital which revealed 91.1% of the study participants had good practice towards infection prevention and control measures [11]. This variation is may be due to difference in sample size, difference in setting and population characteristics and it may be due to not following recommended infection prevention guide lines.

This study revealed that there is significant statistical association in sex of HCWs, working in different units or wards and there also statistically negative association in having of training with infection prevention practice. But the study in Amhara regional state referral hospital showed that there is significant statistical association in age of HCWS, service year and educational status [12]. Also the study conducted in Palestine hospital revealed that there is no statistically significant association between age, years of experience and having of training this discrepancy may be due to difference in setting and population characteristics

## Conclusion

Majority of health care workers' knowledge and attitude toward infection prevention and control measures in Wolaitta Sodo Otona teaching and referral hospital were good and safe enough but practice of health care workers towards infection control were not sufficient. Variables such as, receiving formal training and working in different department has association with infection prevention practice but educational status, work experience and job title has no significant association with infection prevention practice.

## Recommendations

Based on the study finding the following recommendations are forwarded:

Otona teaching and referral hospital should encourage health care workers on application of written guide lines on use of personal protective equipment's encourage health care workers to use personal protective equipment's.

Otona teaching and referral hospital health care workers should apply written guide lines toward infection prevention and control measures responsibly.

The focal person of each department (ward) should follow health care workers closely and should take appropriate measure on HCWs who fails to practice as per guideline and protocol.

Otona teaching and referral hospital administrative bodies should focus on and supervise male health care workers.

Wolaitta Zone health bureau should monitor and supervise health care workers towards infection prevention practice and control measures with the routine services through provision of training and preparing and introducing health care workers infection prevention guidelines, protocol, rules, regulation and opportunities to promote the desired team sprit at all health facility levels are recommended.

## Competing Interest

The authors declare that they have no competing interest.

## Authors' Contributions

SH, EM, WE and FM conceived and designed the study, developed data collection instruments and supervised data collection. SH, WE and FM participated in the testing and finalization of the data collection instruments and coordinated study progress. SH, WE and FM performed the statistical analysis, SH and EM wrote all versions of the manuscript. All authors read and approved the final manuscript.

## Acknowledgement

Our warmest gratitude goes to Arba Minch University for all support and commitment for this research. The authors are great full to all health care professional who participated in the study.

## References

1. Tietjen Let (2011) Infection prevention guideline for health care facilities with limited resource. JHPHIEGO.

2. WHO, Western Pacific Region.

3. Admasu TE, Edward AS, Limndsay ME (2013) Infection control knowledge, attitude and practice among health workers in Addis Ababa, Ethiopia. Infect Control Hosp Epidemiol 34: 1289-1296.

4. Benedetta AL (2017) Infection control in developing nations. A practical guide. WHO 2002.

5. WHO (2017) Health care-associated infections FACT SHEET. Patient safety a world alliance for safer health care.

6. WHO (2017) Infection prevention and control in health care: time for collaborative action. Technical paper, Fifty-seventh Session.

7. Emine AL, Hakan L, Mehmet D, Andreas V (2011) Infection control practice in countries with limited resources. Ann Clin Microbiol Antimicrob 10: 36.

8. Yakob E, Lamaro T, Henok A (2017) Knowledge, attitude and practice towards infection control measures among Mizan-Aman General Hospital Workers, South West Ethiopia. J Community Med Health Educ 5: 370.

9. Mohammed BA, Jaffar AJ (2017) Assessment of nurse's knowledge about nosocomial infection at hospitals in Baghdad City. Journal of Kufa for Nursing Science 4.

10. Hamed S, Abbas B, Nosratollah M, Ebrahim E (2015) Knowledge, attitude and practice of nurses about standard precautions for hospital-acquired infection in teaching hospitals affiliated to Zabol University of Medical Sciences, 2014. Glob J Health Sci 8: 193-198.

11. Imad F, Ahmad A, Faeda E, Lubna H (2015) Nursing department, Arab American University, Palestine. Knowledge and practice of nursing staff towards infection control measures in the Palestinian hospitals. J Educ and Pract 6: 79-90.

12. Freahiywot AT, Eshetu HE, Workie ZW (2015) Knowledge, practice and associated factors towards prevention of surgical site Infection among nurses working in Amhara Regional State Referral Hospitals, Northwest Ethiopia. Surg Res Pract, pp: 1-6.

13. Kelemua G, Gebeyaw T (2014) Assessment of knowledge, attitude and practice of health care workers on infection prevention in Health Institute Bahir Dar City Administration. Sci J Public Health 2: 384-393.

# 6

# Do Practice Nurses in the Caribbean have the Knowledge of the Principles and Concepts of Diabetes Self-Management Education?

Philip Onuoha[1]*, Denis Isreal-richardson[1], Lu-Ann Caesar[1], Chidum Ezenwaka[1] and Michiko Moriyama[2]

[1]The Diabetes & Metabolism Research Group (DMRG), Faculty of Medical Sciences, The University of the West Indies, St Augustine Campus, Trinidad and Tobago

[2]Institute of Biomedical & Health Sciences, Hiroshima University, Japan

*Corresponding author: Philip Onuoha, PhD, MPH, BScN, RNT, RN Director (Ag.), The UWI School of Nursing, Faculty of Medical Sciences, The University of The West Indies, Trinidad and Tobago, E-mailPhilip.Onuoha@sta.uwi.edu

## Abstract

**Aim:** To compare the knowledge of practice nurses on principles and concepts of diabetes self-management education (DSME) before and after a DSME training workshop.

**Methods:** All 150 practice nurses currently studying for a bachelor's degree were invited for a 2-day DSME training workshop. 88 practice nurses (59%) responded. Each participant was requested to complete and return self-assessment questionnaires before and after the training. The pre- and post-workshop knowledge of the nurses were compared using Wilcoxon Signed Rank Test for non-parametric tests in SPSS.

**Results:** The practice nurses were aged between 20 and 62 years and the majority (95.1%) were employed in the public sector. Before the training, 98-100% of the participants knew and agreed with the five articulated princples of DSME and these did not change after the workshop training (all, p>0.05). Similarly, their understanding (96-100%) of the concepts of DSME before and after the training were similar (all, p>0.05).

**Conclusions:** The practice nurses in Trinidad and Tobago have sufficient theoretical knowledge of the principles and concepts of DSME. The transfer of this knowledge to their patients in their care will depend on the educational infrastructure available to facilitate efficient DSME.

**Keywords** Diabetes self-management; Diabetes complications; Diabetes education; Developing countries

## Introduction

Based on the reports of the International Diabetes Federation (IDF), the challenges of diabetes epidemic are more in the developing regions of the world [1]. Although there is considerable regional and international campaign initiatives aimed at preventing diabetes on the entire globe [1], the majority (80%) of diabetes-related deaths take place in the developing countries of the world [2]. Therefore there is the urgent need to focus more on preventing diabetes complications through intensified diabetes self-management education [3]. Although there are reports of low budgetary allocation for healthcare in some developing countries [4], training the patients on diabetes self-management practices would assist in reducing diabetes complications. There are several research studies that have confirmed that non-pharmacological interventions assisted in controlling glycemia in type 2 diabetes patients and subsequently prevent diabetes complications [5-7]. Furthermore, a culturally competent diabetes self-management education (DSME) has been demonstrated to assist in reducing blood glycemia and improve the patients' diabetes knowledge score [8]. It is well recognized that nurses are usually involved in the promotion of diabetes self-care [9], but nurses who have not had acquired the necessary diabetes education may lack the ability to provide such education. For instance, some research studies have shown that nurses' diabetes knowledge score are between 64.3% and 75% [10,11]. A more recent UK research report showed that practice nurses' knowledge score on diabetes increased from 66% pre-education to 86% post-education programme [12]. The previous reports that many patients do not usually get formal diabetes education or encouragement for diabetes self-care might be related to the practice nurses' insufficient diabetes knowledge [13,14]. Therefore, the present study aimed to compare the knowledge of practice nurses on principles and concepts of diabetes self-management education (DSME) before and after a DSME training workshop in a Caribbean Island.

## Methods

### Subjects recruitment

All the 150 practice nurses who enrolled in a bachelor's degree programme of the University of the West Indies, Trinidad and Tobago were invited (through posters and announcements during formal classes) for the 2-day diabetes self-management education (DSME) training workshop. Of the 150 available practice nurses, 88 (representing 59%) registered for the workshop and participated in the training exercise.

### Study Protocol

A questionnaire tool consisting of three sections: (i) Bio-data with seven closed-ended questions, (ii) five questions on the principles of DSME and (iii) six questions on the concepts of DSME were used for the assessment. To preserve the anonymity of the practice nurses, the questionnaires did not contain any personal identifiers except that the questionnaires were serially numbered in duplicate to facilitate matching the pre-workshop and post-workshop knowledge of each participant. During the registration for the workshop, each practice nurse was given two copies (pre- and post-workshop assessment questionnaires) bearing the same number but differentiated with a "pre-" and "post-workshop" mark on top right-hand side of the questionnaire. Each participant was asked to complete and submit the pre-workshop assessment questionnaire before the commencement of the workshop. Two DSME professionals facilitated the workshop using information contained in several published research reports on DSME [5-7,15,16]. The training focused on the principles (frequent and sustained patient contact, patient-healthcare provider's joint decision-making via dialogue, continuous patient education and support, assisting patients in goal-setting etc) and concepts (need for daily/weekly/monthly journal to record self-monitoring activities, patient understanding of physiological and laboratory data, patient self-monitoring of body weight, BP, blood glucose, diet and exercise activities, patient regular consultation with healthcare providers, emphasis on patient acquisition of self-care skills etc) of DSME. It also included the behaviour modification theories, how to enhance self-efficacy necessary skills of DSME and how to follow up evidence-based practice.

The two facilitators each gave 2-hour didactic lectures on DSME (total 4 hours) and subsequently there was small group brainstorming sessions of an hour in groups of 8 to 10 participants. During the small group discussions, the participants were asked to brainstorm (based on their experiences at their places of work) on the provision of DSME and the challenges of such education at their places of work. The two facilitators went from one group to another listening to each group's brainstorming sessions. At the end of the small group discussions, all the groups converged at the large lecture theatre and one representative of each group made a presentation based on their brainstorming session. The presenters dwelled on what they considered as the benefits and challenges of DSME based on their experiences in their places of work. Feedbacks were taken from the facilitators as appropriate. After this large group session, the participants were requested to complete and return the post-workshop assessment questionnaire tool.

### Statistics

The Statistical Package for the Social Sciences (SPSS) was used for the statistical analysis. The participants' knowledge of the principles and concepts of DSME pre- and post-workshop were compared using Wilcoxon Signed Rank Test for non-parametric tests for two related samples. The data were presented as absolute number and percentages (in parenthesis). A p-value less than 0.05 was considered statistically significant.

### Limitations

The workshop participants might show some selection/participant bias given that participants were part of practicing nurses who were undergoing some continuing professional development programme and so may not necessarily represent a typical practicing nurse in Trinidad and Tobago. Also, the authors suspect that many of the nurses might have been exposed to other forms of chronic disease management education programmes in an Island country that is small. Further, many of the question items required a simple Yes/No response. Perhaps it was possible for many of the responses to be responded to correctly through common sense. However, we believe that any information garnered would go a long way in understanding the extent of need of DSME in the Island state.

## Results

Table 1 shows the background characteristics of the participants. Of the 150 practice nurses were invited for the workshop, 88 (representing 59% response rate) registered and participated. Of the 88 participants, eight (10%) did not return their post-workshop assessment questionnaire and were thus excluded in the data analysis. The participants were aged between 20 and 62 years and the majority (95.1%) were employed in the public sector. The majority (60%) of the practice nurses were people of African descent while 17.7% were of mixed ethnicity (Table 1). The participants' knowledge of the principles of DSME before and after the workshop are shown on Table 2. Almost all the participants (98-100%) knew and agreed with the five articulated princples of DSME and these did not change after the workshop (all, p > 0.05). Table 3 shows the participants' understanding of the concepts of DSME before and after the workshop. There were no significant differences in their understanding of the concepts of DSME before and after the workshop (Table 3, all, p>0.05).

| Parameters | participants | | |
|---|---|---|---|
|  | Male | female | Total |
| **Qualifications** | | | |
| Registered Nurses, N (%) | 4 (4.5) | 69 (78.4) | 69 (78.4) |
| Registered Nurse and Midwife, N (%) | - | 15 (17.0) | 15 (17.0) |
| **Employment** | | | |
| Employed, N (%) | 4 (4.5) | 75 (85.2) | 79 (89.8) |
| Not employed, N (%) | - | 9 (10.2) | 9 (10.2) |
| **Work place** | | | |
| Public, N (%) | 4 (4.9) | 74 (90.2) | 78 (95.1) |
| Private, N (%) | - | 4 (4.9) | 4 (4.9) |
| **Ethnicity** | | | |
| African descent, N (%) | 2 (2.4) | 49 (57.6) | 51 (60.0) |
| Indian descent, N (%) | 2 (2.4) | 17 (20.0) | 19 (22.4) |
| Mixed ethnicity, N (%) | - | 15 (17.7) | 15 (17.7) |

**Table 1** : Background characteristics of the participants of the DSME training workshop.

| Parameters | Responses of the participants | | | |
|---|---|---|---|---|
|  | Agree | Don't agree | Not sure | p-value |

| | | | | |
|---|---|---|---|---|
| **The principles of diabetes self-management education encourage frequent and sustained patient contact with diabetes healthcare providers to facilitate behavioral changes.** | | | | |
| Pre-workshop, N (%) | 79 (98.8) | 1(1.3) | - | 0.120 |
| Post-workshop, N (%) | 79 (98.8) | 1(1.3) | - | |
| **The principles of diabetes self-management education emphasis patient's-healthcare provider's joint decision-making process through dialogue.** | | | | |
| Pre-workshop, N (%) | 79 (98.8) | 1(1.3) | - | 0.375 |
| Post-workshop, N (%) | 79 (98.8) | 1(1.3) | - | |
| **The principles of diabetes self-management education emphasis continuous patient education and support initiatives to produce positive effects.** | | | | |
| Pre-workshop, N (%) | 77 (97.5) | 2(2.5) | - | 0.453 |
| Post-workshop, N (%) | 77 (97.5) | - | 2(2.5) | |
| **The principles of diabetes self-management education include assisting patients in goal-setting to facilitate achievement of the self-care effects.** | | | | |
| Pre-workshop, N (%) | 79 (100) | - | - | 1.000 |
| Post-workshop, N (%) | 79 (100) | - | - | |
| **Diabetes self-management education includes results in improved physiological data, the patient's quality of life and reduced diabetes complications.** | | | | |
| Pre-workshop, N (%) | 79 (100) | - | - | 0.630 |
| Post-workshop, N (%) | 79 (100) | - | - | |

**Table 2:** Assessment of the participants' knowledge of the principles of diabetes self-management education (DSME).

| Parameters | Responses of the participants | | | |
|---|---|---|---|---|
| | Agree | Don't agree | Not sure | p-value |
| **A programme of diabetes self-management education includes patient's daily or weekly or monthly journal to record self-monitoring activities.** | | | | |
| Pre-workshop, N (%) | 80(100) | - | - | 0.250 |
| Post-workshop, N (%) | 80(100) | - | - | |
| **A programme of diabetes self-management education includes teaching and interpretation of laboratory and physiological data.** | | | | |
| Pre-workshop, N (%) | 77(96.3) | 1 (1.3) | 2(2.5) | 0.219 |
| Post-workshop, N (%) | 77(96.2) | 1 (1.2) | 2(2.5) | |
| **A programme of diabetes self-management education includes self-monitoring skills in measuring indices such as weight, BP, blood glucose, diet and physical exercise activities.** | | | | |
| Pre-workshop, N (%) | 80 (100) | - | - | 1.000 |
| Post-workshop, N (%) | 80 (100) | - | - | |
| **A programme of diabetes self-management education includes emphasis on regular consultations with physicians/nurses to assist in goal setting and decision making.** | | | | |
| Pre-workshop, N (%) | 80 (100) | - | - | 0.250 |
| Post-workshop, N (%) | 80 (100) | - | - | |
| **A programme of diabetes self-management education employs theoretical strategies such as cognitive behavior therapy, social skills training and cognitive reconstruction method.** | | | | |
| Pre-workshop, N (%) | 77(97.5) | 1 (1.3) | 1 (1.3) | 0.390 |
| Post-workshop, N (%) | 77(97.5) | 1 (1.3) | 1 (1.3) | |

| The overall objective of diabetes self-management education is for the patient acquisition of self-care skills. | | | | |
|---|---|---|---|---|
| Pre-workshop, N (%) | 75(98.7) | 1 (1.3) | - | 0.219 |
| Post-workshop, N (%) | 75(98.7) | 1 (1.3) | - | |

**Table 3 :** Assessment of the participants' knowledge of the concepts of diabetes self-management education (DSME).

## Discussion

This study compared the knowledge of practice nurses on the principles and concepts of diabetes self-management education (DSME) before and after a DSME training workshop. The analysis of the data showed that the majority (96-100%) of the practice nurses knew the theoretical principles and concepts of DSME before the training. These findings are very encouraging especially coming from a developing high-income country [17]. These findings are discussed in relation to provision of DSME in work places in developing countries.

The current findings from an acute research study showed that practice nurses who are doing a bachelor's degree programme have the theoretical knowledge of the principles and concept of diabetes self-management education (DSME). On the basis of these findings, it could be argued that the practice nurses studied are theoretically well equipped to provide DSME to the patients in their work places. This interpretation is made in the context of a previous research report which showed that diabetes patients were poorly managed due to insufficient knowledge of DSME among nurses [18]. Indeed, other workers have also argued that nurses who have not had a specialized training in diabetes education may lack the ability to provide DSME [19]. The preceding argument put together, it is unclear if theoretical knowledge of the principles and concepts of DSME amongst practice nurses would translate to provision of DSME to the diabetes patients in their care. Nurses and dietitians in Trinidad and Tobago have previously opined that inadequate healthcare personnel, economic resources and educational facilities constituted significant barriers to provision of DSME in their places of work [4]. Although Trinidad and Tobago is classified as a high-income economy [17], diabetes education at the primary care clinics does not meet the requirements for effective DSME [15]. In most clinics at the primary care settings (where most patients reside), practice nurses usually conduct generalized diabetes education in non-structured format within a short time frame within the crowded chronic disease clinics. The clinic education class is not tailored to meet individual patient's needs/challenges or set goals for lifestyle modifications or made provision for feedback from the patients in the next clinic (Personal experience). The IDF advisory on DSME emphasized the importance of both DSME and diabetes self-management support (DSMS) in preparing diabetes patients in making well informed decision, coping with the challenges of living with diabetes and assisting in lifestyle modifications that support the patient's self-management efforts [1].

In view of the foregoing, we argue that the knowledge of the principles and concepts of DSME may not necessarily translate to provision of such education to the patients given that the quality of a healthcare system is largely dependent on its healthcare personnel and available economic resources. Diabetes self-management was described as a union between expert clinical care and expert self-care [20]. For a patient in a developing country to acquire the expertise for self-care, the healthcare system must provide educational and material support. For instance, it has been demonstrated that type 2 diabetes

patients who were provided with blood glucose monitoring facilities (glucometer, test strips, lancets, alcohol swabs etc) were able to self-monitor their blood glucose levels and subsequently had improved blood glycemia and reduced coronary heart disease risk profile [19]. Thus, the importance of diabetes self-management support (DSMS) is critical in the provision of DSME. For example while 94% of type 2 diabetes patients that participated in a research study on home blood glucose monitoring acknowledged that self-monitoring of blood glucose assisted in their blood glucose control, 70% indicated that self-monitoring of their blood glucose levels was a very expensive practice [21]. This would suggest that if there is no diabetes self-management support, the application of the theoretical knowledge from DSME will be ineffective. Previous studies have shown that many patients in developing countries have high theoretical knowledge score on the benefits of healthy lifestyle, yet there are high prevalence rates of the risk factors for cardiovascular disease and the metabolic syndrome amongst the same type 2 diabetes patients [22-28].

Thus DSME in developing countries need real material support to be successful. Given the low budgetary allocation to the healthcare sector in developing countries [4], it would appear that many health care systems may not be prepared for DSME [3]. It is recommended that governments of the developing countries should allocate adequate economic resources to the public health sectors to intensify DSME [4]. We therefore conclude that the practice nurses in Trinidad and Tobago have sufficient theoretical knowledge of the principles and concepts of DSME. The transfer of this knowledge to the patients in their care will require adequate educational infrastructure to facilitate the provision of diabetes self-management education.

## Acknowledgement

This study was supported in part by the Japanese Society for the Promotion of Science (JSPS) grant (to Professor Michiko Moriyama), the University of the West Indies School of Nursing and the Department of Para-Clinical Sciences, Faculty of Medical Sciences, The University of the West Indies, St Augustine Campus.

## References

1. World Health Organization, International Diabetes Federation (2000) The western pacific declaration on diabetes. WHO, Western Pacific Regional Office, IDF Western Pacific Region, Secretariat of the Pacific Community and Western Pacific Diabetes Declaration.

2. Roglic G, Unwin N (2010) Mortality attributable to diabetes: estimates for the year 2010. Diabetes Res Clin Pract 87: 15-19.

3. Ezenwaka C, Eckel J (2011) Prevention of diabetes complications in developing countries: time to intensify self-management education. Arch Physiol Biochem 117: 251-253.

4. Self-monitoring of blood glucose improved glycemic control and the 10-year coronary heart disease risk profile of female type 2 diabetes patients in Trinidad and Tobago.

5.   Tharkar S, Devarajan A, Kumpatla S, Viswanathan V (2010) The socioeconomics of diabetes from a developing country: a population based cost of illness study. Diabetes Res Clin Pract 89: 334-340.

6.   Eriksson KF, Lindgärde F (1991) Prevention of type 2 (non-insulin-dependent) diabetes mellitus by diet and physical exercise. The 6-year Malmö feasibility study. Diabetologia 34: 891-898.

7.   Tuomilehto J, Lindström J, Eriksson JG, Valle TT, Hämäläinen H, et al. (2001) Prevention of type 2 diabetes mellitus by changes in lifestyle among subjects with impaired glucose tolerance. N Engl J Med 344: 1343-1350.

8.   Davies MJ, Heller S, Skinner TC, Campbell MJ, Carey ME, et al. (2008) Effectiveness of the diabetes education and self management for ongoing and newly diagnosed (DESMOND) programme for people with newly diagnosed type 2 diabetes: cluster randomised controlled trial. BMJ 336: 491-495.

9.   Brown SA, Garcia AA, Kouzekanani K, Hanis CL (2002) Culturally competent diabetes self-management education for Mexican Americans: the Starr County border health initiative. Diabetes Care 25: 259-268.

10.  Carey N, Courtenay M (2007) A review of the activity and effects of nurse-led care in diabetes. J Clin Nurs 16: 296-304.

11.  Lipman TH, Mahon MM (1999) Nurses' knowledge of diabetes. J Nurs Educ 38: 92-95.

12.  Baxley SG, Brown ST, Pokorny ME, Swanson MS (1997) Perceived competence and actual level of knowledge of diabetes mellitus among nurses. J Nurs Staff Dev 13: 93-98.

13.  Hearnshaw H, Hopkins J, Wild A, MacKinnon M, Gadsby R, Dale J (2001) Mandatory,multidisciplinary education in diabetes care: can it meet the needs of primary care organization? Practical Diabetes International 18: 274-280.

14.  Mensing C, Boucher J, Cypress M, Weinger K, Mulcahy K, et al. (2000) National standards for diabetes self-management education. Task Force to Review and Revise the National Standards for Diabetes Self-Management Education Programs. Diabetes Care 23: 682-689.

15.  Gleeson-Kreig J, Bernal H, Woolley S (2002). The role of social support in the self-management of diabetes mellitus among a Hispanic population. Public Health Nurs 19: 215-222.

16.  Moriyama M, Nakano M, Kuroe Y, Nin K, Niitani M, et al. (2009) Efficacy of a self-management education program for people with type 2 diabetes: results of a 12 month trial. Jpn J Nurs Sci 6: 51-63.

17.  Funnell MM, Brown TL, Childs BP, Haas LB, Hosey GM, et al. (2007) National standards for diabetes self-management education. The Diabetes Educator 33: 599-403.

18.  The World Bank (2012) Countries and Economies

19.  Drass JA, Muir-Nash J, Boykin PC, Turek JM, Baker KL (1989) Perceived and actual level of knowledge of diabetes mellitus among nurses. Diabetes Care 12: 351-356.

20.  Hollis M Glaister K, Lapsley JA (2014) Do practice nurses have the knowledge to provide diabetes self-management education? Contemp Nurse 46: 234-241.

21.  Ezenwaka C, Onuoha P, Sandy D, Isreal-Richardson D (2013) Diabetes self-management education in a high-income developing country: survey of the opinion of nurses and dietitians. Int J Diabetes Dev Ctries.

22.  Henrichs HR (2009) The need for knowledge of self. Diabetes Voice 54: 3

23.  International Diabetes Federation and World Health Organization (2006) The diabetes declaration and strategy for Africa; a call to action and plan of action to prevent and control diabetes and related chronic diseases.

24.  Ezenwaka CE, Olukoga A, Onuoha P, Worrell R, Skinner T, et al. (2012) Perceptions of Caribbean type 2 diabetes patients on self-monitoring of blood glucose. Arch Physiol Biochem 118: 16-21.

25.  Ezenwaka CE, Offiah NV (2003) Patients' health education and diabetes control in a developing country. Acta Diabetol 40: 173-175.

26.  Ezenwaka CE, Nwagbara E, Seales D, Okali F, Hussaini S, Raja B, Wheeler V, Sell H, Avci Eckel J (2007)A comparative study of the prevalence of the metabolic syndrome and its components in type 2 diabetic patients in two Caribbean islands using the new International Diabetes Federation definition.

27.  International Diabetes Federation (2011) Annual Report : A turning point for diabetes.

28.  International Diabetes Federation, World Health Organization (2004) Diabetes action now, the initiatives of World Health Organization and International Diabetes Federation. Geneva: World Health Organization and International Diabetes Federation, 2004.

# 7

# Mapping the Medication System: Weaknesses and Risk Management

**Cris Renata Grou Volpe\*, Diana Lucia Moura Pinho, Marina Morato Stival Lima, Walterlânia Silva Santos, Tania Cristina Santa Barbara Rehen and Silvana S Funghetto**

*Universidade de Brasilia, Brazil*

**\*Corresponding author:** Volpe CRG, Universidade de Brasilia, Faculdade de Ceilandia, Centro Metropolitano, Brazil, E-mail: crgrou@unb.br

## Abstract

Secure systems aimed at preventing medication error are the essential. Our objective was to describe and map the medication system of a large hospital in Brasilia, DF, Brazil and propose risk management strategies for their principal weaknesses. For this cross-sectional, exploratory, and descriptive study, the data was collected with the support of two nurses trained by the researcher. Direct observations and semi-structured interviews of professionals involved in the medication system covered the processes: prescription, dispensing, preparation, and administration of medications. The data collection period was from May 8 to 22, 2012. Eight nursing technicians from this study site, who are responsible for the preparation and administration of medications, participated in the study. We identified 34 activities, undertaken by different professionals, which show the complexity and greater possibility of error. The weaknesses identified include interruptions, displacement, environmental problems, human resources, lack of patient identification, infrastructure, technical problems during preparation and administration, as well as deficiencies in compliance with rules and security protocols. It was concluded that the more the process is computerized the less weaknesses are present. Therefore, implementation of risk management strategies and the use of technologies are needed to detect and reduce risks to ensure the quality of the executed processes.

**Keywords:** Medication errors; Medication systems; Nursing

## Introduction

Error is a phenomenon inherent in human nature, which can occur even in the most perfect systems, including a complex health system. One must assume that despite the training and care of people, errors occur in any process that involves human activity [1].

Thus, it is essential to develop safe and efficient systems to assist in error prevention, as well as identify and minimize its consequences. The opportunity to learn from mistakes is a useful strategy to improve the security of the systems and prevent recurrence. Thus, development is necessary of a non-punitive culture that encourages notification and analysis of errors in the context of the system [2].

In health services, a large number of activities are involved in the medication process. According to literature, a safe number of steps would be between 20 and 30, covering the prescription process, dispensing and administration of the medication [3]. As the system becomes more complex, the risk for errors increases [4].

On the other hand, in developing countries, the increase in medication errors is attributed to several factors, especially the lack of computerization of the health system and limited investment in communication technologies associated with the increasing complexity of therapeutic procedures [5]. The special and assistive character of the health system incorporates advanced technologies and treatments, but at the same time, may not add new procedures to work processes, which are often out of date.

In 2014, the Brazilian Ministry of Health, in partnership with other agencies, published a document that provides information and guidelines for the National Patient Safety Program that was implemented in 2013. This document encourages health care in an effective and error-free manner, with the adoption of protective barriers and establishment of reporting system for events adverse to the patient's health. The National Health Surveillance Agency also has a series of protocols and documents published about the quality and safety of patients in healthcare that can assist in practice [6].

The literature reports several risk management strategies, which can be used in health institutions for system security, including investment in technologies such as implementation of the electronic prescription, use of bar codes, automation of dispensing unit dose and use of smart infusion pumps [7].

In this context, considering that the error in the medication process should be avoided, it is important to understand and contribute information to support the implementation of risk management and preventive measures that reflect the safety and quality of the healthcare.

Therefore, our objective was to describe and map the medication system of a large hospital in Brasilia, to propose risk management strategies for its main weaknesses.

## Materials and Methods

This cross-sectional, exploratory, and descriptive study was performed in a public hospital in the Federal District, in central Brazil, from May 2013 to July 2013.

The present investigation was carried out in the internal medical clinic and the hospital pharmacy, which covers the entire medication system.

The factors that contributed to the selection of the internal medical clinic were: 1) volume of medication; 2) complexity of the medication process (calculation of doses, diversity of injectable medications and variety of infusions); 3) number and diversity of hospitalized patients; and 4) clinical conditions of the users and types of medicines used.

Data collection was performed with the support of two nurses trained by the researcher. Direct observations and semi-structured interviews with professionals involved in the medication system were conducted with the objective of describing and mapping the system for prescription, dispensing, preparation, and administration of medications.

During the data collection period, the activities in the medical clinical unit were carried out by two doctors, six nurses and fourteen nursing technicians, totalling 22 professionals. At the pharmacy unit, seven pharmacists, two nursing technicians, seven administrative technicians, and one assistant, totalled 17 professionals.

The nursing work in the institution is divided according to the model of classic nursing care. Nursing technicians are responsible for the preparation and administration of medications as well as bathing, feeding and primary health care. Nurses are responsible for administrative activities, work schedules and application of dressings and catheters, among other functions, for executing comprehensive care. The work schedules of nursing technicians are organized by the responsible nurse on duty considering the number of patients per professional, and the severity of the patients and care they require.

The inclusion criteria for study participants included professionals directly involved in the steps of the medication process, who accept to participate in the study and were not on vacation or leave for the period of data collection.

Interviews were conducted with the pharmacist responsible for dispensing medications, the director of the hospital pharmacy, two administrative technicians responsible for services at the hospital pharmacy, the nurse technician of the medical clinic responsible for requesting medication from the pharmacy, two nursing assistants, the head nurse of the medical clinic, and the physician responsible for prescribing medications to the patients in the medical clinic.

The participants were interviewed in order to collect information about their socio-demographic profile (age, sex, education, amount of professional experience and their time working in the unit) and workload (hours and number of patients under their care) as well as the operating characteristics of the pharmacy, how many workers per shift, their activities and the routine of the sector. Questions were asked about the routine preparation and administration of the medications and how the system operation. The medical team was asked about the routine activity of prescriptions and operation of the electronic prescription system.

The researcher and research assistants spent 15 days examining the medication system. These observations lasted five days in each step (prescription, dispensing, preparation and administration), distributed in morning, afternoon, and evening shifts. Observations were made on more than one step per day.

Systematic observation was done for each step of the medication system, medical prescription (prescription room), dispensing (dispensing room), preparation (preparation room) and administration (unit wards).

Observations were made of the prescription, dispensation, preparation, and administration of the medications. Adapted from the study of literature, issues examined included: the environment (physical space) where the activities are performed, organization,

lighting, noise level, interruptions; data about the professional responsible for the activity and information about the activity; resources used to develop the activity, such as consultation and prescription context for the completion of prescription (whether electronic or manual); professional responsible for the prescription; record of patient's prior evaluation; number of professionals involved in the observed step; description of prescription situations; quality of prescription printing; routines to control the dispensing of psychotropic drugs; controlled and refrigerated dispensing; and medication monitoring system. In other words, we sought to understand and record in detail of Who? Where? How? and What was done? in the context of the dispensing activity. Finally, variables related to the adequacy of preparation technique and administration of medicine, dilution, labelling, guidance to the patient, verification and record of the procedure were observed.

Each observer recorded observations in a field diary and, when necessary, noted additional comments considered relevant. Records contained information on the environment of each step of the medication process, as well as aspects of the work process.

The data collected was organized into Microsoft Office Excel® spread sheets. Descriptive and inferential analyses were used to examine the differences between the groups. The analysis was performed using the Package for the Social Sciences (SPSS®) software version 18.0.

Categorical variables are reported as absolute and relative frequencies, numerical variables are reported as mean and standard deviation (minimum and maximum).

The development of the study met national and international standards of research ethics involving human subjects.

## Results

The eight nursing technicians that participated in the study were responsible for the preparation and administration of medications at the studied location. They were observed during drug preparation and administration activities in order to describe and track the medication system. The socio-professional data of the participants showed that 6 (75.0%) professionals were females with a mean age of 39.12.

A flowchart was used to map of the medication system. This helped to visualize of the macro process, sub processes and activities carried out in order for the medication to reach the patient.

The macro process of the system is composed of 4 sub processes: prescription, distribution, preparation, and administration of the medication. Figure 1 is the flowchart of the mapped macro process and its sub processes.

The critical points/weaknesses of the sub processes are shown schematically by the symbol and the numerical sequence (1 to 25). Figure 2 shows the critical points (weaknesses) identified in the medication system.

The prescription sub process is performed the prescription room, used by prescribers for this activity. There are 6 computers to carry out the activity.

The furniture does not meet the ergonomic principles. The environment has artificial lighting and ventilation, and it is noisy due to the parallel conversations between professionals and the use of mobile phones. There is a large circulation of people (Figure 2, number 1).

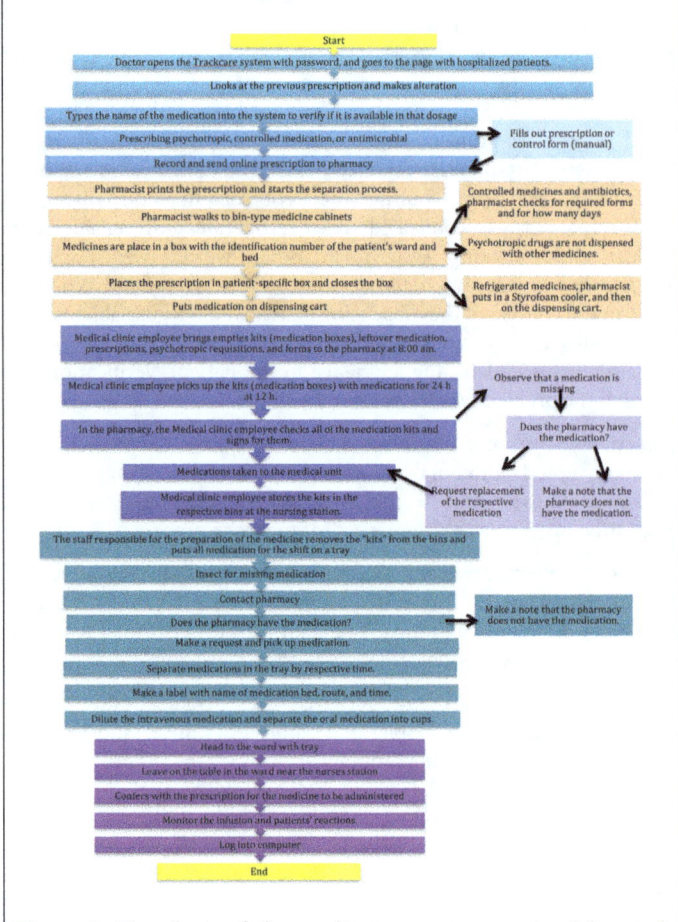

**Figure 1:** Flowchart of the medication system, regional hospital, 2013.

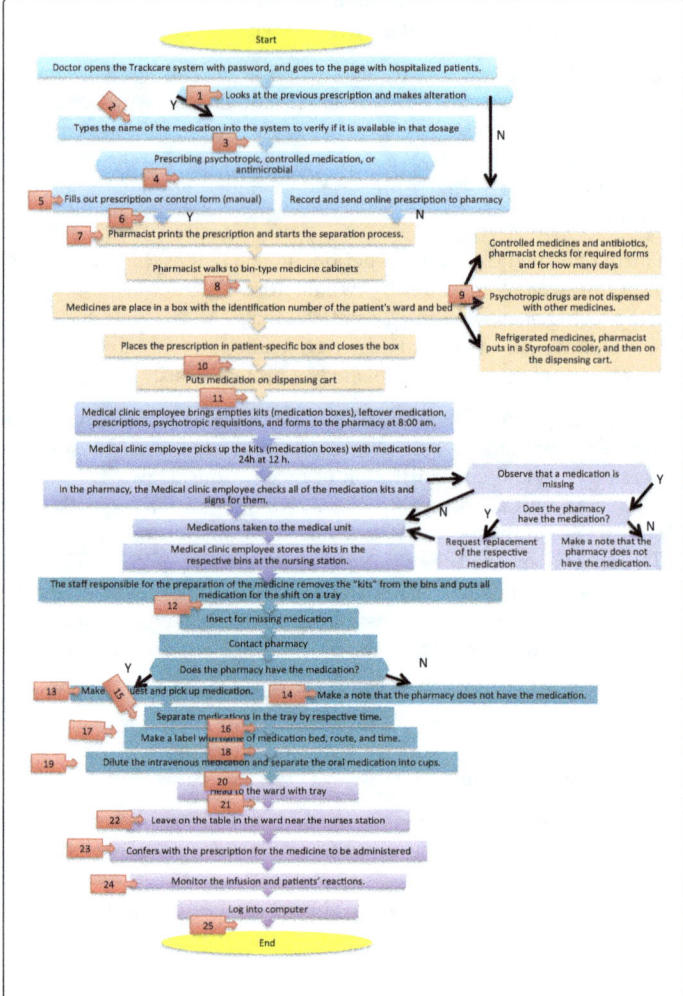

**Figure 2:** Flow chart of the medication system, indicating the weaknesses in the system, regional hospital, 2013.

In this sub process, displacements are frequent to visit patients or to find forms (Figure 2, number 2). The presence of only one professional was observed to make prescriptions for approximately 25 patients daily. The communication between the pharmacy and the clinic is not a good. When it occurs, it is only to report missing medicines, pending requests and problems with prescriptions (Figure 2, number 3).

Interruptions occur during all sub processes, on average a total of six (6) per observation period. These interruptions included attending cell phone and talking with patients' relatives, pharmacy representatives, sector employees with questions about patients, other doctors, residents and students. (Figure 2, number 4).

Prescribers must fill out a large number of forms, such as pharmacy requisitions (psychotropic drugs), non-standard medication form when the family needs to purchase the medication, inpatient examination requests, and medical certifications (Figure 2, number 5).

Other sources of information were not consulted by the medical team to prepare the prescription (Figure 2, number 6).

The sub process of dispensing and distributing medications occurs in the dispensary of the hospital pharmacy, which is adjacent to the storage areas. The lighting is artificial, free of sunlight. The ventilation is also artificial, through central air-cooling and air conditioners.

The physical space for dispensing is small, with many boxes of materials and medicines and, therefore, not adequate for the activity. The inadequacies in the hospital infrastructure were observed. The person in charge of the sector indicated that this area is scheduled to be renovated (Figure 2, number 7).

In the dispensing room, the professionals work on side benches, and on their side is a table with a computer for printing the prescriptions to be dispensed. The furniture also does not meet ergonomic principles. The rack with shelves and drawers are identified according to the active principle. Psychotropic medications are stored in a specific cabinet, not locked and without any control (Figure 2, number 8).

Interruptions occurred to solve problems, to dispense medications to the ICU, or to assist professionals requesting medication. Parallel conversations and extensive circulation of people in the area during the dispensing were observed. Dislocations were frequent, as the pharmacist often had to go to the storeroom to fetch medicines that were missing from the dispensing shelves (Figure 2, number 9).

Other weak points were the lack of diagnostic information in the prescriptions printed at the pharmacy, and the lack of communication between pharmacist and doctor to notify about medicines not provided by the network. There was no double conference about the medications, as recommended in the literature. In addition, no notification was sent to the requesting unit about the lack of medications in the pharmacy and on the collective distribution of medications such as ointment, creams, and eye drops (Figure 2, number 10).

Strengths include the printing of prescription at the pharmacy and the participation of pharmacists in the dispensing with a consultation about the medication before it was taken to the unit.

The sub process of preparation and administration of the drug was carried out in a room adjacent to the nursing station, in an area with a large circulation of people, which poses a risk factor for increased errors (Figure 2, number 11).

Safety failures were observed in the preparation sub process, noting that often the professionals did not observe aseptic principles (hand hygiene), although the location is suitable for it (Figure 2, number 12). They also did not use universal protection barriers, such as procedure gloves, nor comply with basic aseptic procedures, such as disinfection of the ampoule and absence of aseptic access (Figure 2, number 13).

Failure to identify the medication was another observed risk factor. One issue was the labelling of the medications to be administered (on the medication cups, only the bed number was identified and the injectable only contained the bed number and ampoule attached to the syringe) (Figure 2, number 14).

The medications for several patients were often prepared at the same time (Figure 2, number 15). In addition, the number of employees was less than needed (Figure 2, number 16).

Another risk factor was the preparation of the medication near the nursing station (in the ward), without adequate conditions (Figure 2, number 17). Likewise, the medication based on the transcription of the prescribed drugs was prepared in inappropriate places (Figure 2, number 18). Transcription can be considered a critical and precarious aspect, because when transcription is based on memory, it might be copied wrong and thus generate errors such as changing the name of the drug, dose and route.

Preparation and administration of medications were done in advance (Figure 2, number 19), and administration of medications for two different schedules occurred at the same time (14:00 and 16:00 at 14:00) (Figure 2, number 20). The numerous interruptions and the constant noise of telephone, students asking, other professionals talking, television at the nursing station during preparation of the medicine (Figure 2, number 21) were also risk factors observed in this sub process.

Displacements to search for materials and to respond to requests were other verified risk factors, as well as failures to register the administration of medication, which were performed only once, at the end of the shift. In addition, the control of drugs brought from home or purchased by family members for treatment, which were kept at the ward (Figure 2, number 22).

There was a lack of orientation regarding the administration of medication (Figure 2, number 23) and failures in the monitoring of this sub process, with an error in monitoring the infusion (Figure 2, number 24). Another critical point was the registering of the administration of medication, which, due to the distance of the computer or forgetfulness of the professional, was often not performed (Figure 2, number 25).

## Discussion

The system installed in August 2011 was completely electronic. Thus, in the electronic medical records, information was recorded and only available by the system, including prescription of the medication, request and results of exams, registration of nursing professionals, medical progress, and request of materials and medications. In addition to this information, it provides data that facilitate the practice of efficient and safe prescriptions, for example: allergy alerts, duplicate data, drug interactions, dose quantity validation, verification of drug information and therapeutic substitution, dose calculation and BMI.

Several interruptions occur during all the sub processes. These interruptions can divert attention, which affects the concentration and security of the task. However, some protective barriers were observed. Strong points of the prescription sub process included the prescribers' preliminary assessment of the patients and consultation with the previous prescription, as well as the doctor and nurse's evolution before writing the prescription. The electronic system also showed no failures or problems during the observation period. Strengths also present in the sub process include no reuse or contamination of materials and identification of the patient by name. In general, a consultation was made at the time that the medication was administration, either with the prescription, when available, or with the transcript.

In the medication system and its sub processes, 34 activities are performed by different professionals, which show the complexity and great possibility for error.

This study demonstrates that an electronic prescription system is a favourable factors, which is in agreement with the reports in the national and international literature and contributes to the reduction of medication errors [8,9].

Risk factors such as interruptions, dislocations, environmental problems, sufficient human resources, lack of patient identification, poor infrastructure, non-compliance with safety rules and protocols and technical failures during preparation and administration were also described by other authors [9].

The weakness in complying with safety rules and protocols proposed by the Ministry of Health stands out as one of the critical and difficult management points and it is necessary to sensitize professionals to adopt good safety practices. Opting for the unit-dose distribution system and the centralized preparation of parenteral solutions is a management strategy that can help to minimize the risk potential when the space is available exclusively for the preparation of the medication and controlled from external conditions.

The professionals involved in the medication system must understand that this is a complex system. Therefore, they must have the knowledge that allows them to analyze and intervene in order to provide responsible and safe care for both the patient and the medical team [10]. In this and other studies [7], the nurses' performance is still a little distant when it comes to working with process mapping. These professionals supervise their personnel in the process of preparation and administration of medicines, but they lack a more defined action within the system.

According to the US Institute of Medicine Committee on Quality of Health Care in America, to make systems safer, processes must improve to respect human limitations, i.e., not rely on memory or simplify processes by reducing the number of steps. Mechanisms that stimulate actions to prevent errors are necessary, such as not providing medication in the absence of important patient data as weight, height and allergies [5].

Regarding the risk management strategies to avoid relying on just memory, the use of individual electronic devices, such as tablets, associated with the electronic prescription system is recommended to allow the nursing technicians easy and quick access to patient information, both for access to prescription and other user data and for recording their own activities. This conduct would allow a more integrated system and the incorporation of the technology into the sub processes of the preparation and administration of the medication.

Some steps in the system such as checking, documentation, and monitoring were often not observed [11]. However, failure to comply with these actions may result in medication error, because the process, as a systemic organization, begins with the prescription and ends with proper registration and monitoring by the nursing administration [12].

Bedside computers in association with computerized system make this registry faster and with less potential for failures. A study found that implementation of a computerized system, reduces by 30% the time required for documentation, leaving the professional more time available to invest in the nursing process as a whole [13,14].

Other technological strategies that can also be adopted to improve the preparation and administration processes include the use of the smart infusion pumps, which can contribute to system safety, because they have a wide range of acceptable programming parameters. Smart pumps are designed with drug-specific safety software to help nurses solve programming errors [15,16].

Smart pumps with bar code readers are designed to minimize these administration errors. In this case, the pump digitizer can be used to register the bar code on the patient's wristband, nurse's badge, and IV medication label. The bar code pump can detect if the infusion has been given to the right patient. In a fully integrated system, the bar code pump has a server that communicates with the electronic prescription system and/or the pharmacy information system, which guarantees compliance. However, this fully integrated approach is still rare [15,16].

Systems that use information technology, such as electronic prescription, automated distribution, barcoded medication administration, electronic medication reconciliation and personal health records are vital components of broader strategies to avoid medication errors. Therefore, a growing body of evidence calls for its widespread application [17-19].

A computerized distribution system associated with the unit dose would also be a proposal to simplify the preparation step, making it safer. In this system, the medication is dispensed in the exact dose, according to the medical prescription, requiring neither manipulation and/or reconstitution of the medication by neither the nursing team nor the need for mathematical calculations. This system allows the nursing team to administer the correct dose, minimizing the risks of adverse events, as well as reducing the time spent by professionals to prepare medications [8,20,21].

A measure to reduce drug errors, in order to ensure compliance with the nine rights of medication administration (right patient, drug, dose, route, pharmaceutical form, schedule, documentation, action and response), is a barcode system for quick identification of the patient submitted to the procedure [22]. Studies confirm that the use of bar codes can prevent medication errors [23,24]. They reduce errors by 54-87% at this stage [25-27].

In the context of the present study, it was possible to verify that, with the computerization of the prescription, the implementation of these strategies becomes easier. The system itself could block and issue reminders, which would make eliminate the exclusive trust of memory. It could also solve the problem of lack of data, because it could block prescription in the absence of essential information such as weight, height, and allergies.

It was verified that the sub processes that used the computerized system more, such as prescription, dispensing and distribution, presented less weaknesses. This corroborates the fact that these technologies are a management strategy to increase users' safety.

However, the results also found that, even with these advances of the electronic system, there are two systems within the same macro process: electronic, which goes through the sub process of prescription, dispensing, and distribution, and manual, in the sub processes of preparation and management.

In this sense, some measures can be implemented to reduce errors in this institution, in the field of the present research, among them: to form commissions composed of a multi professional team, whose purpose is to provide safe and quality assistance to the users, establishing management plans and thus a culture of risk monitoring.

These results are expected to provide integration of health education institutions and health services, which together can develop drug preparation and administration protocols as well as training programs. They could also promote continuing education of professionals, because information is one of the team's key tools for delivering safe, high-quality care.

A suggested measure to promote risk management is the investment in improvements in electronic prescription, which includes adaptations of the system, standardization of prescription items, and implementation of a unit-dose drug distribution system. It is believed this can improve the preparation and administration of medications, directly helping reduce medication errors and improve patient care.

## Conclusion

The results point to a medication process with critical points, which can be considered unsafe and risky, that compromise the activity of the professionals involved and the safety of their users. The study indicates that implantation of an electronic prescription system reduces risk factors for medication errors.

The processes that use the computerized system more, which include the prescription, dispensing, and distribution system, presented less weaknesses, which corroborates that the use of technologies is a management strategy that can guarantee the safety of users. Even with the advances provided by the electronic system, the study found the coexistence of two systems within the same macro process, the electronic one for sub process of prescription, dispensing, and distribution and the manual one in the sub processes of preparation and administration.

The measures to be taken to reduce errors in this institution include: creating of multi-professional commissions to discuss and establish strategies that can promote patient safety; elaborating protocols for preparation and administration of medication and enforce them and establishing reward plans by creating incentives for professionals who excel in performing their activities.

The findings of the study corroborate some research already existing in the field of Patient Safety and contribute to the elimination of weaknesses in the current system of the medication process. Adoption and fortification of security protocols are clearly indispensable to avoid errors that can occur even with the implantation of a digitized system in the health environment.

Nursing is vitally important to avoid medication errors, because such errors, depending on the situation, may even result in death of the patient. Thus, the adequate training of professionals with current and evidence-based technical-scientific knowledge, as well as ethical commitment and the recognition of their importance in the health system are also fundamental, because professionals act as a protective barrier for the patient.

# References

1. Reason J (2001) Human error. Cambridge (MA): Cambridge University Press.

2. Silva LC, Bohomol E (2015) Medication errors: Notify in theory and in practice be punished. How to change this paradigm? 18: 876-880.

3. Leape LL (2000) Reporting of medical errors: Time for a reality check. Qual Health Care. 9: 144-145.

4. Miasso AI, Grou CR, Cassiani SHB, Silva AEBC, Fakih FT (2006) Medication errors: types, causes and measures taken in four Brazilian hospitals. Rev Esc Enferm USP 524- 532.

5. Kohn LT, Corrignan JM, Donaldson MS. (Eds.) (2001) To err is human: Building a safer health system. Washington: Committee on Quality of Health Care in America, National Academy of Institute of Medicine.

6. Ministry of Health (Brazil) (2013) Approves the Basic Patient Safety Protocols. Official Journal of the Union 24 Sep 2013.

7. Rothschild JM, Keohane CA, Cook EF, Orav EJ, Burdick E, et al. (2005) A controlled trial of smart pumps to improve medication safety in critically ill patients. Crit Care Med. 33: 533-540.

8. Cassiani SHB, Monzani AS, Silva AEBC, Fakih FT, Optiz SP, et al. (2010) Identification and analysis of medication errors in six Brazilian hospitals. Sci Nurs 16: 85-95.

9. Gimenes FRE, Teixeira TCA, Silva AEBC, Optiz SP, Mota MLSM, et al. (2009) Influence of the writing of the medical prescription on the administration of medications at different times than prescribed. Acta Paul Enferm 22: 380-384.

10. Azevedo Filho FM (2013) Safety in the use of drugs in an intensive care unit. Brasília: Faculty of Health Sciences, University of Brasília.

11. Franco JN, Ribeiro G, D'Innocenzo IM, Barros BPA (2010) Perception of the nursing team about causal factors of medication administration errors. Rev Bras Enferm 63: 927-932.

12. Grou Volpe CR, Moura Pinho DL, Morato Stival M, Gomes de Oliveira Karnikowski, M (2014) Medication errors in a public hospital in Brazil. BJN 23: 11.

13. National Coordinating Council for Medication Error Reporting and Prevention (NCCMERP). Definition medication error.

14. Keohane CA, Bane AD, Featherstone E, Hayes J, Woolf S, et al. (2008) Quantifying nursing workflow in medication administration. JONA 38: 19-26.

15. Tang FI, Sheu SJ, Yu S, Wei IL, Chen CH (2007) Nurses relate the contributing factors involved in medication errors. J Clin Nurs 16: 447-457.

16. Trbovich PL, S Pinkney, Cafazzo JA, Easty AC (2010) The impact of traditional and smart pump infusion technology on nurse medication administration performance in a simulated inpatient unit. Qual Saf Health Care 19: 430-434.

17. Ohashi K, Dykes P, McIntosh K, Buckley E, Wien M, et al (2013) Bates evaluation of intravenous medication errors with smart infusion pumps in an Academic Medical Center. AMIA Annu Symp Proc 1089-1098.

18. Agrawal A (2009) Medication errors: prevention using information technology systems. Br J Clin Pharmacol 67: 681-686.

19. Cassiani SHB, Gimenes FRE, Monzani AAS (2010) The use of technology for patient safety. Rev Eletr Enf 1: 413-417.

20. Maaskant JM, Vermeulen H, Apampa B, Fernando B, Ghaleb MA, et al. (2015) Interventions for reducing medication errors in children in hospital. Cochrane Database Syst Rev 3.

21. Avelar AFM, Salles CLS, Bohomol E, Feldman LM, Peterlini MAS, et al, (2010) 10 Steps to Patient Safety. São Paulo: COREN-SP.

22. Elliott M, Liu Y (2010) The nine rights of medication administration: An overview. Br J Nurs 19: 1-7.

23. Silva LD, Camerini FG (2012) Analysis of administration of intravenous drugs in a sentinel hospital. Texto contexto - enferm 21: 633-641.

24. AMIA Podcast (2007) Bar Code Medication Administration Evidence.

25. Cheung KC, Bouvy ML, De Smet PAGM (2009) Medication errors: the importance of safe dispensing. Br J Clin Pharmacol 67: 676-680.

26. Institute of Medicine. Preventing Medication Erros.

27. Bowman S (2013) Impact of electronic health record systems on information integrity: Quality and safety implications.

# 8

# Neonatal Danger Signs: Attitude and Practice of Post-Natal Mothers

**Reena Thakur[1], Rajesh Kumar Sharma[2*], Laxmi Kumar[2] and Sanchita Pugazhendi[2]**

[1]Kol Vally Institute of Nursing, India

[2]Swami Rama Himalayan University, India

*Corresponding author: Rajesh Kumar Sharma, Assistant Professor, Himalayan College of Nursing, Medical Surgical Nursing, Swami Rama Nagar, Jollygtant, Dehradun, Uttarakhand 248140, India, E-mail: rajeshsharma.hcn@gmail.com

## Abstract

**Background:** A mother is the nearest person to a neonate to identify, present and manage the neonates' problem, which ensure that neonate can lead a healthy life. Every year four million babies die in the first month of life and a quarter of these take place in India. About 98% of new-born deaths occur in developing countries, where most new-borns deaths occur at home. The main obstacles in improving new-born survival are that many babies are born at home without skilled attendance. Hence the present study was aimed to assess the attitude and practice of mothers to recognize neonatal danger signs and various household practices followed by mother to identify and to treat danger signs.

**Materials and method:** A descriptive cross-sectional study with quantitative approach was undertaken on 100 post natal mothers by convenient sampling technique with the objective to assess the attitude and practice of post natal mothers regarding neonatal danger signs. Attitude scale and self-reporting practice check-list were used as a data collection tools.

**Results:** Result of the study shows that 61% of mothers had moderate attitude, 39% of mothers had favorable attitude. Whereas, practice level was high among majority (90.56%) of the post natal mothers regarding neonatal danger signs. There was a statistically significant correlation (r=0.401 at 0.01 level of significance) between attitude score and practice score.

**Conclusion:** The study concluded that there is need to improve the attitude and practices of post natal mothers regarding neonatal danger signs either during antenatal visit, post natal period or at community level. Community based educational program should be launched to enhance knowledge, attitude and practice of post natal mothers regarding neonatal danger signs.

**Keywords:** Post-natal mothers; Neonates; Neonatal danger signs; Attitude; Practice; Information booklet

## Introduction

In human life, the period from birth to 28 days of age is known as neonatal period (World Health Organization, 2014). Birth is a major challenge to the new-born to negotiate successfully from intra-uterine to extra-uterine life [1].

Globally 10 million under five children die every year. Majority of them die in their neonatal period. Among them 98% of these deaths occur in developing countries. Almost half of the deaths in under-five-year-olds occur in infancy. About two-thirds of infant deaths occur in the neonatal period. It has also been noted that one-third of all neonatal deaths occur on the first day of life, almost half within 3 days and nearly three-quarters within the first week of life. In developing countries, about 34 of every 1000 live births result in neonatal death [2,3].

Nigeria ranked highest in Africa in terms of number of neonatal deaths and second highest in terms of neonatal deaths worldwide. Estimated neonatal deaths which occurred in Nigeria in 2003, 37% were due to severe infections like pneumonia, sepsis, neonatal tetanus and diarrheal diseases; while preterm births and birth asphyxia accounted for another 49% [4].

In India the neonatal mortality rate (NMR) dropped significantly from 69 per 1000 live births in 1980 to 53 per 1000 live births in 1990 [2]. In recent years, however, the NMR has remained almost static decreasing only from 48 to 44 per 1000 live births from 1995 to 2000 and from 2011 to 2015 it has come down 22 to 28 per 1000 live births. A similar situation has been reported from other developing countries [2]. In Uttrakhand, Rudraprayag district has minimum NNMR (11) whereas Haridwar has maximum NNMR (50) and range is 39/1000 live births. In Dehradun neonatal mortality rate is 32 per 1000 live births.

Lack of specificity of the clinical manifestations of various neonatal morbidities has been noted, resulting in difficulty in making a definitive diagnosis, delay in seeking care and resultant high mortality [4].

The danger signs of severe illness included are 1) history of difficulty feeding, 2) movement only when stimulated, 3) temperature below 35.5°C, 4) temperature above 37.5°C, 5) respiratory rate over 60 breaths per min, 6) severe chest in drawings and, 7) history of convulsions. Assessment of these signs will result in a high overall sensitivity and specificity for prediction the need for hospitalization of a new-born in the first week of life [4].

Health and survival of children is dependent upon the health status of mother along with awareness, education and skills in mother is the best primary health worker. In view of her constant and continued contact with her child, she is the best person to identify the early evidence of illness and major development deviation from normal [5].

## Materials and Methods

A descriptive cross sectional study with quantitative approach was undertaken in Doiwala block, Dehradun District for a period of 1 month (December 2014-January 2015) to assess attitude and practice of post natal mothers regarding neonatal danger signs. Total 100 post natal mothers were selected by convenient sampling technique under following inclusion criteria. (1) All post-natal mothers who were having a baby of one month of age; (2) Mothers who were below the age of 40 years; (3) Mothers who were willing to participate. Only 53 mothers have reported that their neonate had neonatal danger signs. So only these mother practices were assessed. Data were collected by using Attitude rating scale and self-reporting practice check-list. Data were analyzed by using inferential and descriptive statistics.

## Results

| Sample characteristics | Frequency (f) | Percentage (%) |
|---|---|---|
| **Age (years)** | | |
| 20-24 | 57 | 57 |
| 25 and above | 43 | 43 |
| **Education** | | |
| Primary | 20 | 20 |
| Secondary | 33 | 33 |
| Higher secondary | 47 | 47 |
| **Occupation** | | |
| Working | 4 | 4 |
| Non-working | 96 | 96 |
| **Monthly Income** | | |
| 10,000 and below 10,000 | 88 | 88 |
| Above 10,000 | 12 | 12 |
| **Family Type** | | |
| Nuclear | 21 | 21 |
| Joint | 79 | 79 |
| **Living Area** | | |
| Rural | 9 | 9 |
| Semi-urban | 91 | 91 |
| **No. of Children** | | |
| 1 | 56 | 56 |
| 2 | 29 | 29 |
| 3 and more then 3 | 15 | 15 |
| **Pre-Exposure** | | |
| Yes | 24 | 24 |
| No | 76 | 76 |
| **Baby Gender** | | |
| Boy | 49 | 49 |
| Girl | 51 | 51 |
| **Birth month of baby** | | |
| Below 9 month | 5 | 5 |
| At 9 month | 69 | 69 |
| Above 9 month | 26 | 26 |

**Table 1:** Socio demographic profile of the post-natal mothers, (N=100).

The above Table 1 regarding demographic variables of study participants revealed that more than half (57%) of participants were in the age group of 20-24 years, Majority (80%) of participants had secondary and higher secondary education, (96%) non-working, (88%) monthly income less than 10,000, (79%) belonging to joint family, (91%) living in semi-urban area. More than half (56%) had one child, whereas only one fourth (1/4) (24%) of mothers had previous exposure on knowledge regarding neonatal danger signs. The ratio of baby gender among participants was almost equal (51%-49%) and most of (69%) of baby born at full term.

| Aspect | Category | Frequency | Percentage % |
|---|---|---|---|
| Unfavourable | 20-46 | 0 | 0 |
| Moderate | 47-73 | 61 | 61 |
| Favourable | 74-100 | 39 | 39 |

**Table 2:** Frequency and percentage distribution of attitude level of post-natal mothers regarding neonatal danger signs.

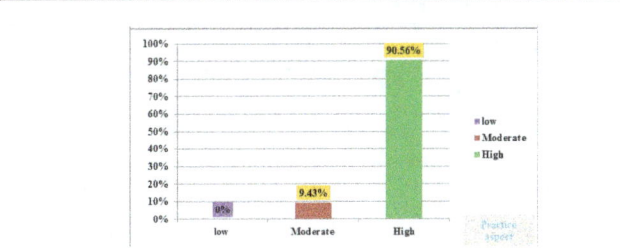

**Figure 1:** Bar diagram showing the percentage distribution of post natal mothers according practice level.

Table 2 reveals that, the attitude level was moderate among 61% of the post natal mothers regarding neonatal danger signs, 39% of the mothers having favorable level of attitude.

In above Figure 1 shows that level of practice among post natal mothers was high (90.56%), shows that majority of mothers are able to recognize the neonatal danger signs and symptoms and takes preventive actions regarding them.

| Aspect | Statement | Max. Score | Mean | SD | Mean% |
|--------|-----------|-----------|------|-----|-------|
| Attitude (N=100) | 20 | 100 | 71.78 | 7.898 | 71.78 |
| Practice (N=53) | 32 | 32 | 25.55 | 2.325 | 79.84 |

**Table 3:** Attitude and practice mean and SD score of post natal mothers regarding neonatal danger signs.

Table 3 reveals that the mean attitude of post natal mother was 71.78. Hence, it is to be interpreted that mothers were having moderate attitude regarding recognize and prevention of neonatal danger signs.

|  | Mean | SD | r-value | P-value |
|--|------|-----|---------|---------|
| Attitude | 70.92 | 7.859 | 0.401 | 0.003 |
| Practice | 25.55 | 2.325 | | |

**Table 4:** Correlation between attitude score and practice score of post-natal mothers regarding neonatal danger signs.

In Table 4, Karl Pearson test was used to find the correlation between the attitude score and practice score among post natal mothers regarding neonatal signs and it was found statistically significant (P<0.003). Hence, it can be interpreted statistically that as positive attitude of postnatal mothers increases, the practice of post natal mothers towards neonatal danger signs also increases.

## Association between attitude score, practice score and selected demographic variables

| Sr. No | Demographic data | Below median (<71) | Above median (71>) | Chi square | df | P-value | Significance |
|--------|------------------|--------------------|--------------------|------------|-----|---------|--------------|
| 1 | **Age** | | | | | | |
| | 20-24 | 26 | 31 | 0.202 | 1 | 0.887 | NS $\chi^2$ |
| | 25 and above | 19 | 24 | | | | |
| 2 | **Education** | | | | | | |
| | Primary | 16 | 4 | | | | |
| | Secondary | 12 | 21 | ----- | 2 | 0.001 | Sig F |
| | Higher secondary | 14 | 30 | | | | |
| 3 | **Occupation** | | | | | | |
| | Non-working | 42 | 54 | ----- | 1 | 0.0416 | Sig F |
| | Working | 4 | 0 | | | | |
| 4 | **Monthly income** | | | | | | |
| | 10,000 and below | 38 | 50 | 0.979 | 1 | 0.322 | NS $\chi^2$ |
| | Above 10,000 | 7 | 5 | | | | |
| 5 | **Family type** | | | | | | |
| | Nuclear | 11 | 10 | 0.585 | 1 | 0.444 | NS $\chi^2$ |
| | Joint | 34 | 45 | | | | |
| | | | | | | | |
| 6 | **Living area** | | | | | | |
| | Rural | 2 | 7 | ---- | 1 | 0.1799 | NS F |
| | Semi urban | 43 | 48 | | | | |
| 7 | **No. of children** | | | | | | |
| | 1 | 23 | 33 | | | | |
| | 2 | 12 | 17 | 3.35 | 2 | 0.188 | NS $\chi^2$ |

| | | | | | | | |
|---|---|---|---|---|---|---|---|
| | 3 or more then 3 | 10 | 5 | | | | |
| 8 | **Pre exposure** | | | | | | |
| | Yes | 6 | 18 | 5.1 | 1 | 0.024 | Sig $\chi^2$ |
| | No | 39 | 37 | | | | |
| 9 | **Baby gender** | | | | | | |
| | Boy | 18 | 31 | 2.65 | 1 | 0.103 | NS $\chi^2$ |
| | Girl | 27 | 24 | | | | |
| 10 | **Birth month of baby** | | | | | | |
| | Below 9 month | | | | | | |
| | At 9 month | 2 | 3 | ----- | 2 | 0.9375 | NS F |
| | Above 9 month | 32 | 37 | | | | |
| | | 11 | 15 | | | | |

**Table 5:** Association between attitude score and selected personal profile of post natal mother, (N=100).

Table 5 shows that there was statistically significant association between attitude score of participants and education (p<0.001), occupation (p<0.0416) and previous exposure (p<0.024) on knowledge regarding neonatal danger signs. Hence it can interpret statistically that the mother who were having higher education they were having positive attitude towards neonatal danger signs. Also the mother who were having previous exposure on knowledge regarding neonatal danger signs and mothers who were non-working they were having relatively positive attitude towards neonatal danger signs.

### Association between practice score and selected personal profile of post natal mother

There was no statistically significance association between practice score and selected personal variables of the participants regarding neonatal danger signs.

### Discussion

In this study it was found that most of mothers were having moderate attitude regarding neonatal danger signs. These findings are parallel to the previous study done by Darling et al. This study findings showed that majority (61%) of mothers were having favorable attitude regarding new-born care [6].

The present study reveals that, the practice level was high among majority (90.56%) of the post natal mothers regarding neonatal danger signs, only 9.43% of the mothers having adequate level of practice and regarding neonatal danger signs and none with low practice level. These findings are supported by a study done by Darling et al. This study finding showed that more than half of the post natal mothers 57% had high practice level, 43% had moderate practice level and none with low practice level [6].

The findings of the present study concluded that there was statistically significant correlation (r=0.401 at 0.01 level of significant) between the attitude score and practice score among post natal mothers regarding neonatal signs. The present study findings are supported by Rodrigo et al. The findings of the study showed that there was a significant correlation between attitude and behavior scores of mothers on neonatal jaundice [7].

The present study findings revealed that there was significant association between attitude score of participants and education, occupation and previous exposure on knowledge regarding neonatal danger signs. The findings of the study are supported by a previous study done by Rabiyeepoor et al. The study findings revealed that Knowledge and attitude scores of mother regarding jaundice were correlated with the past experiences of neonatal jaundice and educational levels [8].

The findings of shows that there was no significance association between practice score and personal variables of the participants regarding neonatal danger signs. The findings of the study are supported by previous study done by Castalino et al. The study findings revealed that Relationship between knowledge and practice score of the mother was not statistically significant at 0.05 level (r=0.276, p=0.140) [9].

### Conclusion

The findings of the study will help the nursing professionals working in hospital and community areas to educate the mothers about the recognition of neonatal danger signs and measure they should take as early as possible to care the baby with danger signs. Health education should be provided during antenatal visits, in post natal wards and Neonatal intensive care unit; before discharging of the mothers from the hospital would be beneficial and helpful to reduce neonatal morbidity and mortality rate.

### Acknowledgement

I would like to express my deepest appreciation to the research committee of Himalayan College of Nursing, Swami Rama Himalayan University, Dehradun for granting necessary permission and consistent support during research project. In addition, I would like to express my gratitude to the mothers of neonates for their full cooperation to make this study possible.

## References

1.  Kanchan B, Raj Kumari SD, Gomathi B (2013) Effectiveness of an 'Instructional Teaching Programme' (ITP) on the knowledge of postnatal mothers regarding new-born care. Hu Li Za Zhi 3: 231-237.

2.  Black RE, Morris SS, Bryce J (2003) Where and why are 10 million children dying every year? Lancet 361: 2226-2234.

3.  United Nations Children's Fund (2002) State of the world's new-borns 2001, Save the Children Publication, Washington, DC.

4.  Nigeria Demographic and Health Survey (2003) Maryland, USA: National Population Commission/ORC Macro, pp: 144-150.

5.  Darmstadt GL, Bhutta ZA, Cousins' S, Adam T, Walker N, et al. (2005) Evidence based, cost-effective interventions: How many new-born babies can we save? Lancet 365: 977-988.

6.  Darling B, Ranjita SW, Bazil AB (2014) New-born care among post natal mothers in selected maternity centers in Madurai, Tamil Nadu. Int J Allied Ed Sci 2: 119-124.

7.  Rodrigo BKNR, Cooray G (2010) The knowledge, attitude and behavior on neonatal jaundice of postnatal mothers in Provincial General Hospital, Badulla, Sri Lanka. J Child Health 40: 164-168.

8.  Rabiyeepoor S, Gheibi S, Jafari S (2013) Knowledge and attitude of postnatal mothers on neonatal jaundice in Motahari Hospital, Iran - Descriptive analytic study. JCM 3: 1-5.

9.  Castalino F, Nayak BS, D' Souza (2014) Descriptive correlational survey to assess knowledge and practice of postnatal mothers on new-born care. NUJHS 4: 98-101.

# 9

# Night Shift and its Impact upon the Quality of Life of Nurses Working at the Teaching Hospitals of the Medical City Complex in Baghdad City, Iraq

Maan Hameed Ibrahim Al-Ameri*

*Psychiatric Mental Health Nursing Department, College of Nursing/ University of Baghdad, Iraq*

*Corresponding author: Al-Ameri MHI, Assistant Professor, Psychiatric Mental Health Nursing Department, College of Nursing, University of Baghdad, Iraq, E-mail: dr.m.alameri@conursing.uobaghdad.edu.iq

## Abstract

**Background:** Nurses are key players in health care delivery, with night shift nurses having a special role in the provision of this health care. Night shift nurses are responsible for patient care with little support in a difficult working environment; under conditions of fatigue and other hardships directly related to working at night.

**Objective:** The present study aims to find out the impact of night shift on nurses quality of life; and to find out any relationship between the quality of life and some demographic characteristics such as age, gender, marital status, level of education and duration of career.

**Methodology:** A descriptive study was carried out to assess the nurses' quality of life. The nurses who work at Teaching hospitals of Medical City Complex were recruited from the 21st of February to 15th of July 2015. A non-probability sample of 70 night shift nurses was selected. The investigator constructed the questionnaire for purpose of the study. This questionnaire consisted of two parts; some demographic characteristics of those nurses and a scale which assess the levels of quality of night shift nurses. Data are analysed using descriptive statistics (frequencies and percentages) and Pearson Chi-Square as an inferential statistical analysis.

**Results:** The study results revealed that the majority of study participants were young and married. About quarter of the number of the nurses have duration of career of five years and less. More than half of nurses had very weak and weak quality of life. Mid-aged nurses had lower levels of quality of life. The results showed that the male nurses had higher levels of quality of life than female nurses did and the married nurses are more likely to have lower levels of quality of life than unmarried did. Finally, there was a significant relationship between levels of quality of life and gender and age.

**Recommendation:** The study recommends that it should provide adequate off-duty hours to let an uninterrupted sleep cycle of at least 8 h a day, which may affect nurses' daily life at home. It should use permanent shift assignments, which may diminish tiredness effects, instead of rotating shift duties.

**Keywords:** Night shift; Impact; Quality; Life; Nurses; Medical; Hospitals

## Background

The term shift work is defined as an arrangement of working hours that uses two or more teams (shifts) of workers, in order to extend the hours of operation of the work environment beyond that of the conventional office hours [1]. Nursing is considered as a stressful occupation [2-4]. Stress has an implication for health and the satisfaction level of the Nurses involved which eventually has an impact on the quality of care for the patients they attend to [5]. The night-shift nurses has rapidly increased worldwide over the last decades and nurses work long-hour night shift have become under conditions of intense stress. In addition, they often suffer from excessive workloads, stress, minimal social support and low quality of life [6]. Long-term night and shift work in nurses becoming more pessimistic and less vicarious as their training progresses, and might be associated with many health-related problems like fatigue, sleep problems, anxiety and difficulties in maintaining regular lifestyles [7].

Research in night shift has identified a number of stressors depending on the area of specialty. However, some common stressors in these specialties include poor working relationship between nurses and other health team members, demanding communication and relationship with patients' relatives, emergency cases, high workload, understaffed and lack of support or feedback from their seniors [8,9]. Working in night shifts creates difficulties in family life and tends to restrict nurses' social and leisure activities [10]. Particularly, working at night, either on permanent or rotating shifts, often produces discordance with the spouse's working hours and free time [11]. Nurses in 12 h shifts reported less social and domestic disruption than workers in 8 h shifts [12,13]. Numerous studies have shown high amounts of psychological distress in nurses and other healthcare professionals working in various situations [14]. Night shift causes an imbalance between desired lifestyle and work, women have a major role to play in the domestic life and they compromise their sleep to undertake the domestic chores such as care to their children and family chores. To find out whether night shift affects the social aspect of nurses or not 60% of respondents stated that their social life is sometimes affected, 33% stated that always their social life is affected that is mean 93% of the nurses are affected and 7% not affected. The aspect of social life involves nurses' families, work relationships and other social groups [6].

## Objective

The present study aimed to find out the impact of night shift on nurses quality of life; and to find out any relationship between the quality of life and some demographic characteristics such as age, gender, marital status, level of education, and duration of career.

## Methodology

Descriptive design with application of assessment approach study was used from 21st of February to 15th of July 2015. A non-probability sample of 70 nurses were recruited at five hospitals of the Medical City Complex which are Baghdad Teaching Hospital, Ghazi al-Hariri Hospital for surgery, Private Nursing Home, Liver and Digestive System Diseases Hospital, and Teaching Hospital for Burns; 20 nurses; 20 nurses; 15 nurses; 10 nurses; and 5 nurses respectively. A questionnaire was constructed and designed to meet the objectives of present study. This questionnaire consisted of two parts: firstly, demographic characteristics of the nurses jointed in the study such as gender, age, marital status, level of education, and duration of career. Secondly a scale was used to assess the levels of quality of life of nurses participating in the study, this scale The Quality of Life (WHOQOL)-BREF [15] that includes five Domains: psychological domain: nine items; physical domain: eight items; spiritual and religious domain: three items; social domain: seven items; and environment and housing: eight items. This scale is self-administered. The total items scores was measured, scored and finally rated on 4-level rating scale [12]. Four levels were determined by applying quartile descriptive analysis. Very weak level is with cut-off point ranged from 57 to 66; weak level is with cut-off point ranged from 67 to 71; intermediate level is with cut-off point ranged from 72 to 76; good level is with cut-off point ranged from 77 to 105. Data were analysed by applying the statistical package for the social sciences (SPASS) for windows, version 19; the descriptive statistical measures of frequency, percent, distribution tables and quartiles; and inferential data analysis: this approach was performed through the application of the-correlation coefficient; Pearson Chi-Square.

## Results

The results of demographic characters of the students, distribution of sample, distribution in level of QoL regarding to age, gender, marital status, education level and duration of career can be shown in the below tables (Tables 1-8).

| Age | | | Marital Status | | |
|---|---|---|---|---|---|
| | f | % | Status | f | % |
| 20-29 | 22 | 31.40% | Unmarried | 27 | 38.60% |

| | | | | | |
|---|---|---|---|---|---|
| 30-39 | 32 | 45.70% | Married | 41 | 58.60% |
| 40-49 | 11 | 15.70% | Divorced | 1 | 1.40% |
| ≥ 50 | 5 | 7.10% | Widowed | 1 | 1.40% |
| Total | 70 | 100.00% | Total | 70 | 100.00% |

| Gender | | | Levels of Education | | |
|---|---|---|---|---|---|
| | f | % | | f | % |
| Female | 47 | 67.10% | Secondary | 24 | 34.30% |
| Male | 23 | 32.90% | Institute | 38 | 54.30% |
| Total | 70 | 100.00% | College | 8 | 11.40% |
| | | | Total | 70 | 100.00% |

| Duration of Career | | |
|---|---|---|
| | f | % |
| ≤ 5 | 26 | 37.10% |
| 06-Oct | 16 | 22.90% |
| Nov-15 | 15 | 21.40% |
| 16-20 | 4 | 5.70% |
| ≥ 21 | 9 | 12.90% |
| Total | 70 | 100% |

**Table 1:** Demographic characteristics of the students participated in the study, Table 1 shows that the highest percentage of the sample age were from (22-23) years old (28.7%), 67.3% were female, 26.0% were from fourth stage, 66.0% reside in Baghdad, and 81.7% were unmarried.

| | | f | % |
|---|---|---|---|
| | Very Weak | 15 | 21.40% |
| | Weak | 21 | 30.00% |
| | Intermediate | 18 | 25.70% |
| Levels of Quality | Good | 16 | 22.90% |
| | Total | 70 | 100.00% |

**Table 2:** Distribution of the sample according to the Levels of quality of life of nurses, 57-66: Very weak; 67-71: Weak; 72-76: Intermediate; and 77-105: Good, The results indicate that regarding the levels of quality of life, about half of them (50.4%) have very weak and weak levels and only 22.9% are with good level of quality life.

| | | | Level of QoL | | | | |
|---|---|---|---|---|---|---|---|
| | | | Very weak | Weak | Intermediate | Good | Total |
| Age | 20-29 | f | 2 | 7 | 5 | 8 | 22 |

| | | | | | | | |
|---|---|---|---|---|---|---|---|
| | | % | 2.90% | 10.00% | 7.10% | 11.40% | 31.40% |
| | 30-39 | f | 7 | 10 | 10 | 5 | 32 |
| | | % | 10.00% | 14.30% | 14.30% | 7.10% | 45.70% |
| | 40-49 | f | 4 | 4 | 3 | 0 | 11 |
| | | % | 5.70% | 5.70% | 4.30% | 0.00% | 15.70% |
| | ≥ 50 | f | 2 | 0 | 0 | 3 | 5 |
| | | % | 2.90% | 0.00% | 0.00% | 4.30% | 7.10% |
| Total | | f | 15 | 21 | 18 | 16 | 70 |
| | | % | 21.40% | 30.00% | 25.70% | 22.90% | 100.00% |

Table 3: Distribution in the levels of quality of life regarding to age of nurses, Table 3 shows that the highest level of QoL is within the age group of (30-39); and the lowest level is within age group (≥ 50).

| | | | Level of QoL | | | | |
|---|---|---|---|---|---|---|---|
| | | | Very Weak | Weak | Intermediate | Good | Total |
| | Male | f | 8 | 18 | 15 | 6 | 47 |
| | | % | 11.40% | 25.70% | 21.40% | 8.60% | 67.10% |
| | Female | f | 7 | 3 | 3 | 10 | 23 |
| Gender | | % | 10.00% | 4.30% | 4.30% | 14.30% | 32.90% |
| | | f | 15 | 21 | 18 | 16 | 70 |
| Total | | % | 21.40% | 30.00% | 25.70% | 22.90% | 100.00% |

Table 4: Distribution in the levels of quality of life regarding to gender of nurses, Table 4 indicates that 25.7% of the male has weak level and only 8.6% have good level of QoL.

| | | | Level of QoL | | | | |
|---|---|---|---|---|---|---|---|
| | | | Very Weak | Weak | Intermediate | Good | Total |
| | Unmarried | f | 4 | 7 | 10 | 6 | 27 |
| | | % | 5.70% | 10.00% | 14.30% | 8.60% | 38.60% |
| | Married | f | 10 | 14 | 8 | 9 | 41 |
| | | % | 14.30% | 20.00% | 11.40% | 12.90% | 58.60% |
| | Divorced | f | 1 | 0 | 0 | 0 | 1 |
| | | % | 1.40% | 0.00% | 0.00% | 0.00% | 1.40% |
| | Widowed | f | 0 | 0 | 0 | 1 | 1 |
| Marital Status | | % | 0.00% | 0.00% | 0.00% | 1.40% | 1.40% |
| | | f | 15 | 21 | 18 | 16 | 70 |
| Total | | % | 21.40% | 30.00% | 25.70% | 22.90% | 100.00% |

Table 5: Distribution in the levels of quality of life regarding to marital status of nurses, Table 5 shows that two third of married nurses have weak and very weak level of QoL and only 8.6% have good level of QoL.

| | | | Levels of QoL | | | | |
|---|---|---|---|---|---|---|---|
| | | | Very Weak | Weak | Intermediate | Good | Total |
| Level of Education | Secondary | f | 6 | 5 | 4 | 9 | 24 |
| | | % | 8.60% | 7.10% | 5.70% | 12.90% | 34.30% |
| | Institute | f | 7 | 15 | 10 | 6 | 38 |
| | | % | 10.00% | 21.40% | 14.30% | 8.60% | 54.30% |
| | College | f | 2 | 1 | 4 | 1 | 8 |
| | | % | 2.90% | 1.40% | 5.70% | 1.40% | 11.40% |
| Total | | f | 15 | 21 | 18 | 16 | 70 |
| | | % | 21.40% | 30.00% | 25.70% | 22.90% | 100.00% |

**Table 6:** Distribution in the levels of quality of life regarding to the levels of education of nurses, Table 6 reveals that most of institute level of education has weak and very weak levels of QoL (31.4%); and only 8.6% have good level of QoL.

| | | | Level of QoL | | | | |
|---|---|---|---|---|---|---|---|
| | | | Very Weak | Weak | Intermediate | Good | Total |
| Duration of Career | ≤ 5 | f | 3 | 6 | 7 | 10 | 26 |
| | | % | 4.30% | 8.60% | 10.00% | 14.30% | 37.10% |
| | 06-10 | f | 5 | 5 | 4 | 2 | 16 |
| | | % | 7.10% | 7.10% | 5.70% | 2.90% | 22.90% |
| | 11-15 | f | 2 | 7 | 5 | 1 | 15 |
| | | % | 2.90% | 10.00% | 7.10% | 1.40% | 21.40% |
| | 16-20 | f | 1 | 1 | 1 | 1 | 4 |
| | | % | 1.40% | 1.40% | 1.40% | 1.40% | 5.70% |
| | ≥ 21 | f | 4 | 2 | 1 | 2 | 9 |
| | | % | 5.70% | 2.90% | 1.40% | 2.90% | 12.90% |
| Total | | f | 15 | 21 | 18 | 16 | 70 |
| | | % | 21.40% | 30.00% | 25.70% | 22.90% | 100.00% |

**Table 7:** Distribution in the levels of quality of life regarding to the duration of career of nurses, Table 7 shows that 14.3% of total nurses have a good level of quality of life within five years of career; and only 1.4% have very weak level within career group of 16-20.

| Duration of Career | 12.99 | 4 | 0.37 |
|---|---|---|---|

| Demographic characteristics | Pearson Chi-Square | | |
|---|---|---|---|
| | $X^2$ | df | Sig. |
| Age | 14.98 | 3 | 0.05 |
| Gender | 13.09 | 1 | 0.01 |
| Marital Status | 10.12 | 3 | 0.34 |
| Level of Education | 9.034 | 2 | 0.17 |

**Table 8:** Association between demographic characteristics and levels of QoL, Table 8 indicates that there is significant relationship between age and level of QoL.

## Discussion and Conclusion

The results of Table 1 show that the majority of nurses are young and mid-aged (20 to 40 years old), this result is supported by Al-Ameri and other studies [16-19] who confirmed that about 68.2 to 72.1% of their studies' samples were with age ranged between 19 to 39 years. About three quarters of the nurses participated in present study were male, this finding was supported by Al-Ameri [16] and Lee and Henderson [20] who found in their studies on psychiatric nurses that 68 to 72% of those nurses were male. These results could be due the difficulties in working during night shift so the male nurses are more suitable to work at night. Concerning the levels of education of the nurses, the results show that about half of the nurses have diploma in nursing which means two years after secondary school. This result is supported by Al-Ameri [16] but this result is not supported by American and European studies because the standard of level of education for nurses is Bachelor in nursing level [21-23]. More than half of the nurses were married; this situation is considered traditional commitment in Iraq to marry at early years of age, in addition the majority of the participants is 20-39 years old so it is usual to find this high percentage of married nurses [16]. The majority of the sample (81.4%) was with more than five years and less than 15 years of career. These different periods of career are normal due to different ages and different levels of education. About half of the nurses took place in the present study have weak and very weak quality of life, that indicates a bad impact of night shift upon the physical, psychological and social status of a large number of nurses working at night shift [2]. The female nurse are under more burdens of night shift than male nurse are. Moreover, the more the nurse is older the less quality of life has [24]. The married nurses (whether male or female) are more likely to have weaker level of quality of life, this might be due to the difficulties of everyday life events which add more burdens on the nurses in addition to night shift burdens [25]. Those who have ten years of career and less are more likely to have weak and very weak levels of quality of life; this is could be because they have not adjusted very well with night shift work.

## Recommendation

The present study recommends that it should provide adequate off-duty hours to let an uninterrupted sleep cycle of at least eight hour a day, which may affect nurses' daily life at home. It should use permanent shift assignments, which may diminish tiredness effects, instead of rotating shift duties. Encourage the nurses to join the special sessions for coping and stress management to lessen and prevent the work-related stress.

## References

1. Knutsson A, Alfredsson L, Karlsson B (2012) Breast cancer among shift workers: Results of the WOLF longitudinal cohort study. Scand J Work Env Health 39: 170-177.

2. Vitale SA, Varrone-Ganesh J, Vu M (2015) Nurses working the night shift: Impact on home, family and social life. J Nurs Educ Pract 5: 70-78.

3. Martin R (2011) Differences in health and well-being of night shift nurses versus day shift nurses [dissertation]. Northern Kentucky University, p: 38.

4. Bonet-Porqueras R, Moline-Pallares A, Olona-Cabases M (2009) The night shift: A risk factor for health and quality of life in nursing staff. Enferm Clin 19: 76-82.

5. Silva-Costa A, Rotenberg L, Griep R (2011) Relationship between sleeping on the night shift and recovery from work among nursing workers: The influence of domestic work. J Adv Nurs 67: 972-981.

6. Buyukhatipoglu H, Kirhan I, Vural M (2010) Oxidative stress increased in healthcare workers working 24 h on-call shifts. Am J Med Sci 340:462-467.

7. Marion da Silva R., Beck C, Guido L (2009) Night shift pros and cons in nursing: qualitative study. Online Brazilian Journal of Nursing 8.

8. Barrientos LA, Suazo SV (2007) Quality of life associated factors in Chilenas hospitals nurses. Rev Latino-Am Enfermagem 15: 480-486.

9. Suzuki K, Ohida T, Kaneita Y, Yokoyama E, Miyake T, et al. (2004) Mental health status, shift work and occupational accidents among hospital nurses in Japan. J Occup Health 46: 448-454.

10. Totterdell P, Spelten E, Pokorski J (1995) The effects of night work on psychological changes during the menstrual cycle. J Adv Nurs 21: 996-1005.

11. Persson M, Martensson J (2006) Situations influencing habits in diet and exercises among nurses working night shift. J Nurs Manag 14: 414-423.

12. Yuan SC, Chou MC, Chen CJ, Lin YJ, Chen MC, et al. (2011) Influences of-shift work on fatigue among nurses. J Nurs Manag 19: 339-345.

13. Shields M (2002) Shift work and health. Health Rep 13: 11-33.

14. Akerstedt T, Kecklund G, Johansson SE (2004) Shift work and mortality. Chronobiol Int 21: 1055-1061.

15. World Health Organization Quality of Life (WHOQOL) Group (1995) World Health Organization quality of life assessment (WHOQOL): Position paper from the World Health Organization. Soc Sci Med 41: 1403-1409.

16. Al-Ameri MHI (2014) Sources of work-related Stress among Nurses Working at Psychiatric Wards in Baghdad City Hospitals. Iraqi National Journal of Nursing Specialties 27: 51-58.

17. Santos SR, Carroll CA, Cox KS (2003) Baby boomer nurses bearing the burden of care: a four-site study of stress, strain, and coping for inpatient registered nurses. J Nurs Adm 33: 243-250.

18. Folkard S, Tucker P (2003) Shift work, safety and productivity. Occup Med (Lond) 53: 95-101.

19. Geiger-Brown J, Trinkoff A (2010) Is it time to pull the plug on 12 h shifts? Part 1. J Nurs Adm 40: 100-102.

20. Lee V, Henderson MC (1996) Occupational stress and organizational commitment in nurse administrators. J Nurs Adm 26: 21-28.

21. Gray P (2000) Mental health in the workplace: Tackling the effects of stress. Mental Health Foundation, London.

22. Chang YS, Wu YH (2011) Impairment of perceptual and motor abilities at the end of a night shift is greater in nurses working fast rotating shifts. Sleep Med 12: 866-869.

23. Schernhammer ES, Kroenke CH, Laden F, Hankinson SE (2006) Night work and risk of breast cancer. Epidemiology 17: 108-111.

24. Tepas DI, Barnes-Farrel JL (2004) The impact of night work on subjective reports of well-being: An exploratory study of heath care workers from five nations. Rev Saude Publica 38: 26-31.

25. Isikhan V, Comez T, Danis MZ (2004) Job stress and coping strategies in health care professionals working with cancer patients. Eur J Oncol Nurs 8: 234-244.

# 10

# Nurses' Knowledge and Practice Regarding Educational Needs for Patients with Leukemia

Nadia Mohamed Taha[*], Howida Kameel Zatton[2] and Hala Ibrahem Zatton[3]

*Department of Medical Surgical Nursing, Faculty of Nursing Zagazig University, Zagazig, Egypt*

[*]**Corresponding author:** Taha NM, Assistant Professor, Department of Medical Surgical Nursing, Faculty of Nursing, Zagazig University, Zagazig city 44511, Egypt, E-mail: dr_nadya_mohamed@yahoo.com

## Abstract

**Aim:** The aim was to assess nurses' knowledge and practice regarding educational needs for patients with leukemia.

**Design:** A descriptive cross-sectional design.

**Methods:** Two tools were used for data collection, namely as self-administered questionnaire and an observation checklist. The study was conducted at the Oncology and Hematology Department in Zagazig University Hospital.

**Sample:** Convenience sample of 30 nurses with the only inclusion criterion of having at least one-year experience in the study setting.

**Results, conclusion and recommendations:** The study demonstrates deficient knowledge and inadequate practices of nurses providing care to patients with leukemia in the study setting. This is most evident in critical areas such as infection control, skin care, and maintaining nutrition. There is also a shortage in training programs for these nurses. Therefore, there is urgent need to arrange continuing education programs for nurses. The study findings could be used as a basis for construction of training endeavors based on identified knowledge and practice gaps to respond to their unmet needs. The main limitation of this study is its small sample size, which would hamper generalization of its results, in addition to the possible observed bias.

**Keywords:** Leukemia; Knowledge; Practices

## Introduction

Leukemia is a malignancy originating in the stem cells of the hematopoietic system, which results in uncontrolled proliferation of white blood cells (WBCs) [1]. The produced WBCs have different grades of immaturity, with inability to perform functions. The is also decreased production of normal red blood cells, white blood cells, and platelets and infiltration of other organs [2]. Leukemia is fatal if left untreated [3].

Leukemia estimated new cases in the United States in 2011 were 44,600 and deaths 21,780 [4]. The number of new cases of leukemia was 13.7 per 100,000 men and women per year. The number of deaths was 6.8 per 100,000 men and women per year. These rates are age-adjusted and based on 2010-2014 cases and deaths [5]. In Egypt, a high incidence was reported, especially in the pediatric population [6]. The National Cancer Registry Damietta Profile [7] registered 52 cases. The cause of leukemia is not known, but multiple factors are thought to be responsible as age, radiation, chemicals, viruses, genetics, cigarette smoking and cancer therapy [8].

Leukemias are classified according to cell line involved lymphocytic or myelocytic, and according to maturity of the malignant cells as acute (immature cells) or chronic (differentiated cells) [9]. In acute leukemia, the onset of symptoms is abrupt, and without treatment, it is fatal within weeks to months. In chronic leukemia, symptoms evolve over a period of months to years, and the disease trajectory can extend for years [10]. Diagnosis is by symptoms [11], confirmed with complete blood count, followed by bone marrow aspiration [12]. Treatment tends to destroy abnormal cells, but can also damage healthy cells and tissues, and it causes side effects [13].

Since the patient with leukemia has many physical and psychological needs, the nursing role is extremely challenging. The diagnosis of leukemia can evoke great fear from death, which makes the patient difficult to manage, and increases his/her need for continued diligent support as well as teaching [14]. Added to this is the patient family need to be informed about treatment and prognosis. Therefore, the nurse must develop a teaching plan with short and long-term goals, specific nursing actions, and periodic evaluation of progress toward goal achievement [15]. The satisfaction of basic human needs enhance wellness conversely [16] whereas the unmet needs can result in a client's altered health status [17]. For nurses, it is imperative that these physical, psychological, social, and educational patients' needs be met [18]. Moreover, they should be sensitive to the information-seeking behavior of cancer patients and their families [19].

## Significance and of the Study

Cancer occupies the second place after heart disease as a cause of death. The researchers observed that a large number of leukemia patients are admitted to the hematology unit where they work. Those patients have knowledge deficit about the disease manifestation, treatment and follow-up care. This indicates a need to know how far the nurses in the setting know and fulfill their roles towards these patients to optimize independence in daily living activities, prevent complications of the disease and its treatment, and attain remission.

## Aim

The aim was to assess nurses' knowledge and practice regarding educational needs for patients with leukemia.

## Methods

### Design

A descriptive cross-sectional design was used which was conducted in Oncology and Hematology Department at Zagazig University Hospital.

### Sample

The study involved a convenience sample of 30 nurses with the only inclusion criterion of having at least one-year experience in the study setting. Since these were all the nurses available in the setting, no sample size could be calculated.

### Data collection

Two different tools were used for data collection, namely as self-administered questionnaire and an observation checklist.

The self-administered questionnaire was designed by the researchers for assessment of nurse's knowledge of the educational needs of the patient with leukemia. It was constructed in Arabic language based on pertinent literature [20]. It included a section for nurse's demographic characteristics as age, gender, nursing qualification, years of experience both total and in oncology department, and previous attendance of training in leukemia. The second section consist of 63 multiple-choice question assessing nurse's knowledge of blood components, definition of leukemia, its causes, types, clinical manifestations and treatment, as well as nurses' role in management of the patient and in meeting patient needs. For scoring, each correct response was scored one and the incorrect zero. For each area of knowledge, the scores of the items were summed-up and the total divided by the number of the items, giving a mean score of the part. These scores were converted into percent scores. The nurse was considered to have satisfactory knowledge if the percent score was 60% or more and unsatisfactory if less than 60%.

The observation checklist was also designed by the researchers to assess nurse's performance of her role in meeting daily needs of the patient with leukemia. It was based on pertinent literature [21]. These needs included the following.

Personal hygiene and skin care: 12 items such as "Use warm water and mild soap for skin care," "Use only approved lotions and creams on the skin."

Prevention and control of infection: 9 items such as "Maintain protective isolation," "Maintain meticulous hand washing before and after every procedure."

Control bleeding and prevent injury: 10 items such as "Instruct patient to avoid gum bleeding hygiene by using soft tooth brushes," "Teach client to avoid forceful coughing, sneezing, and nose blowing."

Maintaining adequate balanced nutrition: 16 items such as "Provide liquids with different textures and tastes," "Offer small frequent meals including low-fat high-calories foods throughout the day."

Control of side effects of lines of treatment: These included small checklists for dealing with anemia (4 items), fatigue (6 items), diarrhoea (10 items), constipation (6 items), alopecia (5 items) and stomatitis (5 items).

The checklist items were checked as either "done" or "not done." For scoring, the items observed "done" were scored one and the items "not done" were scored zero. For each area, the scores of the items were summed up and the total divided by the number of the items, giving a mean score of this part. These scores were converted into percent scores. The nurse's practice was considered adequate if the percent score was 60% or more and inadequate if less than 60%.

Upon preparation of the checklists, they were presented to a panel of five experts (three professors in Medical-Surgical Nursing, Faculty of Nursing, Ain Shams University, and an assistant professor and a lecturer of Oncology Medicine and Hematology, Faculty of Medicine, Zagazig University) for face and content validation. They reviewed the tools for clarity, relevance, comprehensiveness, understanding, applicability and ease of administration. Minor modifications were required.

### Pilot study

A pilot study was conducted on five nurses from another setting for testing clarity, arrangement of items, content applicability, and timeframe. The necessary modifications were done. The pilot subjects were not included in the main study sample.

### Study manoeuvre

After securing all necessary permissions using official channels, the researchers visited the setting and met with the administration to explain the purpose of the study and its procedures. Then, they met with the eligible nurses, explained to them the aim and process of the study and invited them to participate. Those who consented to participate were handed the self-administered questionnaire with instructions in filling it. This took 20 to 30 min from each nurse. Once completed, the form was collected and the nurse was instructed that she will be observed during her routine daily work.

Participant observation technique was used to avoid any observer bias. The process of observation was done during the morning shift and lasted for many days for each nurse to complete all the checklists. Morning shift was suitable for the researchers because it was easy to find the nurses on this shift. Moreover, follow-up and basic care and procedures to patients are mostly done during this shift, and there was no interruption from visitors. Data collection was carried out over three months from August to October 2010.

### Data analysis

Data entry and Statistical analysis were done using SPSS 20.0 statistical software package. Data were presented using descriptive statistics in the form of frequencies and percentages for qualitative variables, and means and standard deviations for quantitative variables. Qualitative categorical variables were computed using chi-square test. Whenever the expected values in or more than one of the cells in 2 × 2 tables was less than 5, Fisher exact test was used instead. Statistical significance was set at p<0.05.

## Results

The nurses in the study sample were mostly (53.3%) in the age group 30-<40 years (Table 1). Only 2 (6.7%) were having a bachelor degree in nursing. Their total experience years ranged between two and 29 years, with mean 12.7 years. The majority (76.7%) was working in oncology for more than three years. Only about one-fourth (26.7%) had previous training in leukemia.

| | Frequency | Percent |
|---|---|---|
| **Age (years)** | | |
| <20 | 3 | 10 |
| 20- | 7 | 23.3 |
| 30- | 16 | 53.3 |
| 40+ | 4 | 13.3 |
| **Nursing qualification** | | |
| Nursing school diploma | 23 | 76.7 |
| Technical school diploma | 5 | 16.7 |
| Bachelor of nursing degree | 2 | 6.7 |
| **Total years of experience** | | |
| <10 | 11 | 36.7 |
| 10+ | 19 | 63.3 |
| Range | 2.0-29.0 | |
| Mean ± SD | 12.7±7.0 | |
| **Experience years in oncology department** | | |
| <=3 | 7 | 23.3 |
| >3 | 23 | 76.7 |
| **Attended training course about leukemia** | 8 | 26.7 |

**Table 1:** Personal characteristics of studied nurses (N=30).

Table 2 demonstrates a wide variation in nurses' knowledge of blood components and functions. While 90.0% of them had correct knowledge of the definition of increased immature WBCs count, only 20.0% knew the number of platelets, and 30.0% knew the functions of WBCs. As regards nurses' correct knowledge of leukemia; it was generally high reaching 100.0% for primary diagnosis, side effects of chemotherapy, and aim of repeated blood transfusion. Conversely, only 13.3% correctly knew the purpose of chemotherapy, and 26.7% knew gender susceptibility.

| Correct knowledge of | Frequency | Percent |
|---|---|---|
| **blood components and functions:** | | |
| Number of WBCs | 13 | 43.3 |
| Functions of WBCs | 9 | 30 |
| Causes natural increase of WBCs count | 26 | 86.7 |
| Definition of increase immature WBCs count | 27 | 90 |
| Number of Platelets | 6 | 20 |
| Functions of Platelets | 26 | 86.7 |
| **Leukemia** | | |
| Definition | 26 | 86.7 |
| Risk factors | 25 | 83.3 |
| Age susceptibility | 14 | 46.7 |
| Gender susceptibility | 8 | 26.7 |
| Manifestations | 26 | 86.7 |
| Primary diagnosis | 30 | 100 |
| Purposes of bone marrow biopsy | 27 | 90 |
| Precautions in bone marrow aspiration in leukemia | 25 | 83.3 |
| Purpose of CBC in leukemia | 28 | 93.3 |
| Precautions after vein puncture in leukemia | 24 | 80 |
| Methods of treatment | 25 | 83.3 |
| **Chemotherapy** | | |
| Definition | 22 | 73.3 |
| Purpose | 4 | 13.3 |
| Routes | 27 | 90 |
| Precautions before | 29 | 96.7 |
| Side effects | 30 | 100 |
| Contraindicated drugs in leukemia | 19 | 63.3 |
| **Bone marrow transplantation** | | |
| Definition | 20 | 66.7 |
| Sources | 27 | 90 |
| **Repeated blood transfusion** | | |
| Aim | 30 | 100 |
| Role of the nurse in blood transfusion | 26 | 86.7 |

**Table 2:** Knowledge of blood components and functions and of leukemia among nurses in the study sample (n=30).

As illustrated in Table 3, nurses' knowledge of their role in the care of patient with leukemia was generally high. The areas with highest percentages of correct knowledge were those of general nursing care (100.0%), nursing role in oral complications (100.0%), nursing care of hyperthermia (96.7%), nursing care of alopecia (96.7%), definition of anemia (96.7%), and patient and family education (96.7%). On the contrary, the lowest percentages of correct knowledge were related to precautions to prevent infection (6.7%) and nursing care for skin complications (23.3%).

| Correct knowledge of nurse role | Frequency | Percent |
|---|---|---|
| **General care** | | |
| Nursing care | 30 | 100 |
| Pain relief | 27 | 90 |
| **Prevention of infection** | | |
| Causes of increase infection susceptibility in leukemia | 27 | 90 |
| Signs and symptoms of infection | 23 | 76.7 |
| Nursing management regarding infection control | 25 | 83.3 |
| Precautions to prevent infection | 2 | 6.7 |
| **Vital signs** | | |
| Most important vital signs measuring for leukemia | 26 | 86.7 |
| Best site to measure body temperature | 15 | 50 |
| Causes of hyperthermia in leukemia | 29 | 96.7 |
| Care of hyperthermia in leukemia | 29 | 96.7 |
| **Nutrition** | | |
| Nutritional requirements for patient with leukemia | 28 | 93.3 |
| Causes of malnutrition in leukemia | 28 | 93.3 |
| Improving nutritional status of patient with leukemia | 27 | 90 |
| **Skin complications** | | |
| Types of skin complications in leukemia | 25 | 83.3 |
| Nursing care of alopecia | 29 | 96.7 |
| Nursing care of skin complications | 7 | 23.3 |
| **Anemia** | | |
| Definition of anemia | 29 | 96.7 |
| Causes of anemia | 25 | 83.3 |
| Symptoms of anemia | 23 | 76.7 |
| Nursing management of anemia | 22 | 73.3 |
| Controlling bleeding in patient with leukemia | 26 | 86.7 |
| **Gastrointestinal complications** | | |
| Types of oral complications in leukemia | 29 | 96.7 |
| Nursing role in oral complications | 30 | 100 |
| Nursing role in nausea and vomiting | 28 | 93.3 |
| Nurse role regarding anal care | 28 | 93.3 |
| Patient and family education | 29 | 96.7 |

**Table 3:** Knowledge of nurse role in leukemia among nurses in the study sample (n=30).

In total, Table 4 demonstrates that the lowest area of satisfactory knowledge was related to blood components and functions (60.0%),

while the highest was related to nursing role (83.3%). Overall, 70.0% of the nurses had satisfactory total knowledge.

| Total satisfactory (60%+) knowledge | Frequency | Percent |
|---|---|---|
| Blood components and functions | 18 | 60 |
| Leukemia | 23 | 76.7 |
| Nursing role | 25 | 83.3 |
| Total knowledge | | |
| Satisfactory | 21 | 70 |
| Unsatisfactory | 9 | 30 |

**Table 4:** Total knowledge of nurse role in leukemia among nurses in the study sample (n=30).

Concerning nurses' practice, Table 5 shows that the lowest percentage of adequate practice was in the area of control of infection (20.0%). Conversely, the area with the highest percentage of practice was that of control of side effects of medications (73.3%). In total, two-thirds of the nurses (66.7%) were having adequate practice.

| Adequate (60%+) performance | Frequency | Percent |
|---|---|---|
| Maintaining personal hygiene and skin integrity | 21 | 70 |
| Control of infection | 6 | 20 |
| Measures for controlling bleeding tendency | 10 | 33.3 |
| Maintaining balanced nutrition | 11 | 36.7 |
| Controlling the side effects of medications: | | |
| Anemia | 25 | 83.3 |
| Fatigue | 21 | 70 |
| Diarrhea | 23 | 76.7 |
| Constipation | 23 | 76.7 |
| Alopecia | 21 | 70 |
| Stomatitis | 19 | 63.3 |

**Table 5:** Performance of nurse role in leukemia as observed among nurses in the study sample (n=30).

Table 6 points to no statistically significant relations between nurses' total knowledge and any of their demographic characteristics. It also indicates no statistically significant association between nurses' total knowledge and practice.

| | Knowledge | | | | Test | p-value |
|---|---|---|---|---|---|---|
| | Satisfactory | | Unsatisfactory | | | |
| | No. | % | No. | % | | |
| **Age (years)** | | | | | | |
| <30 | 6 | 60 | 4 | 40 | | |

| | No. | % | No. | % | Test | p-value |
|---|---|---|---|---|---|---|
| 30- | 15 | 75 | 5 | 25 | Fisher | 0.662 |
| **Nursing qualification** | | | | | | |
| Bachelor | 1 | 50 | 1 | 50 | | |
| Diploma | 20 | 71.4 | 8 | 28.6 | Fisher | 0.999 |
| **Total experience years** | | | | | | |
| <10 | 5 | 45.5 | 6 | 54.5 | | |
| 10+ | 16 | 84.2 | 3 | 15.8 | Fisher | 0.071 |
| **Experience years in oncology** | | | | | | |
| <=3 | 5 | 71.4 | 2 | 28.6 | | |
| >3 | 16 | 69.6 | 7 | 30.4 | Fisher | 0.999 |
| **Attended training courses in leukemia care** | | | | | | |
| No | 16 | 72.7 | 6 | 27.3 | | |
| Yes | 5 | 62.5 | 3 | 37.5 | Fisher | 0.905 |
| **Total practice** | | | | | | |
| Adequate | 15 | 75 | 5 | 25 | | |
| Inadequate | 6 | 60 | 4 | 40 | Fisher | 0.663 |

**Table 6:** Relations between nurses' knowledge of and their personal characteristics and their performance.

Similarly, Table 7 demonstrates no statistically significant relations between nurses' total practice and any of their demographic characteristics. Although more of the nurses who had no previous training in leukemia had adequate practice, the difference did not reach statistical significance (p=0.113).

| | Practice | | | | Test | p-value |
|---|---|---|---|---|---|---|
| | **Adequate** | | **Inadequate** | | | |
| | **No.** | **%** | **No.** | **%** | | |
| **Age (years)** | | | | | | |
| <30 | 6 | 60 | 4 | 40 | | |
| 30- | 14 | 70 | 6 | 30 | Fisher | 0.879 |
| **Nursing qualification** | | | | | | |
| Bachelor | 1 | 50 | 1 | 50 | | |
| Diploma | 19 | 67.9 | 9 | 32.1 | Fisher | 0.999 |
| **Total experience years** | | | | | | |
| <10 | 7 | 63.6 | 4 | 36.4 | | |
| 10+ | 13 | 68.4 | 6 | 31.6 | Fisher | 0.999 |
| **Experience years in oncology** | | | | | | |
| <=3 | 5 | 71.4 | 2 | 28.6 | | |

| | No. | % | No. | % | Test | p-value |
|---|---|---|---|---|---|---|
| >3 | 15 | 65.2 | 8 | 34.8 | Fisher | 0.999 |
| **Attended training courses in leukemia care** | | | | | | |
| No | 17 | 77.3 | 5 | 22.7 | | |
| Yes | 3 | 37.5 | 5 | 62.5 | Fisher | 0.113 |

**Table 7:** Relations between nurses' performance of and their personal characteristics.

## Discussion

Nurses working with patient who have cancer have a significant supportive role in helping the patient and their families to understand various therapies, preventing or managing side effects, and observing for late effects of treatments. Education is a constant feature of the nursing role especially in terms of new treatments, clinical trials and homecare [22]. Adherence to treatment is largely dependent on patient and family teaching [23]. The present study aim was to identify nurses' role regarding educational needs for patients with leukemia. The findings indicate a wide variation in nurses' knowledge and practice, with no relations between them.

The study sample included a majority of diploma degree nurses. This reflects the actual situation in the study setting, where there is a lack of highly qualified nurses. This might be explained by the preference of most bachelor degree nurses to work in academia or in other specialties that could be less distressing. It might also be related to that the majority of the nurses were from an older generation, as the total years of experience exceeding ten years indicate. At that time, the majority of the nurses were diploma-degree ones.

According to the present study findings, only approximately one-fourth of the nurses reported having had training courses related to leukemia care. This might be one of the causes underlying the lack of knowledge and skills among these nurses. Similar findings were described in studies at Ain-shams University Hospitals [24] and at Zagazig University Hospitals [25]. Nonetheless, the present study could not reveal any association of statistical significance between nurses' knowledge and practice from one side and their attendance of training courses from the other side. The lack of statistical significance might be due to the small sample size, but could also be related to the content and process of such training and the willingness of participants to actively share and get the most benefits. Thus, in disagreement with this present study finding, a randomized controlled trial in Japan demonstrated the beneficial effect of a training program on the knowledge and practice of oncology nurses [26].

The current study a wide variability of nurses' knowledge of blood components and functions. This was particularly evident in their lack of knowledge of the number of platelets, and the functions of WBCs. This is expected given the majority of diploma nurses in the study sample, since diploma degree programs may not give much emphasis to basic sciences. However, the number of platelets should be better known since this is a basic investigation for leukemia patients, and they should deal with it in their daily care. Such lack of knowledge has been related to lack of patient adherence and compliance to medications in a study carried out in Australia [27].

Meanwhile, the present study nurses' knowledge of leukemia was generally high. The main areas of deficient knowledge were related to age and gender susceptibility, as well as the purpose of chemotherapy. The lack of knowledge about susceptibility is not as important for these nurses as the lack of knowledge about the purpose of chemotherapy since this is a major part of their care, and they should have better knowledge of it. Nonetheless, the lack of knowledge about susceptibility, causes, and risk factors of leukemia is not directly influencing the quality of care these nurses provide to patients who already have the disease. Moreover, the etiology of leukemia and many other chronic diseases is still not well-established [28].

The present study findings have also demonstrated generally high nurses' knowledge of their role in the care of patient with leukemia. Few areas had low percentages of correct knowledge, and these were concerning the precautions to prevent infection, and nursing care for skin complications. These two areas are critical given the high susceptibility of the patients with leukemia to infection and skin problems. In congruence with this, Lachance et al. [29], in a study in Canada, reported that the patients with chronic lymphocytic leukemia are highly susceptible to infections, which would have negative impacts on their morbidity and mortality. Therefore, these authors suggested immunoglobulin replacement therapy for prevention and management of infections. In agreement with our finding, a recent study in South Africa reported a similarly low level of knowledge about infection control among nurses [30].

Overall, almost three-fifth of the nurses in the current study had total satisfactory knowledge. This is not very comforting finding since still two-fifth have unsatisfactory knowledge, which could have a negative impact on the quality of care they provide to their patients with leukemia. This is why the Leukemia and Lymphoma Society in the United States is deploying efforts in improving professionals' knowledge of leukemia s and other malignant blood diseases. It offers free professional development and education seminars to nurses and other professionals [31].

Moreover, the lack of knowledge was universal among the nurses in the present study sample regardless age, qualification, experience, or previous training as shown by the lack of significant associations with any of these variables. In agreement with this, Sarani et al. [32], in a study in Iran, found no significant relations between nurses' knowledge and any of their personal characteristics. Moreover, Maghawry [33] in a study at Zagazig University Hospital reported that years of experience had no significant relations with nurses' knowledge. Conversely, El Sayed [34] reported a significant association between nurses' knowledge and their years of experience. The lack of significant relation in our study could be due to the small sample size, which is a main study limitation.

The present study has also investigated nurses' practice of their role in caring for patients with leukemia. The main deficient practice was related to their role in the control of infection. This is an alarming finding given the high susceptibility of these patients to infection. This is certainly due to their deficient knowledge in this area as the study findings indicated. This demonstrates the need for educational interventions for these nurses to improve their knowledge of infection control, which would consequently have a positive impact on their related practices. Given the importance of infection control and prevention in cancer patients on chemotherapy, van Dalen et al. [35] in a study in Amsterdam assessed the value of low-bacterial diet for prevention of infection in such patients. However, the issue needs further research.

Totally, two-thirds of the nurses in the study sample demonstrated adequate practice. Their practice was not significantly related to any of their personal characteristics. Moreover, it had no significant relation to their total knowledge. Again, this might be due to the small sample size in our study. However, the findings are in congruence with Mohammed [36] and Saleh [37] who, in two studies at Zagazig University Hospital, found no significant relation between nurse's knowledge and practice. On the same line, studies in Jordan [38] and in Nigeria [39] demonstrated a gap between nurses' knowledge and practice.

## Conclusion and Recommendations

The study demonstrates deficient knowledge and inadequate practices of nurses providing care to patients with leukemia in the study setting. This is most evident in critical areas such as infection control, skin care, and maintaining nutrition. There is also a shortage in training programs for these nurses. Therefore, there is urgent need to arrange continuing education programs for nurses. The study findings could be used as a basis for construction of training endeavors based on identified knowledge and practice gaps to respond to their unmet needs. The main limitation of this study is its small sample size, which would hamper generalization of its results, in addition to the possible observed bias.

## Ethical Aspects and Conflict of Interest

All necessary permissions were obtained from the hospital director and nursing director of Zagazig University Hospital. Official letters were issued to them from the Faculty of Nursing explaining the aim of the study to obtain permission for collection of data. The study proposal was approved by the research ethics committee at the Faculty of Nursing, Zagazig University. An oral informed consent was obtained from nurses to participate in the study. They were assured about their rights to refuse or withdraw at any time. Complete privacy total confidentiality of any obtained information was ensured. The study procedure could not have any harm on participants.

## Author Contribution

The first author (correspondent author): contributed to the conception of the research, the development of the tools, statistical analysis, and commentary on the tables, wrote the discussion and references, prepared the patient protocol and help in data collection. The second author contributed to the sample collection, provided the pre, post and follow-up test, applied the protocol on patients, and participated in the reference collection and analysis data. The third author contributed to the translation of the tools and booklet into Arabic, participated in the reference collection and data collection and administered the protocol.

## References

1. Gale ZD, Charette AJ (2009) Oncology nursing care plans, Linda Skidmore-Roth, Texas, pp. 265-277.

2. Robinson MO, Roberton D (2010) Practical Pediatrics, Churchill Livingstone, Toronto.

3. Brunner and Suddarth's (2010) Textbook of Medical-Surgical Nursing, Lippincott Williams and Wilkins 198-775.

4. The Leukemia and Lymphoma Society (2012) Leukemia facts and statistics.

5. National Cancer Institute (2017) Cancer stat facts: Leukemia.

6.   Khalek ER, Sherif LM, Kamal NM, Gharib AF, Shawky HM (2015) Acute lymphoblastic leukemia: Are Egyptian children adherent to maintenance therapy? J Cancer Res Ther 11: 54-58.

7.   Egypt National Cancer Registry Damietta Profile (2009) Leukemia.

8.   Kerry H, Janice L (2013) Brunner and Suddarth's Textbook of Medical-Surgical Nursing 13th edition, Lippincott Williams and Wilkins 711-715.

9.   Lewis SM, Heitkemper MM, Dirksen SR (2007) Medical-surgical nursing, assessment and management of clinical problems, USA.

10.  Smeltzer SA, Bare BE (2008) Medical surgical nursing, Lippincott, New York.

11.  Yarbro CH, Frogge MH, Goodman MP (2010) Cancer nursing principles and practice, Jones and Bartlett com, USA.

12.  Swearingen P, Ross D (2006) Medical-surgical nursing care, nursing interventions and collaborative management, Toronto: Mosby.

13.  National Cancer Institute (2013) Leukemia, Preparing for Treatment.

14.  The Leukemia and Lymphoma Society (2011) Leukemia, long-term and late effects of treatment.

15.  Bruce GF, Simons-Morton, Walter HJ (2010) Introduction to health education and health promotion, WB Saunders, Philadelphia.

16.  Surhone LM, Tennoe MT, Henssonow SF (2010) Maslow's hierarchy of needs, VDM Publishing.

17.  Bastable SB, Grambet P, Jacobs KG (2011) Health professionals as educator: Principles of teaching and learning, Jones and Bartlett Learning, Sudbury, MA.

18.  Aziz NM, Rowland JH (2011) Trends and advances in cancer survivorship research: Challenge and opportunity. Semin Radiat Oncol 13: 248-266.

19.  Kav S, Tokdemir G, Tasdemir R, Yalili A, Dinc D (2012) Patients with cancer and their relatives beliefs, information needs and information-seeking behavior about cancer and treatment. Asian Pac J Cancer Prev 13: 6027-6032.

20.  Bastable SB (2008) Nurse as educator: Principles of teaching and learning practice, Jones and Bartlett Publishers, Sudbury, MA.

21.  Tannock IF, Hill RP, Bristow RG (2005) The basic science of oncology. Nursing in cancer and practice, McGraw-Hill, New York.

22.  Black JM, Hawks JM (2009) Medical-surgical nursing clinical management for positive outcomes, Elsevier com, USA.

23.  Kahn JM, Athale UH, Clavell LA, Cole PD, Leclerc JM, et al. (2016) How variable is our delivery of information? Approaches to patient education about oral chemotherapy in the Pediatric Oncology Clinic. J Pediatr Health Care 31: e1-e6.

24.  Salem BN (2005) Care of neonates with respiratory distress on mechanical ventilators, Master thesis, Faculty of Nursing, Ain Shams University.

25.  Zatton H (2007) Impact of implementation of health education program in improving nurses' knowledge and performance about care of viral hepatitis patients admitted in Zagazig University Hospital. Doctorate Thesis, Faculty of Nursing, Zagazig University.

26.  Kubota Y, Okuyama T, Uchida M, Umezawa S, Nakaguchi T, et al. (2016) Effectiveness of a psycho-oncology training program for oncology nurses: A randomized controlled trial. Psychooncology 25: 712-718.

27.  Wu S, Chee D, Ugalde A, Butow P, Seymour J, and Schofield P (2015) Lack of congruence between patients' and health professionals' perspectives of adherence to imatinib therapy in treatment of chronic myeloid leukemia: A qualitative study. Palliat Support Care 13: 255-263.

28.  Rappaport SM (2016) Genetic factors are not the major causes of chronic diseases. PLoS ONE 11: e0154387.

29.  Lachance S, Christofides AL, Lee JK, Sehn LH, Ritchie BC, et al. (2016) A Canadian perspective on the use of immunoglobulin therapy to reduce infectious complications in chronic lymphocytic leukemia. Curr Oncol 23: 42-51.

30.  Dramowski A, Whitelaw A, Cotton MF (2016) Healthcare-associated infections in children: Knowledge, attitudes and practice of paediatric healthcare providers at Tygerberg Hospital, Cape Town. Paediatr Int Child Health 29: 1-7.

31.  IAPO Staff (2014) United States - The Leukemia and Lymphoma Society: Working with patients, carers and hospital professionals to improve awareness, treatment and patient choice. World Hosp Health Serv 50: 13-14.

32.  Sarani H, Balouchi A, Masinaeinezhad N, Ebrahimitabas E (2015) Knowledge, attitude and practice of nurses about standard precautions for hospital-acquired infection in teaching hospitals affiliated to Zabol University of Medical Sciences (2014). Glob J Health Sci 8: 193-198.

33.  Maghawry HG (2007) Assessment of nurses' performance in premature units at Zagazig University Hospital. Unpublished Master thesis, Faculty of nursing, Zagazig University, pp. 50-53.

34.  El Sayed RM (2006) Factor affecting self-care for the patient with leukemia, Master Thesis, Faculty of Nursing, Ain Shams University 75-77.

35.  Van Dalen EC, Mank A, Leclercq E, Mulder RL, Davies M, et al. (2016) Low bacterial diet versus control diet to prevent infection in cancer patients treated with chemotherapy causing episodes of neutropenia. Cochrane Database Syst Rev 4: CD006247.

36.  Mohammed GE (2008) Nurses' knowledge about nursing care of leukemia children at Zagazig University Hospital, Master thesis, Faculty of Nursing, Ain Shams University, pp. 77-79.

37.  Saleh MS (2008) Nurses Compliance to standards of nursing care in performing invasive procedures at Zagazig University Hospital. Unpublished Master thesis, Faculty of Nursing, Zagazig University, pp. 99-101.

38.  AL-Rawajfah OM, Tubaishat A (2015) Nursing students' knowledge and practices of standard precautions: A Jordanian web-based survey. Nurse Educ Today 35: 1175-80.

39.  Iliyasu G, Dayyab FM, Habib ZG, Tiamiyu AB, Abubakar S, et al. (2016) Knowledge and practices of infection control among healthcare workers in a Tertiary Referral Center in North-Western Nigeria. Ann Afr Med 15: 34-40.

# 11

# On the Retention of Younger Nurses

**Louise Tourigny**[1*]**, Vishwanath V Baba**[2] **and Terri Lituchy**[3]

[1]*University of Wisconsin-Whitewater, Whitewater, USA*

[2]*McMaster University, Hamilton, ON, Canada*

[3]*CETYS Universidad, Mexico*

[*]**Corresponding author:** Louise Tourigny, Professor of Management, University of Wisconsin-Whitewater, 800, West Main Street, Whitewater, WI, 53190-1790, USA, E-mail: tourignl@uww.edu

## Abstract

**Objective:** In Trinidad and Tobago, younger hospital-based registered nurses are at risk of leaving the hospital and the country altogether. Therefore, there is a need to investigate the factors that contribute to turnover intention among younger nurses. The literature on newcomer adjustment has been predominantly used to study the integration and adjustment of younger nurses. However, we focus here on occupational mental health and job attitudes as antecedents of turnover intention across age groups referring to younger, mid-age and older nurses. The aim is to compare across age groups in order to determine whether younger nurses differ in terms of antecedents of turnover intention. The objective is to identify the reasons as to why younger nurses decide to quit the hospital.

**Methods:** We used a sample of 252 hospital nurses from Trinidad and Tobago. We did a cross-sectional study design and collected survey data using existing instruments. The occupational mental health concepts included role stressors, job stress, burnout, and depression. The job attitudes included organizational commitment, job satisfaction and turnover intention. We divided the sample in three groups: younger nurses, mid-age nurses and older nurses. The analytical strategy includes ANOVA with Post Hoc Bonferroni and stepwise regression.

**Results:** Younger nurses are more at risk of leaving the hospital. We provide detailed statistical findings revealing that high stress levels and feelings of inadequacy for the job are the most important predictors of turnover intention among younger nurses. We further demonstrate that stress, burnout and depression symptoms are significantly higher and that job satisfaction and organizational commitment are significantly lower among younger nurses. We do discuss findings obtained for the two other age groups as well.

**Conclusion:** We highlight the need for training and development programs that do go beyond providing knowledge and skill development by considering the occupational mental health of nurses.

**Keywords:** Nurses; Age; Stress; Burnout; Depression; Job satisfaction; Organizational commitment; Turnover intention; Trinidad; Tobago

## Introduction

The current shortage of nurses is estimated to increase to 29% by year 2020 in the United States alone [1]. Moreover, in hospitals where turnover among nurses is high the quality of patient care and nurse outcomes are negatively impacted [2]. It is known for a fact that turnover among nurses tends to reduce with age thereby suggesting that younger nurses are at risk of leaving the hospital and the profession altogether [3]. Generally speaking, younger nurses come trained in the latest advances in health care. When nurses stay with the hospital, they pick up valuable clinical experience that is good for patient care. The retention of nurses promotes a good social climate in the hospital. Turnover among younger nurses is costly to the hospital. It creates problems with staffing, workload, and succession planning, and increases recruitment and training costs. Consequently, research is needed to understand why younger nurses quit more readily and what can be done to prevent it. This can further lead to the development of effective intervention strategies before they actually leave the hospital.

In the Caribbean, turnover intention among hospital-based registered nurses is high [4]. This is compounded by the fact that countries such as the United States recruit nurses from the Caribbean. The emigration of nurses from the Caribbean is known to impact the socio-economic welfare of the country [5]. Such exile of talents is sustained by an increased shortage of nurses in countries from the West. Thus, the retention of younger nurses is a crucial practical problem in the Caribbean.

While much has been said about the retention of older nurses in the profession [6-8], less is known about the retention of younger nurses. Push factors contributing to turnover among older nurses include increased workload, job dissatisfaction, disillusionment, and demoralization among others. Research highlights that flexible work schedule, and greater autonomy along with reduced working hours close to retirement reduce turnover. But there is evidence that all nurses do not behave the same way. Older experienced nurses approach the work differently than the younger nurses and develop work attitudes that are in alignment with the work context. The younger ones seem to struggle more as the work adjustment literature suggests, experiencing stress and anxiety as they respond to the demands of the workplace. Yet less is known about the retention of younger nurses regardless of where they are. In Japan, younger nurses with less than 11 years of tenure who reported high exhaustion were more likely to quit the job [9]. In Finland, it was estimated that 26% of younger nurses have considered leaving the profession. Turnover intention among Finish nurses was attributed to high job demands, burnout, low job satisfaction, and low commitment among others. However, most research thus far focused on the newcomer adjustment literature revealing that social support at work was crucial to the retention of younger nurses [10-13]. More recently, competence acquisition, opportunities for professional development and socialization were found to reduce turnover intention among younger nurses [14]. Although these factors can enhance newcomers' adjustment and increase the retention of younger nurses within the first two years of employment [14], we do think that the occupational demands experienced by younger nurses may constitute a decisive determinant of turnover intention and reveal some potential areas of intervention in health care management. Consequently, we focus on the occupational stress experienced by younger nurses and related symptoms of burnout and depression.

Stress, burnout and depression are prevalent among hospital nurses [15]. The literature reveals that heavy workload, job strain, stress, and burnout [1,2] are related to higher turnover intention among nurses. In spite of such evidence, the literature did not shed light on the differential impact of such stress on younger nurses. We need to know whether younger nurses are more severely impacted by job stress, burnout, and depression. Besides, the literature also tells us that occupational mental health impacts job attitudes [16]. Therefore, we also need to understand how their job attitudes influence their intention to quit the hospital.

In this study, we will compare younger nurses against mid-age and older nurses in order to assess whether there are significant differences in terms of occupational mental health and job attitudes among these three groups. More specifically, we will analyze the extent to which perceived role stressors, job stress, burnout, depression, job satisfaction, and organizational commitment differ across age groups. Finally, we will determine the relative importance of each of these factors in predicting turnover intention across age groups.

## Conceptual Development

High job demands without adequate resources are detrimental to the mental health of nurses particularly in the absence of organizational support [17]. Hospital nurses have to deal with physical, mental and emotional job demands. When there is an imbalance between the demands and the organizational resources available to meet the demands, nurses are more likely to experience role stressors, which are known antecedents of job stress. Role stressors include role overload, role conflict and role ambiguity. Role overload or feeling overextended as a result of high job demands that exceed one's available resources is detrimental to the mental health of nurses. Role conflict or having to respond to conflictual demands and role ambiguity or feeling uncertain about one's responsibilities can increase job stress. It is known for a fact that nurses who experience job stress and who do not develop effective coping mechanisms are more likely to suffer from burnout [16]. However, work experience facilitates the development of strategies aimed at buffering burnout. Thus, we would expect that older nurses are less susceptible to burnout compared to younger nurses. Job burnout is a syndrome composed of three inter-related dimensions. First, emotional exhaustion consists of a feeling of depletion of one's emotional and physical resources after repeated

exposures to role stressors. Second, depersonalization is a self-protective but counterproductive response to excessive demands. It is associated with one's desire to withdraw from interpersonal interactions. Thus, nurses depersonalize patients and co-workers as a self-protective means from the exhaustive emotional and social demands associated with their roles. Third, diminished personal accomplishment involves feelings of inadequacy in one's roles and responsibilities [18]. Frequent symptoms of burnout have the potential to trigger work-related depression [19]. We refer here to depressive symptomatology among normal subjects. When nurses experience high job stress, frequent symptoms of burnout and depression, they are less likely to develop a positive attitude toward the profession [16,20].

Job satisfaction and organizational commitment can be considered as the most proximal antecedents of turnover intention [21] in the context of job burnout [20,22-24]. Job satisfaction refers to the cognitive evaluation of one's working conditions and affective reaction to such evaluation. Organizational commitment is composed of three dimensions. Continuance commitment refers to what one may lose by leaving the job such as benefits, seniority, and status. Normative commitment is related to the professional norms and whether it is acceptable practice to leave the job. Affective commitment results from the development of a strong identification with the profession and the hospital [25]. We do expect that older nurses with longer tenure have higher job satisfaction and greater organizational commitment compared to younger nurses. Consequently, we propose that younger nurses are likely to experience more role stressors, higher stress levels, more symptoms of burnout and depression and lower job satisfaction and organizational commitment compared to older nurses. We will also investigate whether indicators of mental health and job attitudes predict turnover intention differentially across age groups.

## Methods

We used a sample of 252 hospital nurses from the Caribbean. Questionnaires were distributed to all nurses who were at work at the time the study was conducted provided that they agreed to participate in the study and to complete the survey. Responses were kept anonymous and nurses were instructed not to put their names or any other identifying information on the completed survey. Nurses were given a consent form that explained the purpose of the study in detail. The consent form clearly indicated that they had the right to withdraw from the study at any point in time. Nurses returned the completed survey directly to the researchers.

We divided the sample into three age categories. The youngest group is composed of nurses between the ages of 18 and 35, the mid-age group of nurses between 36 and 45, and the older nurses between 46 and 65 years of age. The literature reveals that nurses under the age of 35 were considered young [26,27]. According to the Idaho Commission of Human Rights, about 50% of the population in the United States is currently over 45 years of age [28]. Although the Age Discrimination in Employment Act of 1967 classifies older workers as age 40 and over, given the current demographics there are more workers age 45 to 55 and this trend will continue to grow. Thus, we selected 45 to 46 years of age as the transition point between mid-age workers and older workers. Moreover, it should be specified that the trend we currently observe in the United States fits the age distribution found in our sample from the Caribbean. We had 81 nurses in the younger category, 53 nurses in the mid-age category, and 92 older nurses. The sample is composed of 21 males and 231 females.

The distribution of nurses reveals that among younger nurses 71% were in their current job for less than 10 years, 16% between 10 and 15 years, and less than 1% for more than 15 years. For mid-age nurses, 28% were in their current job for less than 10 years, 19% between 10 and 15 years, and 53% for more than 15 years. Finally, for older nurses, 22% were in their current jobs for less than 10 years, 2% between 10 and 15 years, and 76% more than 15 years. Older nurses with less than 10 years had either been promoted or were new to the hospital.

## Measures

Role overload, role conflict and role ambiguity were measured with the Beehr et al. [29] instrument using a 5-point scale ranging from 1 (strongly disagree) to 5 (strongly agree). A sample item for role overload is "It often seems I have too much work for one person to do". A sample item for role conflict is "I often have to bend a rule or a policy in order to carry out an assignment". A sample item for role ambiguity is "I feel uncertain about how much authority I have in my job". Items were reverse scored where appropriate such that a high score on the scale indicates high role stressor. The number of items per scale was 5 for role overload, 6 for role conflict, and 4 for role ambiguity. Reliability coefficients were of 0.60, 0.79 and 0.61 for role overload, role conflict and role ambiguity, respectively.

Job stress was measured with the 13 items from the Parker and Decotiis' in 1983 [30] instrument using a 5-point scale ranging from strongly disagree (1) to strongly agree (5). A sample item is "Sometimes when I think about my job I get a tight feeling in my chest." A high score on the scale indicates high job stress. The reliability coefficient is .88.

The Maslach Burnout Inventory was used to measure the three dimensions of burnout using a 7-point frequency scale ranging from 1 (a few times a year) to 7 (every day) [18]. A sample item for emotional exhaustion is: "I feel emotionally drained from my work." A sample item for depersonalization is: "I do not really care what happens to those I deal with at work." A sample item for personal accomplishment is: "I have accomplished many worthwhile things in this job". Mean frequency scores were computed for each dimension of job burnout. A high mean frequency indicates the manifestation of more frequent symptoms. There were 9 items for emotional exhaustion, 5 items for depersonalization, and 8 items for diminished personal accomplishment. The reliability coefficients are 0.91, 0.79, and 0.76 for emotional exhaustion, depersonalization and diminished personal accomplishment, respectively.

Depression was measured with 20 items from the Center for Epidemiological Studies Depression Survey (CES-D) [31] using a 4-point frequency scale ranging from 1 (rarely or none of the time) to 4 (most or all of the time). The CES-D consists of a list of generic symptoms of depression. Respondents were asked to indicate how often they experienced each described statement in the week that preceded the date of the survey. A sample item is: "I thought my life had been a failure." The reliability coefficient is 0.83.

Organizational commitment was measured with the Allen and Meyer's in 1990 [25] instrument composed of 15 items using a 5-point scale ranging from (1) strongly disagree to (5) strongly agree. A sample item is "I really care about what happens to this hospital." Items were reverse scored where appropriate so that a high score on this scale indicates high organizational commitment. The reliability coefficient is 0.84.

Job satisfaction was measured with one global item. Nurses were asked overall how satisfied they were with their present job. A 5-point scale ranging from (1) very dissatisfied to (5) very satisfied was used.

Turnover intention was measured with one item. Nurses were asked to indicate how likely they were going to quit the job in the coming year using a 4-point scale ranging including 1 (not likely at all), 2 (slight possibility), 3 (quite possible) and 4 (almost certain).

## Results

We used ANOVA with Post Hoc Bonferroni to analyze the differences across the groups. Table 1 presents the ANOVA results.

| Variable | Mean | Standard deviation | F-test | Significance level |
|---|---|---|---|---|
| Role Ambiguity | 3.79 | 0.79 | 3 | 0.05 |
| Role Conflict | 3.28 | 0.92 | 5.69 | 0 |
| Role Overload | 2.38 | 0.78 | 3.76 | 0.02 |
| Stress | 2.52 | 0.83 | 4.11 | 0.02 |
| Emotional Exhaustion | 2.02 | 0.83 | 15.71 | 0 |
| Depersonalization | 1.57 | 0.75 | 6.64 | 0 |
| Diminished Personal Accomplishment | 2.16 | 0.81 | 3.85 | 0.02 |
| Depression | 1.49 | 0.4 | 4.68 | 0.01 |
| Organizational Commitment | 3.39 | 0.66 | 13.43 | 0 |
| Global Satisfaction | 3.31 | 1.09 | 4.36 | 0.01 |
| Turnover Intention | 1.67 | 0.85 | 23.46 | 0 |

Table 1: ANOVA.

| Dependent variable | Age category (i) | Age category (j) | Mean difference (i-j) | Significance level |
|---|---|---|---|---|
| Role ambiguity | 1 | 2 | -0.28 | ns |
| | | 3 | -0.26 | ns |
| Role conflict | 1 | 2 | 0.39 | 0.05 |
| | | 3 | 0.44 | 0.01 |
| Role overload | 1 | 2 | 0.32 | ns |

| | | | | |
|---|---|---|---|---|
| | | 3 | -0.01 | ns |
| | 3 | 2 | 0.33 | 0.03 |
| Stress | 1 | 2 | 0.37 | 0.04 |
| | | 3 | 0.31 | 0.05 |
| Emotional Exhaustion | 1 | 2 | 0.71 | 0 |
| | | 3 | 0.63 | 0 |
| Depersonalization | 1 | 2 | 0.42 | 0 |
| | | 3 | 0.33 | 0.01 |
| Diminished Personal Accomplishment | 1 | 2 | 0.32 | ns |
| | | 3 | 0.28 | 0.05 |
| Depression | | | | |
| | 1 | 2 | 0.17 | 0.04 |
| Organizational Commitment | | 3 | 0.16 | 0.02 |
| Global Satisfaction | 1 | 2 | -0.34 | 0.01 |
| | | 3 | -0.49 | 0 |
| Turnover Intention | 1 | 2 | -0.45 | ns |
| | | 3 | -0.44 | 0.03 |
| | 1 | 2 | 0.44 | 0 |
| | | 3 | 0.82 | 0 |

Table 2: Post Hoc Bonferroni. Note: Only results for younger nurses are reported here along with significant results for the other groups; 1=younger group, 2=mid-age group, and 3=older nurses.

As reported in Table 1, the F-tests were all significant at the 0.05 level or lower. The Post Hoc Bonferroni tests are reported in Table 2. Results reveal that older nurses report significantly more role overload compared to mid-age nurses but not younger nurses. Younger nurses report much higher role conflict compared to the two other groups. There were no significant differences across the three groups for role ambiguity. Younger nurses report higher levels of stress compared to mid-age nurses but not older nurses. They also reported more emotional exhaustion and depersonalization compared to both mid-age and older nurses. There were no significant differences for diminished personal accomplishment. Symptoms of depression were higher among younger nurses compared to the two other groups. Job satisfaction was lower for younger nurses compared to older nurses only. However, younger nurses had lower organizational commitment compared to both mid-age and older nurses. Finally, their intention to quit was also much higher compared to the two other groups of nurses. These findings confirm a higher intention to quit among younger nurses.

We did a stepwise regression test for each group to analyze the predictive effect of the mental health factors and job attitudes on turnover intention using the 0.05 level. Results are reported in Table 3. For each group, we report the findings for the variables that had a significant predictive effect and dismiss all excluded variables that were non-significant. Findings were obtained in two steps for each group. We report the significant findings for step 2. For younger nurses, $R^2$ was of 0.27 and the F-test was of 12.55 ($p < 0.01$). Results indicate that for younger nurses high stress levels and diminished personal accomplishment are the two significant predictors of turnover intention. For mid-age nurses, $R^2$ was of 0.36 and the F-test was of 12.71 ($p < 0.01$). Depersonalization increases and organizational commitment decreases turnover intention for this age group. For older nurses, $R^2$ was of 0.22 and F-test of 11.12 ($p < 0.01$). Depersonalization and depression both increase turnover intention among older nurses.

| Younger nurses | B | SE | β | p |
|---|---|---|---|---|
| Stress | 0.36 | 0.1 | 0.37 | 0.01 |
| Diminished personal accomplishment | 0.35 | 0.12 | 0.3 | 0.01 |
| Mid-age nurses | B | SE | β | p |
| Depersonalization | 0.6 | 0.17 | 0.43 | 0.01 |
| Organizational commitment | -0.37 | 0.15 | -0.3 | 0.05 |
| Older nurses | B | SE | β | p |
| Depersonalization | 0.3 | 0.1 | 0.33 | 0.01 |

| Depression | 0.4 | 0.17 | 0.25 | 0.05 |
|---|---|---|---|---|

**Table 3:** Stepwise regression for turnover intention. Note: Solutions were obtained after two steps. We report only the significant findings at step 2.

## Discussion

As expected, younger nurses experienced more job stress and more frequent symptoms of emotional exhaustion, depersonalization and depression and reported more negative job attitudes and higher intentions to quit. Younger nurses who experience high stress levels and diminished personal accomplishment do feel inadequate for the job to the point where they consider leaving the job. These results indicate that training and development is essential for newcomers. However, the presence of psychological distress as exemplified here by more frequent symptoms of depression among younger nurses is a detrimental factor to their retention. Thus, it should be considered as a critical element in the design of newcomer programs.

In comparison, mid-age nurses were in better mental health and reported lower role overload and role conflict, lower levels of stress, emotional exhaustion, depersonalization and depression, and higher organizational commitment compared to younger nurses. It can be concluded that once nurses reach mid-age that they adapt to the demands and develop more productive responses to the role stressors. Mid-age nurses who were committed to the hospital were less likely to quit. However, as for older nurses, depersonalization seemed to be a precursor to their intention to quit.

These findings highlight that older nurses do experience more role overload. However, they cope better with job demands. In fact, they reported lower levels of stress, less symptoms of burnout and depression, and were more satisfied with their jobs as well as more committed to the hospital. However, we do corroborate existing literature by showing here that older nurses who exhibit depersonalization and report frequent symptoms of depression are more likely to quit the job. Thus, feeling demoralized is a key antecedent of intention to quit among older nurses.

There is a need to focus on the retention of younger nurses by analyzing the effectiveness of Human Resource Management training and development programs that focus on newcomer adjustment and the acquisition of knowledge and skills. However, the findings obtained in this study demonstrate that the integration of younger nurses in the profession may require some other types of intervention. For a start, Employee Assistance Programs may be useful in helping nurses develop effective coping strategies to better deal with job stress by providing psychological help when most needed.

Taken together these findings reveal that younger nurses were the most at risk group. Therefore, we do think that researchers should devote more effort to the study of the factors that can contribute to the retention of younger nurses. Mid-age nurses were doing better compared to the two other groups and seemed well adapted. Finally, older nurses who were at risk of leaving the job were more depressed. Older nurses reported higher role overload. Consequently, unless there are changes to the working conditions of these nurses they may also leave the hospital. However, younger nurses are more likely to find opportunities in the countries of the West should they decide to move for better salaries and working conditions. They may also be more mobile and willing to expatriate themselves. In conclusion, the retention of younger nurses in the Caribbean is an important problem that health care managers have to address in order to sustain quality health care.

## References

1. Lavoie-Tremblay M, O'Brien-Pallas L, Gélinas C, Desforges N, Marchionni C (2008) Addressing the turnover issue among new nurses from a generational viewpoint. J Nurs Manag 16: 724-733.

2. Hayes LJ, O'Brien-Pallas L, Duffield C, Shamian J, Buchan J, et al. (2012) Nurse turnover: A literature review - an update. Int J Nurs Stud 49: 887-905.

3. Clendon J, Walker L (2012) 'Being young': a qualitative study of younger nurses' experiences in the workplace. International nursing review 59: 555-561.

4. Lansiquot BA, Tullai-McGuinness S, Madigan E (2012) Turnover intention among hospital-based registered nurses in the Eastern Caribbean. J Nurs Scholarsh 44: 187-193.

5. Schmid K (2003) Emigration of Nurses from the Caribbean: Causes and Consequences for the Socio-Economic Welfare of the Country: Trinidad and Tobago, A Case Study. UN ECLAC Paper 748.

6. Duffield C, Graham E, Donoghue J, Griffiths R, Bichel-Findlay J, et al. (2015) Why older nurses leave the workforce and the implications of them staying. J Clin Nurs 24: 824-831.

7. Moseley A1, Jeffers L, Paterson J (2008) The retention of the older nursing workforce: A literature review exploring factors which influence the retention and turnover of older nurses. Contemp Nurse 30: 46-56.

8. Storey C, Cheater F, Ford J, Leese B (2009) Retention of nurses in the primary and community care workforce after the age of 50 years: database analysis and literature review. Journal of advanced nursing 65: 1596-1605.

9. Shimizu T, Feng Q, Nagata S (2005) Relationship between turnover and burnout among Japanese hospital nurses. J Occup Health 47: 334-336.

10. Baker III HE, Feldman DC (1990) Strategies of organizational socialization and their impact on newcomer adjustment. Journal of managerial issues 198-212.

11. Fisher CD (1985) Social support and adjustment to work: A longitudinal study. Journal of management 11: 39-53.

12. Nelson DL, Quick JC (1991) Social support and newcomer adjustment in organizations: Attachment theory at work? Journal of organizational behavior 12: 543-554.

13. Saks AM and Ashforth BE (2000) The role of dispositions, entry stressors and behavioral plasticity theory in predicting newcomers' adjustment to work. Journal of organizational behavior 21: 43-62.

14. Tomietto M, Rappagliosi CM, Sartori R, Battistelli A (2015) Newcomer nurses' organisational socialisation and turnover intention during the first 2 years of employment. Journal of nursing management, 23: 851-858.

15. Su JA, Weng HH, Tsang HY, Wu JL (2009) Mental health and quality of life among doctors, nurses and other hospital staff. Stress and health 25: 423-430.

16. Baba VV, Jamal M, Tourigny L (1998) Work and mental health: A decade in Canadian research. Canadian Psychology/Psychologie canadienne 39: 94.

17. Bakker AB and Demerouti E (2007) The job demands-resources model: State of the art. Journal of Managerial Psychology 22: 309-328.

18. Maslach C (1986) Jackson S Maslach burnout inventory 2.

19. Cordes CL, Dougherty TW (1993) A review and an integration of research on job burnout. Academy of management review 18: 621-656.

20. Lee RT, Ashforth BE (1993) A further examination of managerial burnout: Toward an integrated model. Journal of organizational behavior 14: 3-20

21. De Gieter S, Hofmans J, Pepermans R (2011) Revisiting the impact of job satisfaction and organizational commitment on nurse turnover intention: An individual differences analysis. International journal of nursing studie 48: 1562-1569.

22.  Blegen MA (1993) Nurses' job satisfaction: a meta-analysis of related variables. Nurs Res 42: 36-41.

23.  Irvine DM, Evans MG (1995) Job satisfaction and turnover among nurses: integrating research findings across studies. Nurs Res 44: 246-253.

24.  Tett RP, Meyer JP (1993) Job satisfaction, organizational commitment, turnover intention, and turnover: path analyses based on meta-analytic findings. Personnel psychology 46: 259-293.

25.  Allen NJ, Meyer JP (1990) The measurement and antecedents of affective, continuance and normative commitment to the organization. Journal of occupational psychology 63: 1-18.

26.  Salminen H (2012) The significance of perceived development opportunities in the context of retention: Comparing ageing and younger nurses. Tuomo Takala, Jyväskylä University School of Business and Economics, Pekka Olsbo, Ville Korkiakangas, Publishing Unit, University Library of Jyväskylä.

27.  Tschannen D, Kalisch BJ, Lee KH (2010) Missed nursing care: the impact on intention to leave and turnover. Can J Nurs Res 42: 22-39.

28.  Idaho Commission of Human Rights 2007.

29.  Beehr TA, Walsh JT, Taber TD (1976) Relationship of stress to individually and organizationally valued states: higher order needs as a moderator. J Appl Psychol 61: 41-47.

30.  Parker DF, DeCotiis TA (1983) Organizational determinants of job stress. Organizational behavior and human performance 32: 160-177.

31.  Radloff LS (1977) The CES-D scale a self-report depression scale for research in the general population. Applied psychological measurement 1: 385-401.

# 12

# Patients' Perspective of Cancer Treatment and Care in Vhembe District of Limpopo Province

**Dorah Ursula Ramathuba**[1,2*], **Ramutumbu Neo Jacqueline**[3] and **Ndou ND**[3]

[1]Department of Nursing, University of Venda, South Africa

[2]Tshilidzini Hospital, Department of Health, South Africa

[3]Department of Nursing, University of Venda, South Africa

*Corresponding author: Dorah Ursula Ramathuba, Department of Nursing, University of Venda, P/Bag X5050 Thohoyandou 0950, South Africa, E-mail: dorah.ramathuba@univen.ac.za

**Abstract:**

**Objective:** The study explored and described the experiences of patients diagnosed with cancer in Vhembe district, Limpopo Province. A qualitative research design which was phenomenological, exploratory, descriptive was used. The aim of the study was to add to the knowledge and understanding of the complex human phenomena.

**Methods:** A purposive theoretical sample of twelve patients who were diagnosed with different cancers within 2-5 years in a regional hospital in Vhembe district of Limpopo Province was obtained. Data was collected through in-depth interviews with eight participants who were in remission phase or undergoing treatment. Data saturation occurred after in-depth interviews with eight participants, field notes were also used during data collection.

**Results:** The findings revealed that cancer patients experienced poor communication and attitudes, experienced body changes, sense of withdrawal and depression and problems with follow-up care.

**Conclusions:** Understanding the cultural perspective of what it is like to have cancer and filling the gaps of patient's expectations and addressing emotional and physical needs.

**Keywords:** Cancer diagnosis; Cancer patients; Cancer support; Perceptions; Uncertainty; Quality of life; Qualitative analysis

## Introduction

Medical advances in cancer screening and treatment has resulted in patients surviving longer with cancer and treated as out-patients. The initial or acute phase encompass the time of diagnosis which lead to psychological distress with the diagnosis and treatment [1].

According to McCann L et al., having a chronic illness causes disorder to an individual's 'normal' daily routines and can cause biographical disruption affecting how patients perceive themselves and or how they believe others to perceive them [2]. Being diagnosed with cancer "immerses the patient into a complex web of interrelated experiences" This disruption can lead to the perception of social isolation and or of being different, compounding in a sense of feeling a failure to fit in [2]. This shows that viewing cancer as a long-term illness individuals affected by cancer need to feel cared for, supported and understood by those around them. A cancer diagnosis is not limited to a person's physical experiences, but also impacts a person's soul and spirit.

Many patients face emotional and spiritual distress and choose different strategies to cope with the situation. Kvale K et al. indicated that denial and cognitive avoidance are common coping strategies among cancer patients, hope and coping were found to be positively correlated, and hope was viewed as an outcome of coping [3]. Simon CE et al. conducted a study with 18 African American Christian women focusing on the role of spirituality throughout their breast cancer experiences [4]. The results indicated that, for most of the survivors, spirituality and faith assisted them throughout their breast cancer experience.

Nurses must be prepared to support the patient and his family throughout the cancer experience. According to Krumwiede KA et al. men diagnosed with prostate cancer spoke of feeling comfortable through the development of trusted connections and the unwavering support they received throughout their experience with prostate cancer [5]. All of the men indicated that support from their family was important and that it allowed them to deal with the difficult circumstances of prostate cancer. The support of family members, friends, and healthcare workers was identified by the participants as an important aspect of living with prostate cancer. Nurses should provide accurate, complete, and consistent information to help patients understand the full implications of the disease process and all treatment options, not just the treatment options available at the facility of care. Cancer diagnosis among African people is not generally accepted, most ethnic groups view the disease as a white man disease and seeking medical attention is a cause for concern as many delay or combine both types of medical treatment, mostly try the indigenous system before resorting to the western medical treatment. The study therefore aims at exploring and describing the patient's perspectives of cancer treatment and care. The study will contribute to the body of knowledge to nursing practice so that the multidisciplinary team should be culture sensitive in dealing with these patients as they are adjusting to the new disease and the treatment regimen that involves a lot of medical complexities in its management.Thus cancer treatment and care should bridge cultural gaps in caring, incorporate cultural differences to enable clients and families to achieve meaningful and supportive caring.

## Methodology

Phenomenological, qualitative research approach was used in order to explore the experiences of cancer patients within the context of their daily lives. Phenomenology is considered a philosophy, approach, and research method that is both inductive and descriptive. Phenomenology allows the investigator to gain access into a person's world and understand the meaning of that person's experiences [6]. Phenomenology refers to knowledge as it appears to consciousness, the science of describing what one perceives, senses, and knows in one's immediate awareness and experience. Purposive and theoretical sampling was used to select participants, the criteria for selecting participants included: non-hospitalised patients, who are above 20yrs and experienced the diagnosis of cancer, and were now receiving treatment on outpatient basis and were willing to communicate their perception regarding cancer experience.

The sample size was twelve participants with seven women and five men; however due to data saturation five women and three men participated in the study, and represented various backgrounds and socio-economic standing. The participants were treated for various types of cancer, e.g. breast, cervical, skin, stomach and bladder. Two participants were in their second year and six have been dealing with cancer for more than five years. The rights of participants were safeguarded through informed consent and confidentiality.

## Data collection

The participants were approached, purpose and objectives were explained to them and rapport was initiated, and were given a choice as to where the interviews would take place, namely at the clinic or at another venue. Participant felt comfortable in their own homes, thereafter appointments were made for the interviews. Data was collected through in-depth unstructured interviews; the interviews lasted for an hour to one and half hours. The interviews were unstructured to allow for an in-depth exploration of the key theme of the study, in particular the perspective of cancer treatment and care. Interviews began with a broadly open-ended question, specific to the purpose of the study: "What is your perception of cancer treatment and care"? This was followed by some more open ended probing questions such as "How has cancer treatment affected the quality of your life? Some questions were provoked by statements made by participants. The researcher maintained neutrality by not letting their personal feelings interfere with the interview process. Audio-recorder was used during the interview and field notes.

## Data analysis

Data was analysed based on Creswell qualitative analysis, during the analysis, oral descriptions of the participants were transcribed verbatim and read separately in order to gain a general understanding [7]. Significant statements and phrases about the objectives of the study were identified. Meanings were formulated from this significant statements and phrases. The formulated meanings were then organised into clusters of themes. Results of data analysis were then integrated into a description of experiences. To increase validity, two participants were selected randomly and contacted again to read the

descriptions and they agreed that the analyses represented their personal experiences. Common themes were created by merging similar statements for every category. The transcriptions were written in their ethnic language following the completion of the study and analysis, thereafter translated into English but retaining the original meaning.

## Trustworthiness

The model of Guba and Lincoln of trustworthiness in qualitative research was used. The following criteria to ensure trustworthiness are truth-value, applicability, consistency and neutrality [8]. Applying strategies of credibility ensured truth-value. The researcher spend 1-2 hours interviewing and kept a reflective journal, and made observations during the interviews, checked the themes and categories of statements with the participants, and focused on their experiences of living with cancer. Applying strategies of transferability ensured applicability. The researcher provided a clear description of the demographics of participants, and gave dense description of the results with supporting direct quotation of the participants. Similarly applying strategies of dependability ensured consistency. A dense description was given of the research methods used in this study. Neutrality was ensured by confirmability. The process undertaken to conduct research was provided [8].

## Ethical Principles

Ethical principles were applied accordingly following the guidelines of the Democratic Nursing Organisation of South Africa [9]. These ethical principles were applied as follows, participants were not identified throughout the study, and they were interview privately in their comfortable places. All participants gave a written consent after full explanation that they can withdraw anytime without penalty. The participants benefited through this research because they were enabled to express their feelings on their needs and plight of cancer patients in rural communities of Vhembe. All participants received feedback on the research results and we were able to form a cancer survivorship program which is in its infancy where the participants and their family members are sharing and supporting each other on improving their quality of life.

## Results

Five themes were identified during analysis in which Creswell qualitative method of analysis was utilized [7]. The themes are: Poor communication and attitudes, experiencing body changes, Sense of withdrawal and depression and problems with follow-up care (Table 1)

### Lack of proper communication and attitudes

Communication is important in cancer diagnosis; patients need concrete information about their treatments, prognosis and outcome of the disease

*"When my results came back, I was just told I had cancer and was given a return date nothing much was explained, I tried to ask for full details the doctor just told me they are not certain"*. Sometimes failing to give proper information may be due to lack of knowledge in a particular field, such as general practitioners. This is supported by Nguyen GT et al. who indicated that participants noted that doctors said little and tended not to speak about cancer specifically, they

addressed only the chief complaints it might be because they do not want their patients to worry too much [10]. Another factor was that a doctor might not be an expert in the medical issue at hand, he might not be able to offer sufficient guidance. It is thus imperative that patients be referred to appropriate experts. However, language and cultural barriers can sometimes affect communication, and patients reluctant to ask and question issues pertaining to their health.

*"Sometimes when I go for check-up, they do investigations and I don't know what they are or if it is the best treatments I should be getting, as long as I can be better from the disease"*

Nguyen GT et al in their study among Vietnamese immigrants reported that patients expressed poor understanding of medical tests that they received, they felt that it is the responsibility of the doctor, that it was not their role to seek information on their own [10].

*"After receiving my first chemotherapy, I felt sick, was vomiting and felt weak, and went to the clinic, the nurses sent me back,, saying were you not told that these treatments does that to a person, its nothing to worry about, I had to go to a private doctor and was given some medication"* This is an indication of bad attitudes by health professionals because nurses should be instrumental in providing health education as well as addressing their emotional needs.

Communicating your illness to your family can also be distressful as breaking the news may affect relationships in the family situation.

*"I didn't want to tell my children that I had cancer, however they definitely noticed the changes in our house. I remember I had purple marks on my chest (for radiation treatments). My skin was pale; my hair was starting to fall out."* Cancer is usually not something children understand or have experienced. They get information and ideas from other children and what they see in everyday life, including what they see on TV. Without the right information, children may fill in gaps with their imaginations many times, what they imagine is far worse than reality.

Communication is an integral role for health professionals involved in cancer care, and should take into account that it should not cause harm, and distress to patients and families; it should be emotion-centered and provide a hopeful and supportive atmosphere. Patients should also be supported in the process on how to break news to their loved ones when they are ready.

| Themes | Subthemes |
|---|---|
| Lack of proper communication and attitudes | Poor communication of diagnosis |
| | Negative attitudes of health professionals |
| Adjusting to body changes. | Acceptance of new self- image |
| | Embarrassment of body changes |
| Symptomatic effects of treatments | Experiences of activity intolerance |
| | Experiencing of embarrassment of body changes |
| Withdrawal and depression | Feelings of emptiness and isolation |
| | Emotional and psychological pain |
| Problems with follow-up care | Interrupted services |
| | Infrastructural problems |

Table 1 : Themes and Subthemes

## Adjusting to body changes

Cancer and its treatment can cause physical changes. Some people feel insecure about how these changes affect their body and their self-image.

*"At least the nurses told me that I must buy a wig, as I will soon lose my hair as I was starting treatment"*

*"I had a urinary catheter on discharge; it was such an embarrassment, it made me feel belittled because I had to keep it for few weeks while strapped on my leg inside my trouser."*

*"Vhone, a zwongo leluwa! (hey it's not easy) condom catheter is really uncomfortable, and if you remove it then you wet the bed which is disgusting as an adult father figure.*

*"When I started treatment, the other patients I found there, they were all dark skined (vho swifhala, vha sa takadzi), and realised, I'm going to look like them, even now, my palm have changed colour"*

Cancer can change your outlook. Other treatments can affect how you feel. Side effects from cancer treatment, such as weight loss or weight gain, hair loss, and skin changes can also change the way you look. Fatigue can make it harder for you to care for your appearance. Body changes from cancer treatment can range from hair loss to the loss of a limb. These kinds of changes can be hard to handle because others can see them. Many people who lose hair choose to wear scarves, wigs or hats.

## Symptomatic effects of treatments

Cancer patients undergoing chemotherapy experience many symptoms which they can manage when given the appropriate amount of information. However, self-management may not be sufficient or plausible for everyone. Participants reported various side effects

*"My whole body was a wreck, I felt weak and pains all over my bones"*

*"The medication is not doing me right, always after treatment I should be vomiting and it usually last for three days or so"*

Cancer patient can become conditioned to being anxious when going to receive treatments. Many patients have had the experience of what psychologists call classically conditioned vomiting. That is, vomiting even before they get to the cancer center because of the anticipation that they will vomit after treatment.

*"Since I don't have appetite after treatment, my bowels don't work well, they become irritable and experience some loose stool, and I can tolerate (delele li a dzula) slippery green vegetable." at least it stays in my stomach"*

*"I am working, but no longer productive as before and my employer is understanding, so I work at the parcel counter due to weakness and loss of memory"*

Side effects such as insomnia, fatigue and difficulties with memory and concentration can also wreak havoc in the lives of patients. Cancer treatment is an ongoing challenge, after treatment, patients do not return to a pre-cancer diagnosis state. Breast cancer patients (n=1051) in the study of Hoybye MT et al., suffered from cancer or cancer treatment-related late effects before they started a rehabilitation program [11]. Many of these patients suffered from fatigue (66%), lack of concentration (46%) and joint or muscle pains (49%), less from digestive- (18%) and urinary problems (11%). Particularly endocrine symptoms may have a substantial impact on quality of life. Some patients experience moodiness or are confused or unclear as to where they are. This may be the result of certain medications. These effects of treatments are called "iatrogenic effects" which is a fancy way of saying treatment-related effects. Many of these effects are temporary and eventually go away. They are not life threatening and the well-being of the patient improves and anxiety is reduced if information is provided about managing the side-effects.

## Withdrawal and depression

Cancer diagnosis affect the quality of life, once diagnosed a person emotional and psychological state becomes disturbed.

*Having cancer or treatment can also affect your body image. When your skin color change and start wasting due to side-effects of treatment, you are said to be having AIDS. You may feel less confident or afraid of rejection.*

*"You may feel numb or confused, angry about the unwanted changes cancer will bring to your life, sometimes you think of taking chances by taking African treatment and mix with hospital treatment because you need to be healed"*

*"When the news broke about my diagnosis, I was shocked and felt afraid and empty, just saw death starring in my face"*

*"I started to be alone, I was reluctant to go out, there was like this thing on my throat that I felt like crying and it was as if I was losing concentration"*

*"I felt sorry for myself, and I could not talk about it, I was just hurting from the inside"*

These narratives indicates the world view of cancer among black communities, cancer is not seen as a disease like any other chronic condition, it's like a death sentence and others delays seeking medical health and consult traditional healers first as the sometimes associate it with sorcery or witchcraft. Literature suggests that acknowledging and responding to the patients' verbal and non-verbal cues is an important focus for health professionals, as patients respond to the news in a variety of ways [12]. Some patients find receiving bad news difficult and react with disbelief, humor, denial, fear, hope (both realistic and unrealistic) guilt, anxiety and prolonged rage. Reactions to specific family members may include shielding and anticipatory grief [13].

## Problems with follow-up care

The participants reported several problems with follow-up care, one participant said *"It's so frustrating because sometimes you go for follow-up and you do not see the same doctor that consulted or treated you before, thinking that he may be able to understand your problems, it's like repeating your complaints time and again with no breakthrough".* Another participant indicated that *"sometimes your files get lost or are misplaced and they open a new file for you with some of the reports missing and the care becomes inefficient and not effective at all".* Furthermore problems of resources were highlighted like *"At times the machines are not working, and no test can be done to assist with further management or the very doctor or surgeon is on leave and one cannot be assisted because he is the only one and even your complaints cannot be addressed".*

Follow-up treatment care causes much anxiety to patients because they need information about the progress of their conditions and be reassured that the prognosis is good, so lack of communication can create problems, issues relating to faulty equipments or those that are not working should be reported early to the referring hospital so that patients cannot travel unnecessary. Oshima S et al. are of the opinion that follow-up should typically focus on detection and early disease recurrence and management of physical and psychological adverse effects. Follow-up treatment is important when done in the same hospital by the same doctors that treated the patients because they will be having an understanding on how patients experience follow-up and post treatment care.

## Discussions

The findings demonstrated that a substantial number of patients still have problems with cancer diagnosis, how it has been communicated, and communication dynamics related to terminology, medical test and the side effects of treatments and adjusting to body changes, all these factors leads to high levels of anxiety, depression and high levels of distress. Some patients felt that it's easier for them to face the reality of something new or scary if they learn as much as they can about it. This is especially true when you are dealing with a complex group of diseases like cancer. There's often a great fear of the unknown and uncertainty about what's going to happen because cancer is usually associated with death and it causes emotional and psychological distress, thinking about the future and one's dependents. Knowledge can help lessen the fear of the unknown. Early and appropriate psychosocial support and physical rehabilitation could enhance the cancer patients' quality of life, facilitate their adjustment process and possibly prevent them from developing chronic psychiatric disease.

The problems associated with treatments such as side-effects of medications has a negative impact of the patient's perspective because HIV in our rural communities has a negative connotation, for women is associated with women of low morals and one is scorned, so being associated with such diseases causes emotional and psychological pain. Furthermore body changes and adjusting to new lifestyle due to cancer its very disturbing, especially for the males, sexually is a very important aspect among Africans since a man must display his manhood by having many wives and off-springs, to be seen as a respectable man in the community. Maintaining the privacy or confidentiality can also be problematic because of the polygamous situation and usually it is the elder woman who must provide the constant support during the illness and can be very burdensome as she is older than the rest of the wives and it's a cultural accepted norm. Hiccups of follow-up care stemming from chemotherapy, surgery, radiation treatment and hormone therapy rarely exist in isolation and care for these problems are fragmented, as some doctors believe certain problems can go untreated, regarding them as minor or will be better with time, such information does not provide emotional comfort for the patient instead causes more anxiety for the patient. Further, oncologists and surgeons are often poorly linked to physical therapists that may be able to help with side effects, so it is important to take care of the needs of the patient and refer for further management. Furthermore patients reported poor service delivery when going for follow-up and finding resources being inadequate or absent; this increases level of anxiety and increases the level of dissatisfaction [14].

## Limitations

The study was exclusively conducted in one district of Limpopo Province. Therefore generalization of findings is not possible.

However, there is a possibility and need for research to be replicated in other districts among other ethnic groups. The sample of participants had limited type of cancers, it may be necessary that a wide range of cancers be included in order to get rich narrative data and participants perspectives regarding their cancers.

## Conclusion

The study reveals opportunities for providing comprehensive cancer care both for cancer patients and their relatives. Patients' psychological problems, depression, burden of suffering and particularly high levels of treatment-related symptoms suggest substantial needs for ongoing supportive care and for well-directed and effective symptom management in clinical follow-up. Sexual problems should be an important issue in counselling. Doctors and nurses should be aware of relatives' high needs for information and support. Therefore, continued assessment of psychological problems of the patients' and relatives' needs and of the patients' symptoms may provide a basis for purposeful counselling and education. Rehabilitation programmes should be developed for patients and their relatives and implemented in their communities, in primary health care settings, to support them in their long-term adjustment process.

Cancer is not a common disease among black communities, even those diagnosed with cancer are reluctant to talk about it, and hence they feel isolated, lonely and secluded. The study recommends intensive educational campaigns and outreach about cancer as a diagnosis, management of different cancers and lifestyle modification, counselling and rehabilitative programmes. Interventions by oncology nurses in teaching the patient and caregivers the physical and psychological care can assist in families adapting to cancer through formation of support groups to provide supportive communication, counselling, and educational support in improving the quality of life. Future study is needed to explore how the indigenous foods and plants have a role in cancer care and easing the symptomatic effects of cancer treatment.

## Acknowledgement

The authors thank the patients and their relatives who participated in this study for their valuable contributions.

## References

1. Golant M, Haskins NV (2008) "Other cancer survivors": the impact on family and caregivers. Cancer J 14: 420-424.

2. McCann L, Illingworth N, Wengström Y, Hubbard G, Kearney N (2010) Transitional experiences of women with breast cancer within the first year following diagnosis. J Clin Nurs 19: 1969-1976.

3. Kvale K, (2007) Do cancer patients always want to talk about difficult emotions? A qualitative study of cancer inpatients communication needs. European Journal of Oncology nursing 11: 320-327.

4. Simon CE, Crowther M, Higgerson HK (2007) The stage-specific role of spirituality among African American Christian women throughout the breast cancer experience. Cultur Divers Ethnic Minor Psychol 13: 26-34.

5. Krumwiede KA, Krumwiede N (2012) The lived experience of men diagnosed with prostate cancer. Oncol Nurs Forum 39: E443-450.

6. Wilson D, Washington G (2006) Retooling phenomenology: Relevant methods for conducting research with African American women. The Journal of Theory Construction & Testing, 11 : 63-66.

7. Creswell JW (2009) Research design: Qualitative and Quantitative Mixed Methods Approaches. Thousand Oaks, California: Sage.

8. Lincoln YS, Guba EG (1985) Naturalistic inquiry. London: Sage.

9. Democratic Nursing Organisation of South Africa. Ethical considerations in nursing (1998) Pretoria: DENOSA.

10. Nguyen GT, Barg FK, Armstrong K, Holmes JH, Hornik RC (2008) Cancer and communication in the health care setting: experiences of older Vietnamese immigrants, a qualitative study. J Gen Intern Med 23: 45-50.

11. Hoybye MT, Dalton SO, Christensen J, Larsen LR, Kuhn KG, Jensen JN, et al. (2008) Research in Danish cancer rehabilitation: Social characteristics and late effects of cancer among participants in the FOCARE research project. Acta Oncol, 1–9.

12. Ryan H, Schofield P, Cockburn J, Butow P, Tattersall M, et al. (2005) How to recognize and manage psychological distress in cancer patients. Eur J Cancer Care (Engl) 14: 7-15.

13. Randall TC, Wearn AM (2005) Receiving bad news: patients with haematological cancer reflect upon their experience. Palliat Med 19: 594-601.

14. Oshima S, Kisa K, Terashita T, Habara M, Kawabata H, et al. (2011) A qualitative study of Japanese patients' perspectives on post-treatment care for gynecological cancer. Asian Pac J Cancer Prev 12: 2255-2261.

# 13

# Photodynamic Therapy, Laser Therapy and Cellulose Membrane for the Healing of Venous Ulcers

Vitoria H Maciel Coelho[1], Luiza D Alvares[2], Fernanda M Carbinatto[3], Antonio E de Aquino Junior[3*], Dora Patricia Ramirez Angarita[3] and Vanderlei S Bagnato[3]

[1]Federal University of Triângulo Mineiro, Department of Physiotherapy, Uberaba-MG, Brazil

[2]UNICEP, Physiotherapy Faculty, Miguel Petroni, Sao Carlos-SP, Brazil

[3]Sao Carlos Institute of Physics, University of São Paulo, Sao Carlos-SP, Brazil

*Corresponding author: Angarita DPR, Sao Carlos Institute of Physics, University of São Paulo, Av. Trabalhador sao-carlense, n°400- Pq Arnold Schimidt, São Carlos-SP, Brazil, Postal Code 369, Brazil, E-mail: antoniodeaquinojr@gmail.com

## Abstract

**Background:** Venous ulcers, characterized as discontinuous areas of epidermis, are caused by venous hypertension and insufficiency of the muscle pump. They can affect the patient's life quality and cause aesthetic deformity, complications and serious sequelae.

**Objective:** This study investigates the combined effects of photodynamic therapy, laser therapy and cellulose membrane on the healing of venous wounds.

**Methods:** Seven patients at an average of 70 years old and with ulcer history for more than one year were selected. The patients received 3 times per week the application of photodynamic therapy and cellulose membrane; and 2 times per week was applied laser therapy.

**Results:** The results show the reduction of area of ulcer in 7 session ($p<0.04$) and 8 session ($p<0.02$).

**Conclusion:** The ulcers treatment proposes can decrease the healing time of venous ulcers and promote higher life quality for patients.

**Keywords:** Curcumin; Laser; Terapia fotodinamica; wound

## Introduction

Venous ulcer, also known as varicose ulcer and characterized as a discontinuous area of epidermis, is caused by venous hypertension and insufficiency of the muscle pump [1]. It is commonly found in the adult population and exerts major social and economic impacts [2] on the society, as it is a public health problem due to its high incidence, recurrence and long treatment periods. It also represents 70% to 90% of lower limbs ulcers [1,3].

The costs of treatment of chronic ulcers in lower limbs in the USA represent 1% of the health budget. They lead to a loss of 6 million of useful days of work [4] and affect over 2.5 million patients per year [5]. Most studies have indicated higher prevalence of ulcers (approximately 4%) in individuals over 65 years old [6].

A study conducted in Brazil [7] showed the prevalence of venous veins in 47% of 1755 patients and presence of ulcers or ulcer scars in 3.6%.

According to Hess [8], another aggravating factor is the long-time of treatment, which exceeds 9 months in 50% of the cases and over 2 years in 20% of patients. Moreover, the lesions may reappear after complete healing in over 60% of patients, because of the non-follow-up of the recommendations and care proposed in cases with vascular alterations [8].

Due to the significant psychosocial and economic impacts and complexity of the disease, we analyzed the combination of three tools for its treatment, namely photodynamic therapy, laser therapy and cellulose membrane, for a better microbiological control of the lesion and acceleration in the healing process and injury reparation. The clinical protocol involves the application of photodynamic therapy (PDT) characterized as an association between light and a photosensitive substance for the decontamination of the injury. PDT involves three basic elements, namely a photosensitive substance that absorbs light for the initiation of a series of chemical reactions, light, for the activation of the substance, and the oxygen present in the target cell, which reacts with the active substance and generates reactive oxygen species responsible for the destruction of microorganisms [9,10]. The photosensitizer used was curcumin, a natural compound extracted from saffron (*Curcuma longa*).

In the PDT process as an alternative antibiotic treatment, the photosensitizer acts on the located superficial infections [11]. The method has been employed for the treatment of various dermatological conditions, as it promotes the microbiological control of the injury and, in a low dosage, interferes in several stages of the healing process, accelerating the tissue repair [12,13].

The use of cellulose membrane was incorporated for enhancing the cell adhesion and protection of the injury. It is produced by a gram-negative bacterium (*Gluconacetobacter xylinus*) and contains a biopolymer that blocks the entry of microorganisms in the injury, prevents the loss of exudate and promotes cell adhesion.

The association of this process with laser therapy enables the biostimulation of the healing process and tissue repair and involves the application of light in a known wavelength [14,15]. It has been used in the treatment of various types of injury and ulceration and has yielded positive results, especially in chronic cases [16].

Since 1971, the laser therapy has been reported as a non-invasive alternative for the treatment of ulcers [17], due to its bio modulator effect for tissue repair and increases in local circulation, stimulation and proliferation of cells and synthesis of collagen [18]. The mechanisms by which the method accelerates the healing process comprehend the local liberation of growth factors [17] and mitochondrial increase of ATP production [19,20].

We have evaluated a new clinical protocol for the treatment of venous ulcers through the combination of three techniques, namely laser therapy, cellulose membrane application and PDT.

## Methods

### Patients

This study was approved by the ethics committee under research protocol number 667752, CAAE: 30625714.2.0000.5380 of May 29, 2014.

Patients were selected through the confirmatory diagnosis of venous ulcer by dermatologists and complied with the inclusion criteria.

**Inclusion criteria:** venous ulcer diagnosis and ulcer located in the lower limbs; patients with venous insufficiency and edema, varicosities, lipodermatoesclerosis and ezcema.

**Exclusion criteria:** Patients allergic to any medicament used in the study; pregnant women; evidence of diseases, such as cellulitis, osteomyelitis and gangrene in the affected place; patients that used antibiotics for 15 days prior to the treatment; patients with arterial impairments, diabetes or other systemic diseases; patients that use corticosteroid or immunosuppressive and cancer patient.

Seven patients at an average of 70 years old were treated during our study.

### Clinical protocol

The venous ulcers were washed only with a 0.9% physiological saline solution. The photosensitizer, i.e., curcumin gel 1.5% (supplied by Pharma PDT) was applied across the ulcer, which was immediately occluded with plastic film, aluminum paper and gauze. 30 minutes after the application of curcumin, both curative and excess gel was removed with a physiological saline solution and gauze.

Photodynamic therapy (PDT) with light emission diode (LED) of 450 nm wavelength and 75 mW/cm$^2$ intensity was applied for 12 min and a total energy dose of 54 J/cm$^2$ was delivered to the tissue. The cellulose membrane (Nanoskin® provided by Innovative technology-Innovatecs) was then placed across the area of the ulcer and a curative was applied. A nurse changed the cellulose membrane every 3 days. Twice a week, the laser therapy (660 nm laser) was applied on the full extension of the ulcer and under the cellulose membrane for 30 s at 10 J/cm$^2$ fluence. The patients underwent weekly sessions that followed the same protocol for 4 weeks or until the complete healing of the ulcer. The procedure is shown in Figure 1.

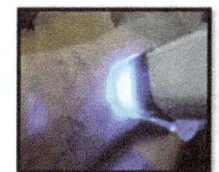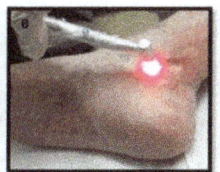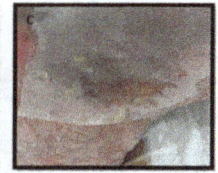

**Figure 1:** Conjugated therapies of venous ulcer treatment. A) PDT; B) Laser therapy; C) Cellulose membrane.

### Follow-up treatment

During all process, a sterilized steel ruler measured the length and width of the ulcer for analysis of the reductions in the lesion size and photographic records were made. The ulcer area was calculated in cm$^2$ through the multiplication of the longest length by the largest width in each session. The session was considered each wound dressing.

### Results

Figure 2 shows the evolution of the venous ulcer reduction. Significant differences were observed between the measurements taken along the treatment. The mean area of the injuries showed statistical differences in comparison with the injuries in the initial session versus session 7 (p<0.04) and initial session versus session 8 (p<0.02). The mean dimension of the initial area was 51 cm$^2$, whereas in sessions 7 and 8, they were 13,6 cm$^2$ and 7,44 cm$^2$, respectively.

The evolution in the venous ulcer (12 years of injury) treatment is shown in Figure 3. Our results are promising, especially regarding the microbiological control of the injury by PDT with curcumin as a photosensitizer. The acceleration of the tissue repair through the association of laser therapy methods and cellulose biomembrane in 7 patients, after 8 sessions, is shown in Figure 2.

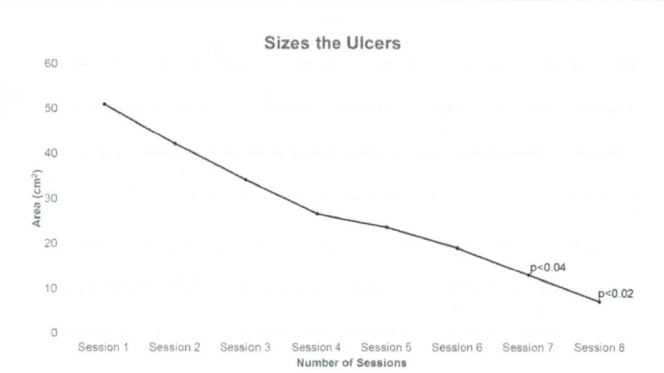

**Figure 2:** Representative graphic of the Area evolution (cm$^2$) of the venous ulcer healing along 8 sessions in the 7 patients treated. Significant statistical differences between Sessions 1 and 7 (<0.04) and between Sessions 1 and 8 (p<0.02).

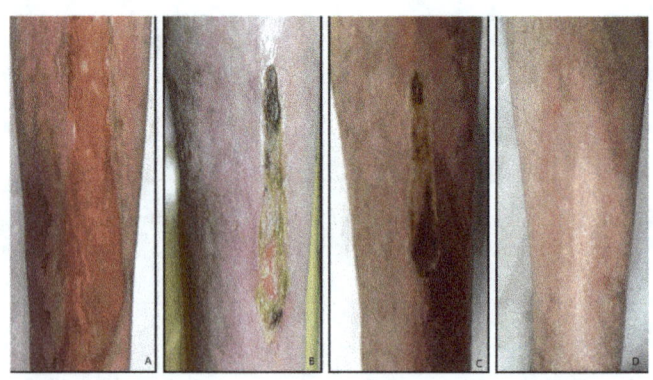

**Figure 3:** Evolution of a venous ulcer during 8 sessions of the treatment (patient with 12 year old injuries), WITH PDT, laser therapy and cellulose membrane. A) Initial injury; B) After session 1; C) After session 6; D) After session 8 end-healing process.

## Discussion

The results showed acceleration in the venous ulcer healing after the eighth session, on average. The combination of laser therapy, cellulose membrane application and PDT improved the wound healing.

Such results can be attributed to the effectiveness of each technique in the wound healing, i.e., laser therapy alone has proven effective in both local and systemic responses, showing an anti-inflammatory effect, reducing pain, accelerating the cell proliferation and optimizing the healing process [21].

In the study realized by Caetano et al. [22] 20 patients and 32 chronic ulcers were used, divided in three groups. In group 1, sulfadiazine cream was used and treated with placebo phototherapy ($<0.03$ J/cm$^3$), group 2 phototherapy was used and group 3 was a control group, only with sulfadiazine cream without phototherapy. The results from this research were that phototherapy promotes healing of chronic venous ulcers, due to treatment with phototherapy healed significantly faster than controls when compared at day 30 (p 0.01), day 60 (p 0.05), and day 90 (p 0.001) and similarly healed faster than the placebo-treated ulcers at days 30 and 90 (p 0.01), but not at day 60.

The cellulose membrane exhibits a distinctive nanofibrillar structure that is a highly nanoporous material that enables the transfer of medicines and is an efficient physical barrier against any external infection. It is a perfect matrix with optimal properties for wound healing [23].

According to Farah [24], a membrane applied under a wound acts as a new skin that can eliminate pain through the isolation of nerve endings, although it may enhance the absorption of exudates in the wound.

In the study realized by Basmaji et al. [25] Nanoskin® was applied in patients with burns and wound naturopathic (Hansen), the results show that Nanoskin® is very effective in promoting autolytic debridement, reducing pain, and accelerating granulation, all of which are important for wound healing.

The PDT process, on the other hand, kills the bacteria through the combination of a photosensitizer and a source of light in an appropriate wavelength, which results in the wound decontamination.

Hamblin et al. [26,27] were the first authors to report on the PDT process in relation to wounds infected in the mouse model. They evaluated the wounds measuring 100 mm$^2$ (8 mm × 12.5 mm), which were made on the backs of mice. The wounds were infected with *E. coli* and *P. aeruginosa* and observed that 90% of the mice infected with *P. aeruginosa* and treated with PDT survived, which demonstrated PDT is a non-invasive technique for the treatment of infected wounds.

Although treatments that use each technique alone (laser therapy, cellulose membrane application and PDT) have shown promising results, the combination of techniques used in this new clinical protocol was more effective regarding reductions in the treatment time due to improvements in the wounds healing.

## Conclusion

The new integrated method can decrease the healing time of venous ulcers, promote higher life quality for patients and generate positive social and economic impacts.

## Author Disclosure Statement

No competing financial interests exist.

## Acknowledgement

This work was supported in part by CNPq (INOF – INCT grant: 573587/2008-6); FINEP (Grant n° 01.13.0430-00) and São Paulo Research Foundation (FAPESP) grant 2013/07276-1 (CePOF)

## References

1. Borges EL (2012) Feridas: Ulceras dos membros inferiores. Guanabara Koogan.

2. Education CM (2006) Management of patients with venous leg ulcer. Abordagem de pacientes com ulcera da perna de etiologia, pp: 509-521.

3. Liu YC, Margolis DJ, Isseroff RR (2011) Does inflammation have a role in the pathogenesis of venous ulcers? A critical review of the evidence. J Invest Dermatol 131: 818-827.

4. Etufugh CN, Phillips TJ (2007) Venous ulcers. Clin Dermatol 25: 121-130.

5. Mostow EN, Haraway GD, Dalsing M, Hodde JP, King D; OASIS Venus Ulcer Study Group (2005) Effectiveness of an extracellular matrix graft (OASIS Wound Matrix) in the treatment of chronic leg ulcers: a randomized clinical trial. J Vasc Surg 41: 837-843.

6. Callam MJ, Ruckley CV, Harper DR, Dale JJ (1985) Chronic ulceration of the leg: Extent of the problem and provision of care. Br Med J (Clin Res Ed) 290: 1855-1856.

7. Maffei FH (1986) Varicose veins and chronic venous insufficiency in Brazil: Prevalence among 1755 inhabitants of a Country Town. Int J Epidemiol 15: 210-217.

8. Hess CT (2002) Tratamento de feridas e ulceras.eds. Reichmann and Affonso Editores, Rio de Janeiro.

9. Dougherty TJ, Kaufman JE, Goldfarb A, Weishaupt KR, Boyle D, et al. (1978) Photoradiation therapy for the treatment of malignant tumors. Cancer Res 38: 2628-2635.

10. Agostinis P, Berg K, Cengel KA, Foster TH, Girotti AW, et al. (2011) Photodynamic therapy of cancer: An update. CA Cancer J Clin 61: 250-281.

11. Bruzell EM, Morisbak E, Tonnesen HH (2005) Studies on curcumin and curcuminoids. XXIX. Photoinduced cytotoxicity of curcumin in selected aqueous preparations. Photochem Photobiol Sci 4: 523–530

12. Choi JY (2010) Molecular changes following topical photodynamic therapy using methyl aminolaevulinate in mouse skin. J Dermatol Sci 58: 198-203.

13. Almeida Issa MC (2009) Immunohistochemical expression of matrix metalloproteinases in photodamaged skin by photodynamic therapy. Br J Dermatol 16: 647-653.

14. Enwemeka CS, Parker JC, Dowdy DS, Harkness EE, Sanford LE, et al. (2004) The efficacy of low-power lasers in tissue repair and pain control: A meta-analysis study. Photomed Laser Surg 22: 323-329.

15. Enwemeka CS (2009) Intricacies of dose in laser phototherapy for tissue repair and pain relief. Photomed Laser Surg 27: 387-393.

16. Kitchen S, Bazin S (1998) Eletroterapia de Clayton. Eds Manole, Sao Paulo.

17. Mester E (1971) Effect of laser rays on wound healing. Am J Surg 122: 532-535.

18. Schindl A (1999) Increased dermal angiogenesis after low-intensity laser therapy for a chronic radiation ulcer determined by a video measuring system. J Am Acad Dermatol 40: 481-484.

19. Karu T (1989) Photobiology of low-power laser effects. Health Phys 56: 691-704.

20. Posten W, Wrone DA, Dover JS, Arndt KA, Silapunt S, et al. (2005) Low-level laser therapy for wound healing: Mechanism and efficacy. Dermatol Surg 31: 334-340.

21. Soares LP (2008) Effects of laser therapy on experimental wound healing using oxidized regenerated cellulose hemostat. Photomed Laser Surg 26: 10-13.

22. Caetano KS, Frade MA, Minatel DG, Santana LA, Enwemeka CS (2009) Phototherapy improves healing of chronic venous ulcers. Photomed Laser Surg 27: 111-118.

23. Czaja W, Krystynowicz A, Bielecki S, Brown RM Jr. (2006) Microbial cellulose--the natural power to heal wounds. Biomaterials 27: 145-151.

24. Farah LFX (1990) Process for the preparation of cellulose film, cellulose film produced thereby, artificial skin graft and its use. Number patents: 4,912,049. United States Patent.

25. Basmaji P, Damiano O, Carlos S (2011) Nanoskin® for medical applications Innovative technology-Innovatecs synthesis of bacterial cellulose scanning electronic microscopy (SEM) and transmission electron microscopy (TEM). Nanoskin® in the Treatment of Chronic Wounds and Burns, pp: 193-196.

26. Hamblin MR, Zahra T, Contag CH, McManus AT, Hasan T (2003) Optical monitoring and treatment of potentially lethal wound infections in vivo. J Infect Dis 187: 1717-1725.

27. Hamblin MR (2002) Rapid control of wound infections by targeted photodynamic therapy monitored by in vivo bioluminescence imaging. Photochem Photobiol 75: 51-57.

# 14

# Preferences and Utilization of Drug Information Resources by Practicing Pharmacists

Bisrat Hailemeskel*, Imbi Drame, Min Choi and Pawvana Pansiri

*College of Pharmacy, Howard University, Silver Spring, USA*

*Corresponding author: Hailemeskel B, Associate Professor and Co-Director of International Projects, Howard University, College of Pharmacy, 2300 4th st, N.W, Washington DC, 20059, United States, E-mail: bhailemeskel@howard.edu

## Abstract

**Objective:** This study was designed to identify preferences and utilization of drug information (DI) resources, and to assess perceived level of drug information skill for pharmacists enrolled in a Non-traditional Doctor of Pharmacy (NTDP) program.

**Background:** The ability to search for, utilize and apply drug information is an essential skill for pharmacists to fulfill their role as the primary source of drug knowledge. However, with exponential growth in the abundance of information, the increasing availability of an array DI resources and as a advocacy measures for provider status and MTM reimbursement intensify, knowing appropriate DI skills has become a challenge for pharmacists. Therefore, understanding the baseline knowledge of practicing pharmacists, such as those in NTDP programs, is crucial for determining how to design effective training measures.

**Methods:** An 18-question survey was distributed to the participants (n=18) to assess their drug resource preferences and perceived skill level. Descriptive statistics were used and Chi-square analysis was performed using IBM SPSS 23.

**Results:** General search engines (55.6%)was the most preferred tool for respondents' drug information search activities, while 72% of respondents frequently used Google for drug information inquiries. However, only 17%of the respondents always cross-checked preliminary search results with other resources, and only 22 percent always verified the authenticity of the websites used. The level of confidence in drug information skills and in the accuracy of information obtained was notably high amongst NTDP students with 72% and 100%, respectively, selecting confident or very confident.

**Conclusion:** Observation from the study suggests that pharmacists should be more aware of the possible risks to patient safety inherent in using Google or other search engines, and should be steered toward utilization of more reputable, evidence-based DI resources.

**Keywords:** Professional training; Education; Counselling; Lay perspectives; Adverse drug reactions; Patient safety; Health promotion; Pharmaceutical public health; Professional practice

## Introduction

The ability to search for, utilize, and apply drug information is an essential skill for pharmacists to fulfill their role as the primary source of drug knowledge [1]. However, with exponential growth in the abundance of information, the increasing availability of an array DI resources, and as a advocacy measures for provider status and MTM reimbursement intensify, knowing appropriate DI skills has become a challenge for pharmacists [2]. Furthermore, the functions afforded by use of drug information skills are numerous and diverse, from ensuring medication safety to evaluation of clinical trials that validate treatment usefulness [1]. The work place setting in general, however, does not allow ample time for pharmacists to respond drug information inquiries, yet current literature purports that pharmacists should be able to anticipate the DI needs at any setting in which they work [2]. This current trend highlights the importance of having a concrete drug information educational foundation at all levels to maintain one's competency as a drug expert [3].

A Non-Traditional Doctor of Pharmacy (NTDP) Program provides an opportunity for practicing pharmacists to earn a doctor of pharmacy degree through coursework that combines distance learning techniques and in-class activities. This design allows institutions to create a more customized experience for pharmacists who are concurrently practicing in a variety of settings. Howard University College of Pharmacy is one of only [4] US pharmacy schools to administer a full-time NTDP program.4Drug information class sessions were designed for Howard University NTDP students to promote effective drug information and evaluation skills, while enabling them to service accurate in-depth information requests using appropriate communication and documentation procedures [4].

This study was conducted to assess the preferences and utilization of drug information resources by pharmacists enrolled in an NTDP program, as well as to determine their perceived level of drug information skill. The study was designed to identify areas for improvement of the drug information coursework administered to the students based upon analysis of study findings.

## Method

A survey consisting of 18 questions was distributed to the NTDP students (n=18) at Howard University. The survey questions were mainly intended: 1) to identify key demographics, such as level of education and number of years in the field; 2) to determine the preferences and utilization patterns for drug information resources; 3) and to identify perceptions about the accuracy of drug information search results confidence level for drug information skill.

Participants were asked to either select the choice with the most suitable description or fill in the blank by writing a specific response, if applicable. For some of the questions, participants were instructed to choose one of the following options under each potential response: Frequent Use (Frequent), Occasional Use (Moderate), Rare Use (Infrequent), and Never Use (Never). Only the percentage calculation for Frequent Use (Frequent) was used to determine the preference based upon each question.

Participants were characterized by years of pharmacy-related experience, less than 10 years (n=8) versus 10 years or above (n=10). Responses from these two cohorts were then compared to determine how the duration of pharmacy experience affects drug information resource utilization habits and the confidence level for search results and abilities.

The data collected from the survey was transferred to IBM SPSS 23 software to compute frequency, and to perform Chi-square and one tailed t-test analysis.

## Results

Among a total of 18 participants, most were in-between the age of 30-39 (44.4%). No participants were less than 30 years of age. The number of female participants was greater than male, 61.1 percent versus 38.9 percent, respectively. When the respondents were asked to identify their educational backgrounds other than pharmacy, the majority (44.4%) percent reported earning a bachelor's degree followed by 27.8% with an associate's degree and 22.2% with a master's degree. The mean number of years of pharmacy-related experience was 15.2 years 10.1 (Tables 1 and 2).

| Variable | Frequency (Percentile) |
|---|---|
| **Age Range** | |
| 20-29 | 0 (0) |
| 30-39 | 8 (44.4) |
| 40-49 | 5 (27.8) |
| >=50 | 5 (27.8) |
| **Gender** | |
| Male | 7 (38.9) |
| Female | 11 (61.1) |
| **Highest Education** | |
| Associate | 5 (27.8) |
| BA/BSC | 8 (44.4) |
| MS/MA | 4 (22.2) |
| Ph.D. | 1 |
| **Working Experience(in Years)** | |
| 0-5 | 4 (22.2) |
| 6-10 | 4 (22.2) |
| 11-15 | 3 (16.7) |
| 16-20 | 1 (5.6) |
| 21-25 | 2 (11.1) |
| 26-30 | 3 (16.7) |
| 31-35 | 1 (5.6) |

**Table 1:** Demography of the participant.

| Q: Which reference resource(s) you normally use when you need drug or health related information? | | | | | |
|---|---|---|---|---|---|
| Category | Frequent Use | Occasional Use | Rare Use | No Use | Omit response |
| Google or other search engines | 55.56 | 33.33 | 0 | 5.56 | 5.56 |
| Textbooks/Journals | 38.89 | 33.33 | 11.11 | 5.56 | 11.11 |
| Package Inserts | 33.33 | 33.33 | 11.11 | 5.56 | 16.67 |
| Other Subscription based database | 27.78 | 33.33 | 27.78 | 5.56 | 5.56 |
| **Q: Which search engine do you normally use to look up for drug or health related questions?** | | | | | |
| Category | Frequent Use | Occasional Use | Rare Use | No Use | Omit response |
| Google | 72.22 | 22.22 | 0 | 0 | 5.56 |
| Yahoo | 27.78 | 5.56 | 5.56 | 27.78 | 33.33 |

| | | | | | |
|---|---|---|---|---|---|
| Bing | 0 | 11.11 | 5.56 | 38.89 | 44.44 |
| Ask/MSN | 0 | 5.56 | 11.11 | 33.33 | 50 |

**Q: Frequency of subscription based drug information reference use (in the past 2 years)**

| Category | Frequent Use | Occasional Use | Rare Use | No Use | Omit response |
|---|---|---|---|---|---|
| Drug Facts and Comparison | 44.44 | 44.44 | 0 | 0 | 11.11 |
| AHFS Drug Information | 22.22 | 27.78 | 22.22 | 0 | 27.78 |
| Micromedex or Clinical Pharmacology | 44.44 | 33.33 | 22.22 | 0 | 0 |
| Physician Desk Reference | 16.67 | 16.67 | 22.22 | 11.11 | 33.33 |

**Q: If you receive a question about a potential adverse effect of a drug from patients, the most likely reference you normally use to answer such question is:**

| Category | Frequent Use | Occasional Use | Rare Use | No Use | Omit response |
|---|---|---|---|---|---|
| Google or general internet search | 33.33 | 27.78 | 5.56 | 0 | 33.33 |
| Package insert | 44.44 | 22.22 | 11.11 | 0 | 22.22 |
| Resources available through your company | 27.78 | 33.33 | 11.11 | 5.56 | 22.22 |
| Textbook | 22.22 | 22.22 | 16.67 | 11.11 | 27.78 |

**Q: If you have searched for medical/health or drugs information, which category is the most common reason(s) for your search?**

| Category | Frequent Use | Occasional Use | Rare Use | No Use | Omit response |
|---|---|---|---|---|---|
| Drug identification | 50 | 16.67 | 16.67 | 0 | 16.67 |
| Indications/Use | 66.67 | 27.78 | 0 | 0 | 5.56 |
| Adverse drug events/Side Effects | 72.22 | 22.22 | 0 | 0 | 5.56 |
| Dosage/Administration | 66.67 | 27.78 | 0 | 0 | 5.56 |

**Q: If a patient calls you to identify a tablet by its shape, imprint or color which reference you normally you use?**

| Category | Frequent Use | Occasional Use | Rare Use | No Use | Omit response |
|---|---|---|---|---|---|
| Google or general internet search | 27.78 | 16.67 | 11.11 | 5.56 | 38.89 |
| Indentidex | 55.56 | 11.11 | 0 | 16.67 | 16.67 |
| Drug-Reaction | 0 | 11.11 | 16.67 | 16.67 | 55.56 |
| The dispensing system at work | 33.33 | 11.11 | 0 | 16.67 | 38.89 |

**Q: A reference source that you normally use to find a US equivalent drug of foreign drugs not available in the US is:**

| Category | Frequent Use | Occasional Use | Rare Use | No Use | Omit response |
|---|---|---|---|---|---|
| Google or general internet search | 27.78 | 27.78 | 5.56 | 5.56 | 33.33 |
| Martindale | 33.33 | 38.89 | 16.67 | 5.56 | 5.56 |
| Drug Facts and Comparisons | 22.22 | 22.22 | 5.56 | 5.56 | 44.44 |
| Index Nominum | 0 | 16.67 | 22.22 | 22.22 | 38.89 |

**Table 2:** The preferences assessment.

Most respondents researched drug/health-related information multiple times a day (44.4%), followed by once a day (27.8%). For amount of time spent on a drug information search, most spent less time, with 1 to 5 minutes ranked highest (38.9%), followed by 6 to 10 min (33.3%).Respondents with 10 years or more of pharmacy experience demonstrated slower processing time, with 22.2% spending more than 15 min vs. 5.5% of respondents with <10 years of experience (p=0.0006).

To the questionnaire also assessed the participants' preferences for search tools used to address drug information inquiries. Google or other general search engine (59.5%) received the highest percentage of "Frequent Use" ratings. Twenty-four percent preferred package inserts, followed by textbooks/journals (22.2%). Subscription-based databases were the least favored among all categories (18.3%).

When asked which specific search engine was preferred for responding to DI inquiries, Google was the most preferred, receiving a "frequent use" rating from 72% of respondents, and considerably outperforming other high traffic search engines such as Yahoo (27.2%). Bing and Ask/MSN were not preferred by any respondents.

Despite the hazard associated with disseminating largely unverified information provided by search engines, only 17% of the participants responded that they "always" cross-check or verify their preliminary search results with other resources. A lower verification rate was observed from those with less than 10 years of pharmacy experience (12.5%) versus those with greater than 10 years of experience (20.2%; p=0.18).

Participant were also asked whether they verify the authenticity of the website or check the website sponsors before using the information obtained. Only 22% of respondents indicated that they "always" verify the authenticity of the website. Nearly three quarters of respondents indicated that they "sometimes" verify or chose "never/I do not remember." Though differences were not significant, the less experienced cohort demonstrated weaker verification efforts than on the more experienced cohort, 25% and 30%, respectively (p=0.37).

The most preferred subscription-based drug information references were Drug Facts and Comparisons and Micromedex and/or Clinical Pharmacology, with each category receiving a rating of "frequent use" from 44.4% of respondents. . Although the "frequent use" rate was identical, the "never use" rate was higher for the Drug Facts and Comparisons (22.2%) compared to Micromedex and/or Clinical Pharmacology (0%). Physician Desk Reference (PDR) and AHFS Drug Information were rated the lowest at 22.2% and 16.7% respectively.

Adverse drug events (72.2%) were the most common reason for a drug information search by pharmacists according to survey results. Other reasons for drug information search, such as indications/use, drug identification, and dosage/administration, also demonstrated relatively high rates "frequent use" at50.0%, 66.7% and 66.7%, respectively.

A follow-up questionnaire was administered to further assess preferences for resources used for investigating adverse events for a specific drug. About 44.4% responded that package insert was their preferred source, followed by Google or other general internet search engine (33.3%), and resources provided by their employers (28.2%). Textbook was the least favorable resource with, only 22.2% citing "frequent use".

About 55.6% of the respondents cited "frequent use" of Identidex as their reference source when identifying an unknown tablet or capsule by its imprint or color. The dispensing system provided by the employer was the second most frequently used resource (33.3%), followed by Google or general internet search (27.8%).

No resources received significantly higher "frequent use" rating than another for researching a US equivalent drug. However, Martindale was used slightly more than other resources (33.3%).The confidence level for the accuracy of search results was high, 100% signified that they felt confident about the accuracy of search results The confidence level for their drug information skills was also very high, with only 27% of the respondents feeling "not fully confident" about their searching skill.

The two major limitations of the study are the small sample size and the fact that the participants were in the non-traditional doctor of pharmacy program. Although it was difficult to make a strong conclusion given these limitations, the study is an indication of the trend of drug information preferences among pharmacists which may stimulates a larger and more compressive study.

## Discussion

General search engines were the most preferred tool employed by the participants for the purpose of obtaining information for drug information inquiries. Not surprisingly, Google was the most preferred search engine at a 72% "frequent use" rate, as since Google takes holds a 64.1% market share in the U.S. according to the market research by comScore in 2015 [5]. The quality of search results from Google is questionable, however, due to Google's PageRank algorithms, ranking websites based on popularity (the number visits per search term) versus the verifiable accuracy and quality of the information provided [6]. The information retrieved using Google or any of the search engines is seldom verified by appropriate and credible authorities, lacking the evidence-based feature coveted by individuals with any level of scientific training.

Perhaps the most concerning study finding was that despite the high use of Google and other general internet search engines, results indicated that survey participants were unlikely to verify the authenticity and/or cross-check preliminary search results with other resources. This practice was observed at a higher rate in participants with less pharmacy experience, which can place patients at undue risk of harm, as these individuals may have an even greater need to cross-check information than their more experienced counterparts. A study conducted by Cardoni on how drug information service impacts patient care, warned of the importance of accurate information for the sake of patient's safety [3]. It should be noted, however, that the data in the study at hand was not statistically significant, likely due to the small sample size.

Participants also demonstrated a high level of confidence on their drug information skill (87%) and the quality of search results (92%). These findings may be a worrisome indicator because pharmacists might not be aware of what appropriate drug information skills entail. They will also be more likely to confidently disseminate or utilize inaccurate information that can result in patient harm and reduced pharmacist credibility to other members of the healthcare community.

The most common reason for drug information search was adverse events or ADE (72%). Although package insert was the most preferred resource in obtaining information on adverse drug events, there one-third of the participants still frequently used search engines. Because ADE is a particularly delicate area of pharmacy knowledge, meaning that "getting the data wrong" is more likely to result in morbidity and mortality, liability issues, and lost trust, than other knowledge areas, it can be particularly troubling when pharmacists are not using the most appropriate resources.

The majority of the participants rated Identidex as most preferred for identifying unknown tablet or capsule by its imprint or color, followed by Google and dispensing systems provided by employers. Martindale was preferred for finding a US equivalent drug of foreign drugs, though findings were not statistically significant. These results demonstrate that pharmacists may be using more appropriate resources for searching questions related to topics with lesser consequences if incorrect information is provided versus ADEs.

## Conclusion

Google was a widely-accepted resource for drug information search activities by pharmacists enrolled in the NTDP program for various purposes, including investigating adverse events. Google and other searching engines, by design, are not set up for close monitoring of the information put forth. Although the measures for ensuring information accuracy are strongly recommended for pharmacists for those reasons, as evidenced by results of this study, educational efforts have not been sufficient enough to minimize use of such search engines as primary resources. Pharmacists should be more aware of the possible risks to patient safety inherent in using Google or other search engines, and should be steered toward utilization of more reputable, evidence-based DI resources. However, further study is needed on a larger scale to verify the accuracy of these findings.

## References

1. Gora-Harper M, Lea M, Russell JM (2013) Introduction to the concept of drug information. In: Drug Information: A Guide for Pharmacists.

2. Bernknopf AC, Karpinski JP, McKeever AL (2009) Drug information: from education to practice. Pharmacotherapy 29: 331-346.

3. Cardoni AA, Thompson LJ (1978) Impact of drug information services on patient care. Am J Hosp Pharm 35: 1233-7.

4. American Association of Colleges of Pharmacy (2016) Non-traditional students: Post-BS programs.

5. Top 15 Most Popular search Engines 2015.

6. Adams C (2016) What is Google Page Rank, How is it earned and does It Matter in 2016? Bruce Clay Inc.

# 15

# Prevalence of Premarital Sexual Practice and Associated Factors among Adolescents of Jimma Preparatory School Oromia Region, South West Ethiopia

**Ayanos Taye[1]\* and Iyobe Asmare[2]**

[1]Department of Nursing, College of Health Sciences, Jimma University, Ethiopia

[2]Department of Nursing, College of Health Sciences, Debreberhan University, Ethiopia

\*Corresponding author: Taye A, Department of Nursing, College of Health Sciences, Jimma University, Ethiopia, E-mail: ayanostm@gmail.com

## Abstract

**Background:** Sexual activities among adolescent have been reported to be increasing worldwide. Several studies in Sub-Saharan Africa have also documented increasing premarital sexual activities among adolescents.

**Objective:** To assess the prevalence of premarital sexual practice and associated factors among adolescent of Jimma preparatory school, Jimma zone, south west Ethiopia.

**Methods:** Cross-sectional study was conducted in Jimma preparatory school from Feb 1-27, 2014. Simple random sampling was used. Data was collected through self- administered questionnaire and analyzed using frequency, percentage and chi-square. The study was conducted till June, 2014.

**Result:** In this study a total of 352 students give their response to the questions asked, and the response rate was 92.5%. Of this 197 (56%) males and 157 (44%) female adolescents were participated in the study. About 25% of the participants had had premarital sex at the time of survey. Among those adolescents who had had premarital sexual intercourse the main reason for initiation was falling in love which accounted for 47.7%. This study also revealed age ($x^2$ = 12.2, p < 0.001), place of residency at ($x^2$ = 23.1, p < 0.001), attending religious activity at ($x^2$ = 59.4, p < 0.0002), mothers' literacy at ($x^2$ = 18.2, p < 0.001) and fathers, literacy at ($x^2$ = 25.5, p< 0.001) were associated with their involvement in premarital sexual practice.

**Conclusion and Recommendation:** Considerable amount of school adolescents had started premarital sexual activity that may predispose them to different sexual and reproductive health problem. Alcohol drinking, seeing sexual related film, peer influence, etc. were found to be contributing factor to the practice. Therefore un integrated effort needs to be initiated to address such adolescents' sexual and reproductive health problems through establishing and strengthening school anti HIV/AIDS clubs, sensitizing parents, community members and the public focusing on parent-child communication and discussion on sex related issues.

**Keywords:** Adolescent; Premarital sexes; Prevalence

## Background

World Health Organization (WHO) defines adolescent people as those between the ages of 10-19 years [1]. Adolescent is the time of transition from childhood to adult hood during which young people experiencing following puberty and human beings faced once in their life time [2].

The world today is experiencing a rapid increasing in the number of young people. Today adolescents constitute approximately one-fifth of the world's population with more than four-fifth in developing countries [3].

Premarital sex is penetrative vaginal or sexual intercourse performed between couples before marriage. Some people who advocate virginity and abstinence argue that those people engaged in such sexual practice may have sex with many sexual partners and may have high number of life time sexual partners. As a result, they may be liable to acquire STIs including HIV. Beside, females, particularly adolescent girls may end up with unwanted pregnancy, abortion, teenage deliveries and various complications of these including death. Moreover, the girls may drop out from school to rare their children and in most cases they become economically dependent upon their parents [4].

The trend in sexual activity of adolescents at younger age increase in the world. In many countries the majority of young people are sexually active before age of 20, premarital sex is common among 15-19 years old [5].

The sexual activities in which young people engaged are risky which can result in HIV infection including other sexually transmitted disease or unwanted pregnancies. Different studies suggested that many young people have got the necessary information from different sources with regard to HIV and AIDS; they do not bring behavioral change in different groups of the population [6].

However the major problem is to bring about behavioral changes in different groups of the population. Adolescents in many developing countries rarely discuss about sexual matter with their parents [7]. Peer pressure and economic problem forces young adult to engage in sexual activity at earlier age [8].

Studying sexual behavior and its associated problems have been one national agenda of many researchers today. This is because many adolescents and young adults are sexually active at the age of 20s. They are highly affected by sexual related problem and the prevalence of HIV/AIDS, early child bearing and early onset of sexual activity among people in different countries of the world [9].

The premarital sexual activity of young people can expose them to the risk of unintended pregnancy, abortion and STDs [10]. Sub-Saharan Africa remains the most affected region in the global AIDS epidemic. Although just over 10% of the world's population live in this region, more than two out of three (68%) adults and nearly 90% of children infected with HIV live there. more than three out of four (76%) of global death is due to AIDS related illnesses in 2007, occurred in sub-Saharan Africa .this proportion is clear evidence of the unmeet need for antiretroviral treatment in the region [11].

Several studies in Sub-Saharan Africa have also documented high premarital sexual practice among adolescents [12]. However, viewing adolescents as a specific group with their own needs is a relatively recent practice, especially in developing countries [13].

Because of cultural taboos, adolescents in many developing countries rarely discuss sexual matters explicitly with their parents. Most information for their patchy knowledge comes from peers of the same sex who may themselves lack adequate information or are incorrectly informed [14].

School adolescents are a group of young people who came from different areas with different family background. Many gaps between adolescents' background may make them to be involved in premarital sexual activity and expose to HIV/AIDS and high rate of STIs. It is known that there is no effective cure of HIV/AIDS and the only effective treatment is prevention. This can be achieved largely through changing behavior related to sexuality by studying why people are driven into premarital sex. The effect of premarital sexual practice on adolescents is not only being risk of HIV/AIDS but also it includes effects like: early pregnancy, abortion and other sexually transmitted disease so this study will play an important role on creating awareness about these risks.

Since large numbers of adolescents are involved in unprotected sexual activities with their teenage, studying premarital sexual behavior beginning from teenagers is necessary. Therefore, this study will play invaluable role on inspiring teenagers about the risk of premarital sexual practice so as to prevent themselves from these risks.

Since there is no baseline survey related to school adolescents' sexual behavior in the area, this study will also provide baseline information to undertake further study on large scale. So this research will have its own contribution for those who will conduct another research.

## Methods and Materials

A School based cross-sectional study design was conducted in Jimma town at Jimma preparatory school from February 1-27, 2014. Jimma town is located in Oromia National Regional State, in Jimma zone, Jimma Woreda at a distance 356 Km from Addis Ababa. Its astronomical location is 7o4` North Latitude and 36o5` East Longitude. Jimma town was founded in 1837. Jimma is one of the reform towns in the region and has a city administration; municipality and 13 kebelles. The towns have a structure plan prepared in 2009. The study was conducted till June, 2014.

Based on the 2007 Census conducted by the CSA, this Zone has the three largest ethnic groups reported in Jimma were the Oromo, Amhara and Yem. Oromiffa was spoken as first language by 90.43% and 5.33% spoke Amharic; the remaining 4.24% spoke all other primary languages reported. The majority of the populations were Muslim, Ethiopian Orthodox Christianity and Protestantism respectively. Currently there are 1 preparatory school, 2 high school, 8 elementary school and 1 university which have 4 campus.

### Sample size determination and sampling technique

To determine the sample size for the study, the following assumption is considered, due to the presence of related studies in the area, assume 50% of school adolescent are sexually active (ever had sex before marriage) and this is taken as (p = 0.05), margin of error (0.05) and standard normal distribution value for the 95% confidence interval (1.96) are considered. The final sample size was 186. After calculating the sample size, the study subject was selected by using simple random sampling technique. Proportion allocation to the section was used grade as strata and stratified into two strata grade 11 and 12.

### Data collection procedure

Different data collection tools were used to collect relevant information based on the study objectives. Pre-test of the questionnaire for clarity and consistency of the questions was done one week prior to the actual data collection. Then necessary correction was made based on the feedback of the data collectors.

By using self-administer questionnaire, information about students about premarital sexual practice, socio demographic characteristic of the respondents, major factor contributing for the involvement of the respondents into premarital sexual activity and another related data will be collected. The principal investigator was coordinating the overall activity of the study.

Data was collected, cleared, edited and analyzed using frequency, percentage and chi-square. The result was presented using tables and diagrams as needed.

The quality of data was ensured through proper training of data collector and pre-test of the questionnaire and close supervision of data collectors. All collected data was checked for completeness, accuracy and consistency by the principal investigator and communicated to the data collectors on the next day.

### Ethical consideration

Formal letter was written from Jimma University Nursing department office to Jimma preparatory school by explaining objectives of the study and its significance, relevant permission will be asked to obtain desirable cooperation and necessary information during data collection.

At individual level the purpose of the study was discussed with all participants prior to their participation in this study. Furthermore, investigate or was informed that their participation in the study is voluntary and that they are not obliged to answer any question with which they are uncomfortable and are also free to withdraw their participation from the study at any time they want. Participants were assured that confidentiality was maintained.

## Results

Among the total of 352 participants, 186 were males and majority 253 were between 15-17 years with mean age of 17 years. About three fifth were attending 12th grade during the study period. Nearly all respondents 341 were unmarried majority of the respondents 149 were orthodox followed by protestant 105 (Table 1).

| Variables | Characteristics | Frequency | Percentage |
|---|---|---|---|
| Sex | Male | 195 | 55.4 |
| | Female | 157 | 44.6 |
| Age | 15-17 years | 253 | 71.8 |
| | ≥18 years | 99 | 28.2 |
| Grade level | 11th | 166 | 47.1 |
| | 12th | 186 | 52.9 |
| Religion | Orthodox | 149 | 42.3 |
| | Protestant | 105 | 29.8 |
| | Muslim | 78 | 22.1 |
| | Catholic | 13 | 3.7 |
| | Others | 18 | 5.1 |
| Ethnicity | Oromo | 197 | 55.9 |
| | Amhara | 81 | 23 |
| | Tigre | 31 | 8.8 |
| | Others | 43 | 12.2 |
| Marital status | Unmarried | 341 | 96.8 |
| | Married | 11 | 3.2 |
| Place Of residence | Urban | 277 | 78.9 |
| | Rural | 75 | 21.1 |
| Source of Income | Family | 323 | 92.7 |
| | Relatives | 3 | – |
| | Friends | 7 | – |
| | Husband/wife | 11 | 3.1 |
| | Others | 8 | – |
| Attending religion | Always | 150 | 42.6 |
| | Often | 76 | 21.6 |
| | Sometimes | 53 | 15 |
| | Never | 73 | 21 |

**Table 1:** Socio-demographic charactestics of the study population, Jimma preparatory school, Jimma town, Oromia region, 2014.

Oromo is the predominant ethnic group of the study population and 274 were living with both parents during the study period.

| Variables | Characteristics | Frequency | Percentage |
|---|---|---|---|
| Mother alive | Yes | 335 | 95.17 |
| | No | 17 | 4.83 |
| Mother education level | Literate | 319 | 90.6 |
| | Illiterate | 33 | 9.4 |
| Occupation of mother | House wife | 86 | 24.4 |
| | Merchant | 109 | 30.9 |
| | Employer | 127 | 36 |
| | Others | 30 | 8.5 |
| Father alive | Yes | 331 | 94.3 |
| | No | 41 | 5.7 |
| Father education level | Literate | 329 | 93.4 |
| | Illiterate | 23 | 6.6 |
| Occupation of father | Daily laborer | 28 | 7.9 |
| | Merchant | 79 | 22.4 |
| | Employer | 173 | 49.14 |
| | Farmer | 49 | 13.9 |

**Table 2:** Description of parents of the study population by life, level of education, occupation, Jimma preparatory school, Jimma town, Oromia region 2014.

| | | | |
|---|---|---|---|
| | At least twice a week | 13 | 3.6 |
| | Less than twice a week | 27 | 7.6 |
| | Never | 312 | 88.6 |
| Types of drug (n=164) | Chat | 75 | 45.7 |
| | Cigarette | 49 | 29.8 |
| | Hashish | 0 | 0 |
| | Alcohol | 40 | 24.39 |
| | Other | 0 | 0 |
| Frequency of using this drugs | Every day | 0 | 0 |
| | At least twice a week | 47 | 13.3 |
| | Less than twice a week | 64 | 18.18 |
| | Never | 241 | 68.6 |

**Table 3:** Description of study population about alcohol drinking, types of drug use, and frequency of using drugs, Jimma preparatory school, Jimma town, Oromia , 2014.

Among the total 352 participants 335 respond as their mother is alive and most the respondents' mothers are literate (90.6%) and being employer and merchant are the leading occupation of mothers. The same is true for the father 311 (94%) are alive and most of them are literate and employer in their occupation (Table 2).

Most (88.6%) of the respondents were free from alcoholic drink and 75 of the participants were using Khat 49 were cigarette smoker (Table 3,4).

## Sexual history of adolescents

89 (25.4%) adolescents reported having had premarital sexual intercourse at the time of survey of which 63 (70.78%) were males. Among those adolescents who had premarital sexual intercourse, the majority 79% had their first sexual intercourse between 18 -19 years. The main reasons for initiation of sexual intercourse is due to physical pleasure (fell in love) 47%, followed by for financial reward 25.8%. When respondents were asked about the reason not having had sexual intercourse they responded fear of parents 52.47% followed by fear of pregnancy 31%.

| Watch film | Often | 122 | | 34.65 |
|---|---|---|---|---|
| | Sometimes | 165 | | 46.9 |
| | Never | 65 | | 18.46 |
| Have sexual intercourse | Yes (n = 89) | Sex | males | 63 | 70.78 |
| | | | females | 26 | 29.3 |
| | | Grade | 11th | 32 | 36 |
| | | | 12th | 57 | 64 |
| | No | 263 | | 74.71 |
| Age at first sex (n = 89) | <18 | 18 | | 20.2 |
| | >18 | 61 | | 79.81 |
| Reason to start sex (n = 89) | Physical pleasure | 42 | | 47.19 |
| | For financial reward | 23 | | 25.84 |
| | Peer pressure | 11 | | 12.45 |
| | Rape | 5 | | - |
| | Drug influence | 8 | | - |
| Reason not to start sex (n = 263) | Fear of parents | 138 | | 52.47 |
| | Fear of pregnancy | 82 | | 31.17 |
| | Fear of stis HIV/ AIDS | 72 | | 27.37 |
| | Religious | 60 | | 22.8 |
| Discus with father | Often | 139 | | 39.5 |
| | Sometimes | 167 | | 47.4 |
| | Never | 36 | | 10.2 |

| | Often | 85 | | 24 |
|---|---|---|---|---|
| Discus with mother | Sometimes | 136 | | 38.36 |
| | Never | 130 | | 36.9 |
| | Often | 110 | | 31.25 |
| Discus with close friends | Sometimes | 210 | | 59.6 |
| | Never | 32 | | 9.2 |

**Table 4:** Distribution of sexual history of respondents in Jimma preparatory school, Jimma town, Jimma zone, Oromia region, 2014.

| Variables | | Premarital sex | | Total | $x^2$ | p- value |
|---|---|---|---|---|---|---|
| | | yes | no | | | |
| Sex | Male | 63 (32.3%) | 132 (63.7%) | 195 | 11.4 | 0.001 |
| | Female | 26 (19%) | 131 (81%) | 137 | | |
| Age | <18 | 18 (13.3%) | 127 (86.7%) | 135 | 12.2 | 0 |
| | >18 | 61 (38.6%) | 158 (61.4%) | 219 | | |
| Grade | 11th | 32 (23.9%) | 134 (75.1%) | 166 | | |
| | 12th | 57 (44.2%) | 129 (55.8%) | 186 | | |
| Residence | Urban | 54 (22.2%) | 223 (77.8%) | 277 | | |
| | Rural | 35 (46.6%) | 40 (53.4%) | 75 | | |
| Attending religion | Regularly | | 199 (88%) | 226 | | |
| | Not regularly | 62 (49.2%) | 64 (50.8%) | 126 | | |
| Alcohol drink | Yes | 25 (62.5%) | 15 (37.5%) | 40 | | |
| | No | 64 (25.8%) | 248 (74.2%) | 312 | | |
| Watch film | Yes | 68 (23.7%) | 219 (76.3%) | 287 | | |
| | No | 21 (32.3%) | 44 (67.7%) | 65 | | |
| Peer influence | Yes | 77 (24.1%) | 243 (85.8%) | 320 | | |
| | No | 7 (19%) | 25 (78.12%) | 32 | | |
| Mother's literacy | Literate | 38(12%) | 281 (88%) | 319 | | |

| | | | | | | |
|---|---|---|---|---|---|---|
| | Illiterate | 13(39.4%) | 20 (70.6%) | 33 | | |
| Father's literacy | Literate | 36(11%) | 293 (54%) | 329 | 25.5 | |
| | Illiterate | 11(47.8%) | 12 (52.2%) | 23 | | |

**Table 5:** Variables evaluated for possible association with premarital sexual inter course among adolescents of Jimma preparatory school, Jimma Zone, Oromia, 2014.

As can it can be seen from Table 5 the chi-square test indicates the relationship between respondent's socio cultural and demographic variables with the dependant variables.

**Respondent's sex:** The data shows that sex has an association with premarital sexual intercourse of the respondents, so that 26 (19%) of females and 63 (32.3%) of were males. The proportion of respondent who ever had sexual intercourse vary with sex, at ($x^2 = 11.4$, p = 0.001). This might be the exposure of males to different alcoholic and other sexual enhancing conditions than females.

**Respondent's sex:** As it can be seen clearly from the Table 6 age has a relationship with premarital sexual intercourse of the respondents so that 18(13.3%) students are below 18 years of age. The proportion respondents who ever had sex increase with age, about 38.6% of students are in the age group 18-19 years at ($x^2 = 12.2$, p = 0.000). The result of this study indicates that premarital sexual practice increase with age.

**Educational level:** As a survey revealed that, educational level of respondents associated with premarital sexual practice of school students with ($x^2 = 6.000$, p = 0.000). The proportion school adolescents ever had sex increase as their educational level increase from 11th to 12th, 32 (23.9) and 55 (44.2%) respectively. The data clearly shows that educational attainment is associated with elevated likely hood of being exposed to sexual relation.

**Residence:** The data clearly shows that, pace of residence is associated with premarital sexual intercourse of school adolescents with ($x^2 = 23.1$, p = 0.000). This revealed that school adolescents who were from rural 35 (46.6%) were sexually active than those from urban 54 (22.2%). This may be due to poor family control low religious activity.

**Religiosity:** Respondents attending their religion activities are very statistically associated with premarital sexual practice of school students with at ($x^2 = 59.4$, p = 0.000). This revealed school adolescents premarital sexual practice increase among those who do not attend their religious activity regularly 62 (49.2) than who followed their religion contniously 27 (12%). Thus, adolescent people who attend religion activities frequently are expected to inter into sexual intercourse than those who do not attend regularly.

**Alcohol drinking:** The Table 6 above indicates that school adolescents who ever had had taken alcohol were more likely involved into sexual activity than their counterparty who had not taken alcoholic substance at ($x^2 = 21.36$, p = 0.244). This revealed that Alcohol drinking was associated with adolescents' involvement in sexual activity.

**Seeing pornographic film:** It is clearly shown in the above table 6 that the exposure of school adolescents to sex film is significantly associated with adolescents' involvement in sexual activity at ($x^2 = 2.08$, p = 0.149). They are more sensitive to peer pressure and adolescent sexually exploited areas.

**Peer influence:** Talking on sexual related issue with close peer is associated with adolescents involvement in sexual activity premarital at ($x^2 = 2.78$, p = 0.095). Adolescents who talk with their peers about sex related issue 77 (24.1%) were more likely involved premarital sexual activity than those who do not talk 7 (19%). Peer influence on sexual initiation reflects the idea that adolescents decisions about whether or not initiate sexual activity are strongly bound to social context.

**Parents' education:** As the Table 6 above displays the parents' education is associated with sexual involvement of school adolescents. The proportion of school adolescents those from un educated mother 13 (39.42%) were more involved premarital sexual activity as compared to respondents mother who were educated 38 (12%) at ($x^2 = 18.2$, p = 0.000) and so father' education status at ($x^2 = 25.5$, p = 0.000). Thus the proportion school adolescents premarital sexual activity decrease as educational level of parents is increased. This may be due to educated parents give more attention to their children discouraging sexual activity.

## Discussion

The overall prevalence of premarital sexual practice in the study population was 28.2%.The proportion of male adolescents who were involved in premarital sex 63 (17.89%) was about twice the proportion female adolescents 26 (7.38%). This finding is relatively low compared to other prior study study findings in the country. In Addis Ababa proportion was 39.8% for males and 5.6% for females [15].

The study conducted in Nekemte showed that among those adolescents who had premarital sex, the majority (57.2%) had their first sexual intercourse between the ages of 15 and 17 years [16]. Early and premarital sexual practice is becoming common and one of the risky sexual behaviors of adolescents and young people. The current study showed that among those preparatory school adolescents who had premarital sex, 18 (20.2%) and 61 (79.8%) reported having had first sex before 18 years [15-17] and at age of 18 and above respectively.

Although adolescents sexuality is often affected by hormonal influences, the role of psychological factors is not insignificant .The desire to maintain relationship with friends peer pressure , lack of guidance poor modeling of elders ,living with single parents or nether and poor religious activity are important in term of influencing adolescents sexuality [17-19]. In this study , the main reason claimed by adolescents for starting the first sexual intercourse were falling in love or physical pleasure 42 (47.19%), for material gift or financial reward 23 (25.84%). In addition watching pornographic films and alcohol drinking are major contributing factors to premarital sexual practice in the study area.

In this study being male, twelfth grade student and age 18 and above were found to be positively and significantly associated with premarital sex in the study area. Similar studies showed that a much higher percentage of young men reported having had premarital sex than young women [20].

This may be due to cultural norms that encourage and approve sexual experimentation of boys and the value given to virginity for girls. Ageless than18 and regular attending religious activity were found to be protective against premarital sex.

Various studies have shown that younger girls enter into sexual relationship with older wealthy men who can assist them school related expenses, or purchase of material goods [21].The current study showed that 23 (25.84%) of adolescents were involved in sex for material gift or financial support.

## Conclusion

Premarital sexual practice of adolescents and associated factors has been examined.

- The study found that about 25.4% of school adolescents practiced premarital sexual practice.
- A love affair was the most prominent factor that precipitated the first sexual intercourse.
- Parents education, parent-adolescents discussion about sex and peer influence were found to be significantly associated with adolescents sexuality. Discussion on sex related issue between adolescents the main objective of the study was to asses' premarital sexual practice among preparatory school adolescents and to identify the major socio-cultural, demographic and parental educational status influencing premarital sexual practice in Jimma preparatory school, Jimma town Jimma zone. Accordingly and parents help the adolescents to develop a clear personal position regarding their sexuality.
- Adolescents in the age group of 18-19 years were more likely to have sexual intercourse as compared to those age group 15-17 years.
- Use of alcohol is possibly associated with adolescents' premarital sex.

## Recommendations

Based on the finding this study, an integrated effort need to be initiated to address adolescents' sexual and reproductive health problems through Establishing and strengthening school anti AIDS clubs, youth reproductive unit/ club in different facilities and empowering women, Discouraging the use of substances /drug among adolescents and sensitizing parents, community members and the public focusing on parent child communication and discussion about sex related issue.

## Acknowledgments

Authors would like to acknowledge Jimma University Department of nursing and Midwifery for the support it rendered for conducting this study.

## Authors contributions

AT and IA designed the study, analyzed the data drafted the manuscript and critically reviewed the article. All authors read and approved the final manuscript and do not have conflict of interest.

## References

1. UNDO/UNFP/WHO (2003) Special Program of Research Development and Research Training in Human Reproductive Health (HRP): Progress in Reproductive Health Research.

2. (2000) Strengthening the Provision of Adolescent-Friendly Health Service to meet the health and development Needs of adolescent in Africa: A consensus. Harare, Zimbabwe.

3. UNFPA (2005) HIV/AIDS and Adolescent: State of World Population

4. UNFAP (2006) The State of World Population. Geneva.

5. Rweng M (2000) Sexual risky behavior among Young People in Bamenda, Cameroon: International Family Planning Perspectives 26: 118-121.

6. National HIV/AIDS Prevention and Control Office (2000) AIDS in Ethiopia: Federal Ministry of Health, Addis Ababa, Ethiopia.

7. Kelly H (2004) Socio economic Disadvantage and Unsafe Sexula Behavior among Young Women in South Africa: Policy Research Division counsel.

8. WHO (2004) Risk and Protective Factors Affecting Adolescent's Reproductive Health in Developing countries: Analysis of Adolescent Sexual and Reproductive Health Literature around the World. Geneva.

9. Chala F (2009) Creating a Better Future for Ethiopian Youth: A conference on Adolescents Reproductive health. The David and Lucile Packard Foundation, Ethiopia.

10. UNAIDS (2008) Preventing HIV/AIDS in Young People: A Systemic Review of the Evidence Global HIV/AIDS Epidemic.

11. Department of Family Health (2001) Five Year Action Plan document for adolescent Reproductive Health in Ethiopia: Federal Ministry of Health, Addis Ababa.

12. Sederowitz J (1999) Making Reproductive Health Service Youth Friendly: Research Program and Policy series.

13. Bongaarts J, Cohen B (1998) Adolescent reproductive behavior in the developing world. Introduction and review. Stud Fam Plann 29: 99-105.

14. Gorge R, Yansane ML, Marks M, MIllomounou D (1998) Sexual behavior and attitude among unmarried urban youths in Guinea. International Family Planning Perspectives 24: 65-71

15. Temin Miriam FE, Okonofau FO, Morodion O, Renne EP, Coplan P, et al. (1997) Perception of sexual behavior and knowledge about STDs among Adolescent in Bennei City, Nigeri: Family Planning Perspectives 54: 186-187.

16. Teshager S (2005) Determinants of Risky Sexual Behavior in Bahir Dar among adolescents: Unpublished Msc thesis, Addis Ababa University.

17. Adeye (2012) Prevalence of Premarital sex and factor influencing it among in private atetterritory institution in Nigeria, International Journal of Psychology And Counciling 4: 6-9.

18. Karim AM, Magnani RJ, Morgan GT, Bond KC (2003) Reproductive health risk and protective factors among unmarried youth in Ghana. Int Fam Plan Perspect 29: 14-24.

19. Bonnel C, Allen E, Stran (2005) Influence of Family type and Printing behavior on teenage sexual behaviors and conceptions: Journal of Epidemiology Community Health pp: 502-506.

20. Seme A, Wirtu D (2008) Prevalence of Premarital sexual practice among school adolescents of Nekemte Town: Ethiop J Health Dev 22: 167-173.

21. Upchurch D, Anshensel C, Sucoff C, Storems L (1999) Neighborhood and Family Context of Adolescent sexual activity: Journal of Marriage and Family 21: 151-172.

# 16

# Leader-Member Exchange (LMX) and Psychosocial Factors at Work among Healthcare Professionals

Jan Johansson Hanse[1,2*], Ulrika Harlin[3], Caroline Jarebrant[3,4], Kerstin Ulin[5,6] and Jörgen Winkel[7,8]

[1]Professor, Nordic School of Public Health NHV, Sweden

[2]Professor, Department of Psychology, University of Gothenburg, Sweden

[3]Industrial researcher, Swerea IVF, Mölndal, Sweden

[4]PhD student, Department of Sociology and Work Science, University of Gothenburg, Sweden

[5]Senior lecturer, PhD, Institute of Health and Care Science, Sahlgrenska Academy, University of Gothenburg, Sweden

[6]Senior lecturer/nurse, Sahlgrenska University Hospital, Gothenburg, Sweden

[7]Senior professor, Department of Management Engineering, Technical University of Denmark, Denmark

[8]Senior professor, Department of Sociology and Work Science, University of Gothenburg, Sweden

*Corresponding author: Professor Jan Johansson Hanse, Nordic School of Public Health, Box 12133, SE-40242 Gothenburg, Sweden, E-mail: jan.johansson.hanse@nhv.se

### Abstract

Aim: The study aims to examine the associations between leader–member exchange (LMX) and psychosocial factors at work.

Methods: A questionnaire-based cross-sectional study was undertaken at four units in two not-for-profit hospitals in southwestern Sweden. The study sample included 240 employees.

Results: Significant correlations were found between LMX items and most of the psychosocial domains and dimensions. The strongest correlations were found between the LMX item affect and rewards/recognition, role clarity and predictability, and the LMX item loyalty and rewards/recognition. In sum, high-quality LMX was associated with good psychosocial work conditions experienced by the employees.

Conclusions: The results support possible ways for managers and employees to strengthen their relationships and this may in turn lead to more sustainable systems in health care.

**Keywords :** COPSOQ; Leadership; LMX; Psychosocial

## Introduction

European Agency for Safety and Health at Work [1] has emphasized managerial significance and role in improving the psychosocial work environment among workers. In this study, leadership is based on leader–member exchange quality (LMX). Leader–member exchange quality (LMX) is about the quality of the dyadic, work relationship between an employee and her/his leader (supervisor) in terms of the interrelated dimensions of trust, respect and mutual obligation [2]. LMX theory argues that when the supervisor provides resources in a way that is perceived to be beneficial and fair, the employee will view the relationship positively and reciprocate via increased commitment and effort-resulting in a high quality relationship. It suggests that leaders relationships with subordinates can range from those based solely on the formal employment contract (low quality LMX) to those that are characterized by mutual trust, respect and reciprocal influence (high quality LMX) [3]. Previous studies indicate that LMX relationships establish rather quickly and stabilize [4]. Past research has demonstrated that LMX is correlated to a number of important outcomes for employees. The quality of LMX has been found to be associated with job satisfaction, positive work attitudes, wellbeing, organizational commitment and performance [5-8]. Previous studies also have shown that adverse psychosocial workplace factors can increase the risk of ill-health (e.g. musculoskeletal disorders, stress-related disorders, burnout, sickness absence, labor turnover) among workers in general [9,10] and among healthcare workers [11]. Healthcare workers report high levels of workplace stress and are at a higher risk of mental health problems than many other occupational groups [12]. Therefore the present study aims to examine the associations between leader–member exchange (LMX) and psychosocial factors at work among healthcare professionals. The study reports findings from the Swedish part of a Nordic Multicenter Study regarding performance and wellbeing in Lean rationalization processes at hospitals [13].

## Methods

### Procedure and participants

A questionnaire-based cross-sectional study was undertaken at four units in two not-for-profit hospitals in southwestern Sweden. The study was based on questionnaires carried out at the hospital units during working time. The subjects answered the questionnaire anonymously. Oral and written information was given regarding the confidentiality of the survey process, noting that all results would only be reported back to the organization in aggregate for the unit as a whole. The study sample included 240 employees.

## Measures

### Demographic and employee-related variables

This part consisted of items concerning sex, age (6-point response scale; younger than 20 years, 20-29 years, 30-39 years, 40-49 years, 50-59 years, 60 years or older), years of employment at the hospital unit (4-point response scale; less than 3 months, 3-12 months, 1-3 years, more than 3 years) and job title/profession (5-point response scale; registered nurse, enrolled nurse, secretary, physician, another position).

## Leader-member exchange (LMX)

The quality of the supervisor-employee ('follower') relationship was measured according to the Leader – member exchange (LMX) theory [14]. In the current study, employee-rated LMX was measured using four items from Liden and Maslyn´s LMX-scale [15]: affect, loyalty, contribution and professional respect. These four items represent four sub-dimensions to measure the employees´ perception of the quality of relationship with their supervisors. In the current study we used a short version of the employee-rated LMX [15] with one item for each dimension:

- • 'Affect': My supervisor is a lot of fun to work with.
- • 'Loyalty': My supervisor would defend me to others in the organization if I made an honest mistake.
- • 'Contribution': I am willing to apply extra efforts, beyond those normally required, to meet my supervisor's work goals.
- • 'Professional respect': I respect my supervisor's knowledge of and competence on the job.

Each item was rated using a seven-point Likert-type scale where higher scores represent higher quality exchanges, i.e. high-quality LMX (1 = strongly disagree to 7 = strongly agree). In the current study, Cronbach alpha reliability for the LMX global scale was .87.

## Psychosocial factors at work

The psychosocial work environment was measured with scales from the Copenhagen psychosocial questionnaire (COPSOQ) [16]. The COPSOQ has been used in more than 10 years as a tool for assessing the psychosocial work environment [9] and is a suitable instrument to measure the psychosocial work environment among hospital workers [11]. Reliabilities estimates with Cronbach's alpha, Green's test-retest alpha and intraclass coefficient (ICC) are according standard guidelines adequate to good [17].

The following domains and dimensions (scales) were used [16], where high scores represent good psychosocial work conditions:

Domain: 'Demands at work', with the following dimensions:

- 'Quantitative demands' (4 items, each item had five fixed response alternatives): Is your workload unevenly distributed so it piles up? How often do you not have time to complete all your work tasks? Do you get behind with your work? Do you have enough time for your work tasks?

- 'Tempo/Work pace' (3 items, each item had five fixed response alternatives): Do you have to work very fast? Do you work at a high pace throughout the day? Is it necessary to keep working at a high pace?

Domain: 'Work organization and job contents', with the following dimension:

- 'Influence at work' (4 items, each item had five fixed response alternatives): Do you have a large degree of influence concerning your work? Do you have a say in choosing who you work with? Can you influence the amount of work assigned to you? Do you have any influence on what you do at work?

Domain: 'Interpersonal relations', with the following dimensions:

- 'Predictability' (2 items, each item had five fixed response alternatives): At your place of work, are you informed well in advance concerning for example important decisions, changes, or plans for the future? Do you receive all the information you need in order to do your work well?
- 'Rewards/Recognition' (2 items from the short version, each item had five fixed response alternatives): Is your work recognized and appreciated by the management? Are you treated fairly at your workplace?
- 'Role clarity' (3 items, each item had five fixed response alternatives): Does your work have clear objectives? Do you know exactly which areas is your responsibility? Do you know exactly what is expected of you at work?

Domain: 'Values at workplace level', with the following dimensions:

- 'Trust regarding management' ('vertical trust') (2 items, each item had five fixed response alternatives): Does the management trust the employees to do their work well? Can you trust the information that comes from the management?
- 'Justice and Respect' (2 items, each item had five fixed response alternatives): Are conflicts resolved in a fair way? Is the work distributed fairly?
- The COPSOQ item 'Job satisfaction' was also included in the current study: Regarding your work in general. How pleased are you with your job as a whole, everything taken into consideration? (four fixed response alternatives).

## Data analyses

Descriptive statistics and reliabilities (Cronbach's alpha) were calculated. The data were analyzed using Pearson correlation and hierarchical linear regression analysis to assess the association between LMX items and psychosocial factors at work. In the hierarchical linear regression analysis the variables were entered in two (or more) steps in the following order: demographic variables (method enter), LMX variables (method stepwise).

The level of significance was set at $p<.05$. The size of the effect was determined according to conventions by Cohen [18]. Cohen defined effect sizes for correlations of around 0.10 as 'small', around 0.30 as 'medium' and around 0.50 as 'large'. In multiple regression analysis (R-square) the effect classes are around 0.02 for 'small', around 0.13 for 'medium' and around 0.26 for 'large'.

SPSS version 21.0 for Windows was utilized to perform the statistical analyses.

## Results

### Demographic and employee-related variables among healthcare professionals

The sample (n=240) consisted of 59 per cent registered nurses, 24 per cent enrolled nurses, 10 percent secretaries and 6 per cent physicians. Of the respondents, 82 per cent were females and 18 per cent were males. Twenty-three per cent were younger than 30 years, 62 per cent were between 30-49 years and 15 per cent were 50 years or older. As regards the period of employment at the hospital unit, 23 per cent had less than one year employment, 17 per cent between one and three years and 60 per cent had more than three years of employment.

### Bivariate associations between LMX and psychosocial factors at work

Significant correlations were found between LMX items and most of the psychosocial domains and dimensions. High-quality LMX was associated with good psychosocial work conditions experienced by the employees.

The strongest correlations were found between LMX and the domains interpersonal relations (r between 0.31-0.51, p<0.001) and values at workplace level (r between 0.31 - 0.42, p<0.001). At dimension level, the strongest correlations were found between the LMX item affect and rewards/recognition (r=0.51, p<0.001), role clarity (r=0.47, p<0.001) and predictability (r=0.47, p<0.001) respectively, and the LMX item loyalty and rewards/recognition (r=0.48, p<0.001).

Somewhat lower correlations were found between LMX and the domains work organization and job contents (r between 0.19 - 0.23, p<0.01) and demands at work (r between 0.03 - 0.29). Within the domain demands at work there were no significant correlations between LMX items and the dimension tempo/work pace (r between 0.03 - 0.08, ns).

The findings also reveal that the quality of the LMX has significant relationships with job satisfaction (r between 0.29 - 0.45, p<0.001). The strongest correlations was found between the LMX item affect and job satisfaction (r=0.45, p<0.001). The higher quality of LMX, the higher job satisfaction was experienced by the staffs.

### Multiple associations between LMX and psychosocial factors at work

Next, we examined the relationship between LMX items and psychosocial domains, after controlling for demographic variables in step 1 (Tables 1-5).

As shown in Table 1 in the hierarchical regression analyses, we found that one (professional respect) of the four LMX items in the models was significantly associated with demands at work ($\beta$=0.19, p<0.01). The LMX items affect, loyalty and contribution were not significantly associated with this psychosocial domain, when entered with other variables (demographics and LMX).

| Variable | Model 1 | | | Model 2 or 3 (last model) | | |
|---|---|---|---|---|---|---|
| | B | SE(B) | $\beta$ | B | SE(B) | $\beta$ |
| Age | 0.04 | 0.04 | 0.08 | 0.04 | 0.59 | 0.08 |
| Sex | 0.11 | 0.09 | 0.09 | 0.09 | 0.28 | 0.08 |
| Years of employment | -0.01 | 0.04 | -0.02 | 0.00 | 0.07 | 0.13 |
| Professional respect [a] | | | | 0.07 | 0.02 | 0.19** |
| Adjusted R[2] | 0.01 | | | 0.03 | | |
| F for change in R[2] | 0.67 | | | 7.20** | | |

**Table 1:** Hierarchical multiple regression analysis for LMX items (independent variables) on Demands at work (dependent variable). Demographic variables were entered in step 1 (n=240).

Note:    *p<0.05; **p<0.01; ***p<0.001

a = Model 2

b = Model 3

Examination of the data in Table 2 show that one (contribution) of the four LMX items in the models was significantly associated with the domain work organization and job contents ($\beta$=0.22, p<0.01). The LMX items affect, loyalty and professional respect were not significantly associated with this psychosocial domain, when entered with other variables (demographics and LMX).

| Variable | Model 1 | | | Model 2 or 3 (last model) | | |
|---|---|---|---|---|---|---|
| | B | SE(B) | $\beta$ | B | SE(B) | $\beta$ |
| Age | 0.04 | 0.05 | 0.07 | 0.05 | 0.05 | 0.08 |
| Sex | -0.14 | 0.12 | -0.09 | -0.14 | 0.11 | -0.09 |
| Years of employment | -0.04 | 0.05 | -0.06 | -0.06 | 0.05 | -0.10 |
| Contribution [a] | | | | 0.10 | 0.03 | 0.22** |
| Adjusted R[2] | 0.00 | | | 0.04 | | |
| F for change in R[2] | 1.07 | | | 9.53** | | |

**Table 2:** Hierarchical multiple regression analysis for LMX items (independent variables) on Work organization and job contents (dependent variable). Demographic variables were entered in step 1 (n=240).

Note: *p<0.05; **p<0.01; ***p<0.001

a = Model 2

b = Model 3

Table 3 shows that that two (affect & professional respect) of the four LMX items in the models was significantly associated with the domain interpersonal relations ($\beta$=0.40, p<0.001 & $\beta$=0.28, p<0.001). The LMX items loyalty and contribution were not significantly associated with this psychosocial domain, when entered with other variables (demographics and LMX).

| Variable | Model 1 | | | Model 2 or 3 (last model) | | |
|---|---|---|---|---|---|---|
| | B | SE(B) | $\beta$ | B | SE(B) | $\beta$ |
| Age | -0.04 | 0.04 | -0.07 | -0.05 | 0.03 | -0.11 |
| Sex | -0.15 | 0.10 | -0.11 | -0.15 | 0.08 | -0.11 |

| Variable | B | SE(B) | β | B | SE(B) | β |
|---|---|---|---|---|---|---|
| Years of employment | -0.01 | 0.04 | -0.01 | -0.02 | 0.03 | -0.04 |
| Affect [b] | | | | 0.15 | 0.03 | 0.40*** |
| Professional respect [b] | | | | 0.11 | 0.03 | 0.28*** |
| Adjusted $R^2$ | 0.00 | | | 0.36a / 0.40b | | |
| F for change in $R^2$ | 0.95 | | | 115.22a*** / 13.76b*** | | |

Table 3: Hierarchical multiple regression analysis for LMX items (independent variables) on Interpersonal relations (dependent variable). Demographic variables were entered in step 1 (n=240).

Note: *p<0.05; **p<0.01; ***p<0.001

a = Model 2

b = Model 3

As can be seen in Table 4 two (loyalty & professional respect) of the four LMX items in the models was significantly associated with values at workplace level (β=0.30, p<0.001 & β=0.21, p<0.01). The LMX items affect and contribution were not significantly associated with this psychosocial domain, when entered with other variables (demographics and LMX).

| | Model 1 | | | Model 2 or 3 (last model) | | |
|---|---|---|---|---|---|---|
| Variable | B | SE(B) | β | B | SE(B) | β |
| Age | -0.04 | 0.05 | -0.06 | -0.05 | 0.04 | -0.08 |
| Sex | 0.01 | 0.11 | 0.00 | 0.02 | 0.10 | 0.01 |
| Years of employment | 0.00 | 0.05 | 0.00 | -0.02 | 0.04 | -0.03 |
| Loyalty [b] | | | | 0.13 | 0.03 | 0.30*** |
| Professional respect [b] | | | | 0.09 | 0.04 | 0.21* |
| Adjusted $R^2$ | 0.00 | | | 0.17a / 0.20b | | |
| F for change in $R^2$ | 0.23 | | | 46.12a*** / 6.24b* | | |

Table 4: Hierarchical multiple regression analysis for LMX items (independent variables) on Values at workplace level (dependent variable). Demographic variables were entered in step 1 (n=240).

Note: *p<0.05; **p<0.01; ***p<0.001

a = Model 2

b = Model 3

Examination of the data in Table 5 demonstrate that one (affect) of the four LMX items in the models was significantly associated with job satisfaction (β=0.43, p<0.001). The LMX items contribution, loyalty and professional respect were not significantly associated with this psychosocial domain, when entered with other variables (demographics and LMX).

| | Model 1 | | | Model 2 or 3 (last model) | | |
|---|---|---|---|---|---|---|
| Variable | B | SE(B) | β | B | SE(B) | β |
| Age | 0.03 | 0.04 | 0.06 | 0.01 | 0.04 | 0.02 |
| Sex | 0.04 | 0.10 | 0.03 | 0.03 | 0.09 | 0.02 |
| Years of employment | -0.02 | 0.04 | -0.04 | -0.02 | 0.04 | -0.05 |
| Affect [a] | | | | 0.16 | 0.02 | 0.43*** |
| Adjusted $R^2$ | 0.00 | | | 0.17 | | |
| F for change in $R^2$ | 0.20 | | | 45.18*** | | |

Table 5: Hierarchical multiple regression analysis for LMX items (independent variables) on Job satisfaction (dependent variable). Demographic variables were entered in step 1 (n=240).

Note: *p<0.05; **p<0.01; ***p<0.001

a = Model 2

b = Model 3

## Discussion

LMX is multi-dimensional measure [15]. This measure assesses a global score for the exchange as well as for the four sub-dimensions of affect, loyalty, contribution and professional respect. Affect measures the employees liking for the supervisor, loyalty measures the degree of loyalty the respondent feels from the supervisor, contribution measures the amount of the respondents own effort exhibited in achieving work goals, and professional respect measures the respondents professional esteem for the supervisor. The most striking result to emerge from the data is that at least one (sometimes several) LMX-item(s) was significantly associated with almost all psychosocial factors at work. The only non-significant association was found between LMX-items and the dimension tempo/work pace.

In previous studies LMX has been found to be significantly associated with psychosocial factors at work (e.g. job satisfaction, work attitudes, wellbeing, organizational commitment) [5-8]. The results from the current study are consistent with those of other studies and suggest that LMX and psychosocial factors are related also among healthcare professionals. The strongest correlations were found between LMX and the domains interpersonal relations (r between 0.31 - 0.51, p<0.001) and values at workplace level (r between 0.31 - 0.42, p<0.001). These effect sizes are 'medium' to 'large' according to Cohen [18]. LMX focuses on the unique relationships that may develop between supervisors and individual employees within an organization. Each sub-dimension of LMX emphasizes a unique aspect of leader-employee (follower) relationship. Each aspect has the potential to help increase our understanding of which aspects that are significantly associated with various psychosocial factors at work. It seem reasonable to conclude that a good relationship with the supervisor (high LMX) relates to the meaningfulness of work, as staffs could get more interesting work and more understanding of their role within the hospital organization. By improving psychosocial factors at work, it is possible to promote employee health as well as to prevent employee ill-heath [19].

Another important finding was that the higher quality of LMX, the higher job satisfaction was experienced by the staffs. The effect sizes of these associations are 'medium' to 'large' according to Cohen [18]. The strongest association was found between the LMX-item affect and job satisfaction. The LMX-item affect measures the employees liking for the supervisor. This association was expected as job satisfaction is an affective response (the emotional response to a situation) based upon the degree to which a job fulfills various factors, both intrinsic and extrinsic, that are valued by the individual employee. In previous studies job satisfaction has been found to be is an important factor influencing the health of workers [20]. Achieving a high level of job satisfaction among healthcare professionals is an important objective since it may positively impact organizational efficacy, make the staff motivated and feel that they are a part of the organization [1,21].

## Limitations and Future Research

Although our study contributes to social exchange relationships and its associations with psychosocial factors at work among healthcare professionals, several limitations must be recognized. The data were cross-sectional. The cross-sectional nature of the data calls into question any inferences one makes concerning the directionality of relationships, which implies the relationships observed cannot be interpreted causally. Therefore, we recommend longitudinal research. Another potential limitation of the study is same-source data—increasing concern for common method variance problem. However, by using multiple measures (questions) of each domain/dimension tends to reduce the effect of measurement error [22]. Moreover, this study is limited in its applicability to other employment settings. The findings may not be consistent with studies conducted within industries. It is recommended that research in the future employs diverse sample so that the generalizability of findings to other settings can be enhanced.

In the current study, as well as in previous studies LMX have mostly been measured by taking only the employee (follower) perspective. This may be a weakness, but previous studies shows that LMX agreement (i.e. the extent to which leader and employee ratings of LMX are intercorrelated) are rather low [6]. It seems that employee and leader perspectives measure different aspects of the relationship. In the current study, focus was upon employees' perspective as regards social exchange relationships.

## Acknowledgements

Financial support for this research was provided by AFA Insurance and Region Västra Götaland in Sweden. The authors would like to thank the participating health care professionals and our collaborators at the hospital units.

## References

1. European Agency for Safety and Health at Work (2013) Healthy workplaces. Manage stress. campaign guide. Managing stress and psychosocial risks at work.

2. Graen GB, Uhl-Bien M (1995) Relationship-based approach to leadership: Development of leader – member exchange (LMX) theory of leadership over 25 years: Applying a multilevel multi-domain perspective. Lead Quart 6: 219-247.

3. Liden RC, Graen G (1980) Generalizability of the vertical dyad linkage model of leadership. Acad Manag J 23: 451-465.

4. Liden RC, Wayne SJ, Stilwell D (1993) A longitudinal study on the early development of leader-member exchanges. J Appl Psych 78: 662-674.

5. Cropanzano R, Mitchell MS (2005) Social exchange theory: An interdisciplinary review. J Manag 31: 874–900.

6. Gerstner CR, Day DV (1997) Meta-analytic review of leader–member exchange theory: Correlates and construct issues. J Appl Psych 82: 827–844.

7. Randall ML, Cropanzano R, Bormann CA, Birjulin A (1999) Organizational politics and organizational support as predictors of work attitudes, job performance, and organizational citizenship behavior. J Org Behav 20: 159-174.

8. Schyns B, Paul T, Mohr G, Blank H (2005) Comparing antecedents and consequences of LMX in German working context to findings in the US. Europ J Work Org Psych 14: 1-22.

9. Kristensen TS, Hannerz H, Høgh A, Borg V (2005) The Copenhagen Psychosocial Questionnaire--a tool for the assessment and improvement of the psychosocial work environment. Scand J Work Environ Health 31: 438-449.

10. Nieuwenhuijsen K, Bruinvels D, Frings-Dresen M (2010) Psychosocial work environment and stress-related disorders, a systematic review. Occup Med (Lond) 60: 277-286.

11. Aust B, Rugulies R, Skakon J, Scherzer T, Jensen C (2007) Psychosocial work environment of hospital workers: validation of a comprehensive assessment scale. Int J Nurs Stud 44: 814-825.

12. Peterson U, Demerouti E, Bergström G, Samuelsson M, Asberg M, et al. (2008) Burnout and physical and mental health among Swedish healthcare workers. J Adv Nurs 62: 84-95.

13. Winkel J, Birgisdóttir BD, Dudas K, Edwards K, Gunnarsdóttir S, et al. (2012) A Nordic work environment complement to value stream mapping (VSM) for sustainable patient flows at hospitals – A NOVO multicenter study. Proceedings of the 6th NOVO Symposium: Sustainable Health Care: Continuous Improvement of Processes and Systems. Karolinska Institute, Stockholm Sweden. November 15-16, pp 57-58. ISBN: 978-91-637-2380-3.

14. Graen GB, Scandura TA (1987) Toward a psychology of dyadic organization. Res Org Behav 9: 175 – 208.

15. Liden RC, Maslyn JM (1998) Multidimensionality of leader-member exchange: An empirical assessment through scale development. J Manag 24: 43-72.

16. Pejtersen JH, Kristensen TS, Borg V, Bjorner JB (2010) The second version of the Copenhagen Psychosocial Questionnaire. Scand J Public Health 38: 8-24.

17. Thorsen SV, Bjorner JB (2010) Reliability of the Copenhagen psychosocial questionnaire. Scand J Pub Health 38 (Suppl. 3): 25-32.

18. Cohen J (1988) Statistical power analysis for the behavioral sciences. 2nd ed. Hillsdale, NJ: Lawrence Earlbaum Associates.

19. Lohela M, Björklund C, Vingård E, Hagberg J, Jensen I (2009) Does a change in psychosocial work factors lead to a change in employee health? J Occup Environ Med 51: 195-203.

20. Faragher EB, Cass M, Cooper CL (2005) The relationship between job satisfaction and health: a meta-analysis. Occup Environ Med 62: 105-112.

21. Bhatnagar K, Srivastava K (2012) Job satisfaction in health-care organizations. Ind Psychiatry J 21: 75-78.

22. Kline RB (1998) Principles and practice of structural equation modelling. The Guilford Press, New York.

# 17

# Relationships among Health Locus of Control, Psychosocial Status and Glycemic Control in Type 2 Diabetes Adults

**Shu-Ming Chen*** and **Huey-Shyan Lin**

*Professor, Fooyin University, Kaohsiung city, Taiwan*

*Corresponding author: Shu-Ming Chen, Fooyin University, No 151, Chin-Hsueh Rd, Ta-Liao District, Kaohsiung City 83102, ROC, Taiwan, E-mail: ft036@fy.edu.tw

## Abstract

**Background:** Although a common thread among diabetic behavior is the importance of perceived glycemic control, little is known of the factors that lead to psychosocial status in this population.

**Purpose:** We determine whether the psychosocial factors of health locus of control, self-efficacy, self-care behavior, and depression relate to glycemic control in type 2 diabetes.

**Method:** We used a descriptive correlational design. In total, 285 subjects were enrolled from diabetic outpatient clinics in Southern Taiwan. We applied the health locus of control, self-efficacy, self-care behavior and depression questionnaires. Glycemic control was assessed by HbA1c.

**Results:** The internal health locus of control was significantly positively correlated with self-efficacy and self-care behavior, and significantly negatively correlated with depression. Combined depression and self-efficacy partly mediated the relationship between internal locus of control and self-care behavior (P.01), and completely mediated the relationship between external health locus of control and self-care behavior (P.01). Depression and initial HbA1c directly and significantly affected final HbA1c value. Higher depression had the worst HbA1c.

**Conclusion:** Internal health locus of control was partly mediated the relationship between depression and self efficacy. The finding could form a basis for caring people with type 2 diabetes and provide a reference for further research.

**Keywords** Health locus of control; Psychosocial factors; Glycemic control; Type 2 diabetes

## Intoduction

Diabetes is becoming an increasingly important issue due to it rising prevalence, complications, and mortality. Previous diabetes studies have shown that tight control of a patient's glycemic levels reduces serious complications of type 2 diabetes [1]. The glycosylated hemoglobin (HbA1c) level is the indicator of glycemic control, but several problems identified in the literature relate to an understanding of how to motivate people to "control" diabetes self-care behavior. Numerous diabetes self-care studies have explored how challenging it is for diabetic patients to improve or maintain their diabetes [2]. Zulman et al. found that particular psychosocial factors appear to act as important personal barriers or facilitators to diabetes self-care and diabetes status [3]. However, little information is available regarding the relationships among these variances with glycemic control. Weng et al. indicated that health locus of control changes precedes changes in self-care behavior, which consequently lead to changes in glycemic concentrations [4].

The multidimensional health locus of control was developed based on social learning theory and represents an outcome of behavior [5]. The health locus of control construct holds that people view the attainment of a particular outcome as either within their control (internal) or outside of their control (external). Health locus of control is the potential for a behavior to occur in a given situation and the expectation that the behavior will lead to a particular outcome. This construct contends that external health locus of control perceives chance expectations such as fate or luck, and control by powerful others such as family members or physicians. In contrast, in internal health locus control, people believe that attaining a particular outcome is under their control. In perceived internal health locus of control, people take responsibility for their own actions and engage more readily in health-promoting behaviours [5,6]. The literature review presents perceived internal health locus of control to be associated with better adjustment to diabetes, better adherence to self-care regimens, and better glycemic control [4,7] however, certain reviews are pessimistic [8,9]. Exploring interactions between health locus of control and affecting factors, such as self-efficacy and depression.

Self-efficacy is a powerful predictor of diabetes self-care behaviors. Numerous studies have found self-efficacy to be positively related to improved self-care outcomes [7,10,11]. O'Hea et al. determined that psychological factors such as self-efficacy, health beliefs, and emotional distress are significantly associated with diabetes self-care behaviors. Aljasem et al. stated that self-efficacy is a powerful predictor of self-care behavior in controlling diabetes and HbA1c. Self-efficacy is behavior specific and dynamic and focuses on beliefs of personal abilities in a specific setting or to a particular behavior such as a positive effect on behavior change and positively influencing long-term glycemic control [12]. An increase in self-efficacy showed significant improvements in health behavior and health status [13]. However, how self-efficacy and locus of control work together to predict health-related behaviors is particularly important. Previously published results have indicated that the internal health locus of control is positively associated with self-efficacy and learning how to be self-motivated [4,14,15].

Diabetes patients have a two times higher risk for depression than the general population [16]. Diabetes accounts for 13.17% of mild depression levels [17], as do common diabetic complications, which also put patients at high risk for depression. Trief et al. stated that poorer diabetic control is associated with psychological facets of depression [18]. Therefore, although emotional distress is required to motivate diabetes patients to maintain proper self-care behavior, the glycemic control of these patients can decline. According to the literature review, numerous psychological distresses, including emotional distress and depression, affect glycemic control [13,19]. Therefore, health locus of control may be an important factor in psychosocial issues influent to facilitate patients to make behavior changes to change glycemic levels [20].

Little information is available regarding the relationships among the health locus of control, comorbid depression, and self-efficacy of adults with type 2 diabetes. This community-based clinical study provides an approach for determining the predictors of self-care behavior among people with diabetes. Enhanced understanding of the relationships among health locus of control, self-efficacy, and depression in diabetes and help to identify the potential effects of these factors on self-care behaviors and glycemic control. This information should help diabetes health providers plan evaluations that are more effective and possibly conduct a more productive intervention program. Thus, we determine the relationship between health locus of control, self-efficacy, depression, self-care behaviors and glycemic control in type 2 diabetes patients.

## Methods

### Study design

This study was a cross-sectional design with a descriptive correlation approach. Data were collected using permission regarding use of structured questionnaires and face-to-face interviews.

### Sample and setting

Participants were recruited from endocrinology departments at a community-based clinical teaching hospital in Southern Taiwan. Participants were required to meet the inclusion criteria: (a) age 18 years and able to communicate in Chinese; (b) diagnosed with type 2 diabetes; (c) do not have history of critical disease or mental disease; (d) voluntary participation. The exclusion criteria were (a) having type 1 diabetes, gestational diabetes, or types of diabetes with other causes; and (b) having complications that would interfere with the ability to participate in the study (e.g., vision problems, end-stage renal disease and renal dialysis, cognitive impairments, diabetes ketoacidosis). The sample size was calculated based on the power analysis. Using a moderate effect-size for statistic power analysis for a probability level of 0.05 and 0.80 power, a sample size of 250 participants was deemed adequate. An attrition rate of 20% was anticipated based on the literature review [21]. Of the 300 participants approached, 10 people refused to participate, and 5 did not complete the questionnaires. In total, 285 participants were included in the analyses for the present study.

### Ethical considerations

Human research ethics committees at a regional hospital provided ethical approval for the study. Signed informed consent was obtained from all participants prior to beginning the study. Anonymity and confidentiality were ensured, and the participants were informed that they could withdraw from the study at any time.

### Instruments

The personal-information questionnaire included participant demographic data and medical condition data (age, gender, marital status, education level, income status, religion, duration, HbA1c, hypertension, lipemia, cardiomyopathy, nephropathy, and neuropathy).

The Multidimensional Health Locus of Control Scale (MHLC), developed by Wallston, Wallston and DeVellis in 1978, was applied to determine situational and perceived internal health locus of control and external health locus of control. The health locus of control scale consists of 18 items. A high score of internal health locus of control is correlated with a high level of participant-perceived internal personality. A high score of external personality trait is correlated with a high level of participant-perceived external personality. Yang tested the reliability and validity of the Chinese version and obtained a Cronbach's α value of 0.83 [22].

The Self-Efficacy Scale, developed by Chen et al. consists of four dimensions and 19-items, including general (5-items), diet (5-items), exercise and foot care (4-items), and medication (5-items). The Self-Efficacy Scale was applied to determine perception and abilities. Responses were graded on a Likert 11-point scale, ranging from 0 (can't handle the situation at all) to 10 (can handle the situation) [23]. A high score correlates with a high level of participant-perceived self-efficacy. Cronbach's α values in the Chinese version obtained 0.87.

The 21-item self-report Depression Anxiety Stress Scale (DASS-21) was developed by Lovibond and Lovibond with the aim of assessing depression, Anxiety and stress. Responses were graded on a 4-point Likert scale, ranging from 0 (did not apply to me at all) to 3 (applied to me very much, or most of tie). A high score is correlated with a high level of participant-perceived depression. The internal consistency for the DASS-21 subscales has been reported to be 0.91 (depression), 0.84 (anxiety), and 0.90 (stress). The Chinese version of the instrument been used by Taouk, Lovibond and Laube in a study with 729 Hong Kong Chinese speaking people. The internal consistency reported in this Chinese population for the DASS-21 was 0.92 (depression), 0.94 (anxiety), and 0.91 (stress) [24,25].

The Diabetes Self-Care Behavior Scale, developed by Hsu et al., consists of four dimensions and 14-items, including wound care (4-items), nutrition (3-items), medication (4-items), and SMBG (3-items). The Diabetic Self-Care Behavior Scale was applied to self-care behaviors. Responses were graded on a Likert 5-point scale, ranging from 1 (can't handle the behavior at all) to 5 (can handle the behavior). A high score is correlated with a high level of participant-perceived diabetic behavior. Cronbach's α values in the Chinese version obtained 0.87 [26].

## Data collection

After the participants provided informed consent, data were collected in individual face-to-face interviews by using structured questionnaires (Personal-information, MHLC, Self-Efficacy, DASS-21, Diabetes Self-Care Behavior). Data on the patients' initial and final HbA1c levels were gathered from their medical records.

## Data analysis

The SPSS software version 18.0 for Windows, and Amos software version 18.0 were used for statistical analyses. The interval data were expressed as means and standard deviations (SD), and the categorical data as frequency and percentage. A path analysis was adopted to describe relationships among variables using a structural equation model (SEM) with only measured variables. The path analysis specifies a model based on expected relationships among variables and tests if the observed variable relationships fit model expectations, thereby allowing simultaneous relationship testing among numerous variables. A path analysis was used to explore simultaneous relationships among demographic variables and health locus of control, self-efficacy, depression, self-care behavior and glycemic control. The CFI, TLI, and NFI values greater than 0.90, the normed 2 less than 5.0 [27], and the RMSEA value less than or equal to 0.08 indicated a good model fit. A P value less than 0.05 was considered statistically significant.

## Results

### Sample characteristics

The final study consisted of 285 participants with type 2 diabetes. The participant ages ranged from 19 to 83 years, (mean= 60.44; SD = 10.99 years), 181 (63.5%) were women, and 238 (82.1%) were married. Among these, 175 (61.4%) had primary school education or lower, 166 (58.3%) had a monthly income under NT$19,999, and 233 (81.8%) held religious beliefs. The disease duration of the participants ranged from 1 to 45 years (mean = 8.66, SD= 6.30). Complication was defined as the occurrence of syndromes related to diabetes, including hypertension 167 (58.6%), lipemia131 (46.0%), cardiomyopathy 21 (7.2%), nephropathy 116 (40.7%), and neuropathy 140 (49.1%). The HbA1c ranged from 4.6% to 14.5% (mean= 8.5%, SD = 2.14%).

Prior to analysing the means and SD of the internal health locus of control (mean= 26.99, SD = 3.05) cronbach's α values obtained 0.78, self-efficacy (mean=140.17, SD = 19.00) cronbach's α valuesobtained0.82, depression (mean= 5.49, SD = 5.56) cronbach's α valuesobtained0.83, and self-care behavior (mean= 54.19, SD = 9.60) cronbach's α values obtained 0.87, the findings indicated that most participants had a high sense of control over their behavior (Table 1).

| Items | n (%) | Mean | SD | Range |
|---|---|---|---|---|
| Age(year) | | 60.44 | 10.99 | 19-83 |
| Gender | | | | |
| male | 104 (36.5) | | | |
| female | 181 (63.5) | | | |
| Marital status | | | | |
| single | 47 (17.9) | | | |
| married | 238 (82.1) | | | |
| Education | 64 (22.5) | | | |
| No education | 16 (5.6) | | | |
| Literacy | 95 (33.3) | | | |
| Primary school | 46 (16.1) | | | |
| High school | 45 (15.8) | | | |
| Vocational education | 19 (6.9) | | | |
| Bachelor or more | | | | |
| Income (per month) | 80 (28.2) | | | |
| 9999 or below | 86 (30.1) | | | |
| 10,000 - 19,999 | 102(35.9) | | | |
| 20,000-49,999 | 17(5.8) | | | |
| 50,000 or more | | | | |
| Religion | 233 (81.8) | | | |
| yes | 52 (18.2) | | | |
| no | | | | |
| HbA1c(%) | | 8.52 | 2.14 | 4.6-14.5 |
| Disease duration(year) | | 8.66 | 6.30 | 1-45 |
| Hypertension | 167 (58.6) | | | |
| yes | 118 (41.4) | | | |
| no | | | | |
| Lipemia | 131 (46.0) | | | |
| yes | 154 (54.0) | | | |
| no | | | | |
| Cardiomyopathy | 21 (7.2) | | | |
| yes | 264 (92.8) | | | |
| no | | | | |
| Nephropathy | 116 (40.7) | | | |
| yes | 169 (59.3) | | | |
| no | | | | |
| Neuropathy | 140 (49.1) | | | |
| yes | 145 (50.9) | | | |
| no | | | | |

**Table 1:** Demographic variables and disease status (n = 285)

## Relationships among health locus of control, self-efficacy, depression and self-care behavior

### Direct effects

Figure 1 shows the estimated standardized path coefficients, indicating that internal health locus of control was significantly positively correlated with self-efficacy (β=0.32, P < 0.001) and self-care behavior (β=0.17, P < 0.001), and significantly negatively correlated with depression (β=-0.18, P < 0.01). External health locus of control was significantly positively correlated with depression (β=0.24, P < 0.001) and self-efficacy (β=0.32, P < 0.001). No significant correlation existed between external health locus of control and self-care behavior (β=0.06, .05).

Depression had a significant negative correlation with self-care behaviors (β=-0.07, P < 0.05), and self-efficacy was significantly correlated with self-care behavior (β=0.70, P < 0.001; Figure 1).

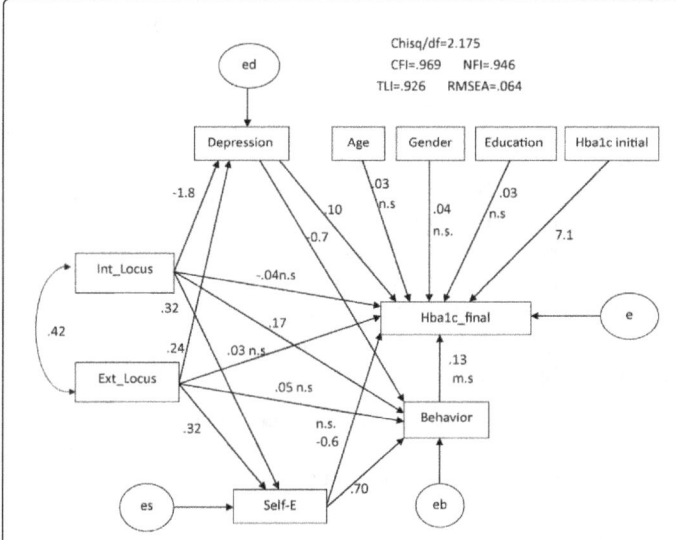

**Figure 1:** Path analysis model of determinants for glycemic control in type 2 diabetes.

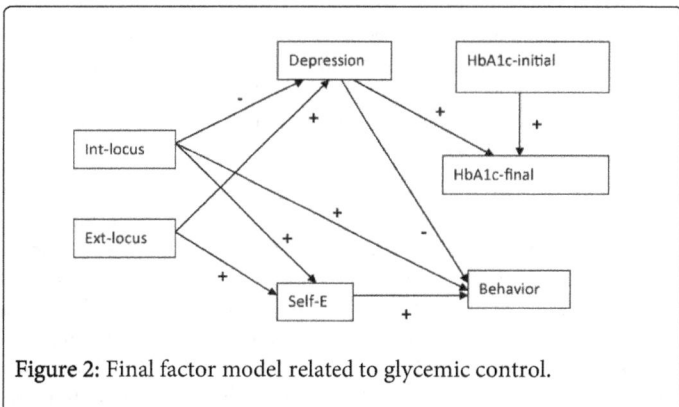

**Figure 2:** Final factor model related to glycemic control.

## Indirect effects

Based on the path analysis results, combined depression and self-efficacy partly mediated the relationship between internal health locus of control and self-care behavior (P < 0.01), and completely mediated the relationship between external health locus of control and self-care behavior (P < 0.01).

## Factors contributing to glycemic control

The normed chi-square for the overall path analysis model was 2.175, indicating that the model fit the data well. The root mean square error of approximation (RMSEA) was 0.064, suggesting exact model fit. The comparative fit index (CFI) was .969 and TLI = 0.926, NFI = 0.946, further supporting a good model fit.

In the path analysis model, both depression and the initial HbA1c value directly and significantly affected the final HbA1c value. A high level of depression was associated with the highest final HbA1c value (β=0.10, P0.05). Low initial HbA1c levels (high level of glycemic control) were associated with low final HbA1c levels. No correlations of HbA1c existed with internal health locus of control, external health locus of control, self-efficacy, gender, and age (P.05; Figure 2).

## Discussion

The purpose of the current study was to examine the relationships among the health locus of control, self-efficacy, self-care behavior, depression, and glycemic control of adults with type 2 diabetes. People with strong internal locus of control beliefs are most likely to engage in positive health behaviors, where as people with external locus of control beliefs, which are controlled by influential people or by chance, are not likely to engage in positive health behaviours [3,5,13,14].

Using the SEM, we observed direct relationships among the health locus of control, self-efficacy, depression, and self-care behavior. This finding is partially supported by Zulman et al. and Shi et al., who observed a positive correlation between the internal health locus of control and self-efficacy and high scores in health-related behavior [3,13]. People with internal health beliefs attribute health outcomes to their own actions and engage readily in positive health behaviors [28]. Moreover, people with an internal health locus of control who experience emotional distresses such as depression are likely to motivate themselves to maintain proper self-care behavior [7].

In addition, external health locus of control was directly and positively correlated with self-efficacy and depression. Henninger et al. observed that patient with severe medical complications tend to have an external health locus of control; thus, they perceive that they exert little personal control over their environment and circumstances [29]. Therefore, self-efficacy might be a crucial factor for people with an external health locus of control. Chen et al. offered an explanation for this observation, stating that patients with an external health locus of control depend on chance and medical professionals, such as physicians and nurses, to manage their diabetes and to enhance their self-efficacy [30]. Therefore, when planning interventions, health providers should be considered powerful people.

We observed that an external health locus of control is a direct factor of depression. This finding might be attributed to the fact that most of the data in this study were collected from elderly people (mean=60.44). Most elderly people live with their children and are financially supported [31]. Therefore, psychosocial support and recognition from the younger population are considered to be major requirements for depression among elderly Taiwanese people with diabetes [32]. However, because questions remained unanswered, additional research and discussion on this topic are required to examine other crucial factors that are associated with depression in elderly people with diabetes.

In addition, we observed the indirect effects by conducting a path analysis. Although the health locus of control was significantly correlated with self-efficacy and depression, no significant correlation existed between an external health locus of control and self-care behavior. The findings of Macaden and Clarke partially support these findings [20]. The Taiwanese diabetes patients who exhibited an external health locus of control managed their diabetic regime, believed thHat their diabetes was due to fate and bad luck, and engaged in poor glycemic control. Patients must be responsible for diabetes management, but limitations such as stress and depression affect diabetes control [32]. Moreover, fate and luck cause patients to believe that they cannot control their health outcomes, leading to depression. The correlation between an external health locus of control and self-efficacy observed in this study indicated that most Taiwanese people with type 2 diabetes attributed the responsibility of glycemic control to influential people and depended on healthcare providers for support [2].

Similarly, Macaden and Clarke indicated that patients in a South Asian context expected physicians to provide solutions to all problems and make all decisions [20]. Patients tended to depend on healthcare providers to control their glycemic levels, transferring the responsibility of managing their disease to the doctor rather than recognizing it as their own [29]. Thus, an external health locus of control is positively correlated with self-efficacy, but not with self-care behavior. Future research must consider the cultural differences among people with type 2 diabetes.

We observed that both depression and the initial HbA1c value were directly and significantly associated with the final HbA1c value, but were only marginally significantly associated with self-care behavior. Although the reason for this interaction is unclear, we speculate that, when diabetic people perceive events as beyond their personal control, they believe that doctors should help them control glycemic levels by using medication [20]. Further research is required to clarify the reason for the aforementioned association. However, the results provided evidence that, when caring for diabetic people, nurses should conduct assessments to collect initial data on the glycemic levels of their patients [4].

No correlations between HbA1c levels and the health locus of control, self-efficacy, gender, education, and age were observed. Moreover, our investigation of the relationship between the initial HbA1c value, the final HbA1c value, the health locus of control, self-efficacy, gender, education, and age yielded inconclusive findings. Although we observed a significant relationship, this became a trend when controlling other variables; thus, the relationship was weak. A stronger relationship could be masked by limited variability in the final HbA1c value, the health locus of control, self-efficacy, gender, or age, leading to the conclusion that the relationships among these variables were weak in this sample. Further research must be conducted to determine whether the results differ in type 2 diabetes populations belonging to other culture groups [30-34].

## Limitations

The current study has limitations. First, because this study used a cross-sectional design, cause-effect determinations could not be established based only on the data; thus, future longitudinal or experimental studies are required to evaluate the direction of causality. Second, the sample analyzed in this study consisted only of people attending a community-based clinic hospital for diabetes treatment. Thus, this sample was not a representative sample of all diabetic patients.

## Implications

The findings of the current study provide relevant information for future programs and studies conducted to improve self-care behavior and glycemic control among type 2 diabetes populations. Intervention programs can be tailored to people's specific health locus of control beliefs. People with external locus of control beliefs tend to rely on the health opinions provided by health care providers; thus, health care providers can establish guidelines for active self-care behavior, provide

strong guidance and supervision, and hold structured activities to improve these patients' perspectives toward their treatment regimens.

## Conclusion

The current study indicated that depression and self-efficacy mediate the associations among health locus of control, self-care behavior, and glycemic control. However, additional studies are required to investigate the health locus of control in various cultures and the diversity among diabetes populations. These studies must involve a longitudinal follow-up to determine how the health locus of control affects self-care behavior and glycemic control.

## Acknowledgement

The authors wish to thank all participants and GPs involved in this study, including diabetes manager, and the staff at the general clinic practice, for their assistance during this study.

## References

1.  American Diabetes Association (2014) Standards of medical care in diabetes--2014. Diabetes Care 37 Suppl 1: S14-80.

2.  Chen G, WuY, Wang T, Liang J, Lin W, et al. (2012) Association between serum endogenous secretory receptor for advanced glycation end products and risk of type 2 diabetes mellitus with combined depression in the Chinese population Diabetes, Technology & Therapeatics 14: 936-42.

3.  Zulman DM, Rosland AM, Choi H, Langa KM, Heisler M (2012) The influence of diabetes psychosocial attributes and self-management practices on change in diabetes status. Patient Educ Couns 87: 74-80.

4.  Weng HC, Hung CM, Chi SC (2010) Psychosocial and biological factors associated with glycemic control for patients with type 2 diabetes: an application of structural equation modeling analysis. Pan-Pacific Management Review 13: 33-47.

5.  Wallston KA, Wallston BS, Smith S, Dobbins CJ (1987) Perceived control and health. Current Psychological Research and Reviews 6: 5-25.

6.  Chen YM (1999) Relationships among health locus of control, self-efficacy and self-care of the elderly with hypertension. Journal of Nursing Research 7: 504-517.

7.  O'Hea EL, Moon S, Grothe KB, Boudreaux E, Bodenlos JS, et al. (2009) The interaction of locus of control, self-efficacy, and outcome expectancy in relation to HbA1c in medically underserved individuals with type 2 diabetes. J Behav Med 32: 106-117.

8.  Hummer K, Vannatta J, Thompson D (2011) Locus of control and metabolic control of diabetes: a meta-analysis. Diabetes Educ 37: 104-110.

9.  Graco M, Hutchinson A, Barker A, Lawlor V, Wong R, et al. (2012) Glycemic outcome not predicted by baseline psychological measures in a diabetes management program. Population Health Management 15: 163-7.

10. Heisler M, Piette JD, Spencer M, Kieffer E, Vijan S (2005) The relationship between knowledge of recent HbA1c values and diabetes care understanding and self-management. Diabetes Care 28: 816-820.

11. Krichbaum K, Aarestad V, Buethe M (2003) Exploring the connection between self-efficacy and effective diabetes self-management. Diabetes Educ 29: 653-662.

12. Aljasem LI, Peyrot M, Wissow L, Rubin RR (2001) The impact of barriers and self-efficacy on self-care behaviors in type 2 diabetes. Diabetes Educ 27: 393-404.

13. Shi Q, Ostwald S K, Wang S (2010) Improving glycaemic control self-efficacy and glycaemic control behaviour in Chinese patients with type 2 diabetes mellitus: randomized controlled trial. Journal of Clinical Nursing, 19: 398-404.

14. Van der Heijden MM, Pouwer F, Romeijnders AC, Pop VJ (2012) Testing the effectiveness of a self-efficacy based exercise intervention for inactive people with type 2 diabetes mellitus: design of a controlled clinical trial. BMC Public Health 12: 331.

15. Rydiewska A, Krzysztofik J, Libergal J, Rybak A, Banasiak W (2013). Health locus of control and the sense of self-efficacy in patient with systolic heart failure: a pilot study. Patient Prefer Adherence, 7 : 337-343.

16. Cosgrove MP, Sargeant LA, Griffin SJ (2008) Does depression increase the risk of developing type 2 diabetes? Occup Med (Lond) 58: 7-14.

17. Tsai KW, Chiang JK, Lee CS (2008) Undiagnosed depression in patients with type 2 diabetes and its associated factors. Tuzi Medicine 20: 44-48.

18. Trief PM, Morin PC, Izquierdo R, Teresi J, Eimicke JP, et al. (2006) Depression and glycemic control in elderly ethnically diverse patients with diabetes: the IDEATel project. Diabetes Care 29: 830-835.

19. Bai YL, Chiou CP, Chang YY, Lam HC (2008) Correlates of depression in type 2 diabetic elderly patients: a correlational study. Int J Nurs Stud 45: 571-579.

20. Macaden L, Clarke CL (2010) The influence of locus of control on risk perception in older South Asian people with Type 2 diabetes in the UK. Journal of Nursing and Healthcare of Chronic Illness 2: 144–152.

21. Kotrlik JW, Williams HA. (2003) The incorporation of effect size in information technology, learning and performance research. Information Techmology, Learnng and Performance Journal 21: 1-7.

22. Yang K (2003) Factors Related to the Medical Seeking Behavior of Cervical Positive Clients in Taipei. Unpublished master's thesis, Taipei Medical University, Taipei, Taiwan.

23. Chen ZT, Chang M, Lin YC (1998) The relationship between self-efficacy, social support and self-care behaviors in diabetes mellitus patients. Journal of Nursing Research 6: 31-43.

24. Lovibond PF, Lovibond SH (1995) The structure of negative emotional states: comparison of the Depression Anxiety Stress Scales (DASS) with the Beck Depression and Anxiety Inventories. Behav Res Ther 33: 335-343.

25. Taouk M, Lovibond PF, Laube R (2003) Psychometric properties of a Chinese version of the 21-item depression anxiety stress scales (DASS-21). University of New South Wales, New South Wales, Australia.

26. Hsu HC, Weng HC, Chen SM, Lee PJ, Lee JM, et al. (2004) Stratified case management for diabetes mellitus patients, the effectiveness and efficiency. Paper presented at the Diabetes Propaganda and Diabetes Management Conference Taipei.

27. Olobatuyi OE (2006) A user's guide to path analysis. University Press of America Inc, Maryland USA.

28. Lou JH, Chen SH, Yu HY, Li RH, Yang CI, et al. (2010) The influence of personality traits and social support on male nursing student life stress: a cross-sectional research design. J Nurs Res 18: 108-116.

29. Henninger DE, Whitson HE, Cohen HJ, Ariely D (2012) Higher medical morbidity burden is associated with external locus of control. J Am Geriatr Soc 60: 751-755.

30. Chen SH, Acton G, Shao JH (2010) Relationships among nutritional self-efficacy, health locus of control and nutritional status in older Taiwanese adults. J Clin Nurs 19: 2117-2127.

31. Wongpakaran N, Wongpakaran T, van Reekum R (2012) Social inhibition as a mediator of neuroticism and depression in the elderly. BMC Geriatr 12: 41.

32. Wu AM, Tang CS, Kwok TC (2004) Self-efficacy, health locus of control, and psychological distress in elderly Chinese women with chronic illnesses. Aging Ment Health 8: 21-28.

33. Rydlewska A, Krzysztofik J, Libergal J, Rybak A, Banasiak W, et al. (2013) Health locus of control and the sense of self-efficacy in patients with systolic heart failure: a pilot study. Patient Prefer Adherence 7: 337-343.

34. Wallston KA, Wallston BS, DeVellis R (1978) Development of the Multidimensional Health Locus of Control (MHLC) Scales. Health Educ Monogr 6: 160-170.

# 18

# Reliability and Validity Testing of Pilot Data from the TeamSTEPPS® Performance Observation Tool

**Mary Beth Maguire**[*], **Marie N Bremner** and **Daniel J. Yanosky**

*Kennesaw State University, Kennesaw, United States.*

[*]**Corresponding author** : Mary Beth Maguire, Kennesaw State University, Kennesaw, United States, E-mail: mmaguir5@kennesaw.edu

## Abstract

**Background:** The TeamSTEPPS® Performance Observation Tool (TPOT) is an instrument used in the evaluation of team performance: however, no assessment of the tool's reliability or validity exists among nurse educators.

**Methods:** A convenience sample of 31 nurse educators completed the TPOT to assess the reliability and validity of the instrument.

**Results:** Using Cronbach's alpha, the TPOT demonstrated a strong internal consistency coefficient. Through cross-group analysis of scoring between undergraduate and graduate nursing faculty, some evidence for convergent validity was confirmed.

**Conclusion:** This pilot study establishes the internal consistency reliability and convergent validity of the TPOT instrument when used by nurse faculty.

**Keywords** TeamSTEPPS® performance observation tool; Simulation team training; Reliability

## Reliability and Validity Testing of Pilot Data from the TeamSTEPPS® Performance Observation Tool

Fifteen years have passed since the Institute of Medicine first published To Err is Human [1]. This groundbreaking work described hospital errors as the eighth leading cause of death among patients in the United States. Many of the hospital errors identified were not a result of technical incompetence but rather human factors. Today, such medical errors persist and as recently as 2010, 180,000 deaths were attributed to them [2].

## Background

### TeamSTEPPS®

One way to improve human factors and minimize medical errors is through the TeamSTEPPS® curriculum. TeamSTEPPS® stands for Team Strategies and Tools to Enhance Performance and Patient Safety. TeamSTEPPS® is a comprehensive set of materials and training curriculum which seeks to improve patient safety through the use of team-based principles. The TeamSTEPPS® program was created by the Agency for Healthcare Research and Quality (AHRQ) and the Department of Defense (DOD). The curriculum is an evidence-based program based on 25 years of research related to teamwork, team training, and culture change [3]. TeamSTEPPS® was adopted as the national standard for healthcare team training in November 2006 [4]. However, despite TeamSTEPPS® set as the gold standard for health care team training, to date there has not been testing for reliability and validity of a tool that measures team performance based upon the curriculum.

The TeamSTEPPS® program is comprised of four primary teamwork skills: leadership, communication, situation monitoring, and mutual support. The TeamSTEPPS® curriculum reinforces the use of behaviors such as Situation-Background-Assessment-Recommendation (SBAR), check-back, and huddle which seek to improve team performance [3]. The implementation of TeamSTEPPS® principles has proven to reduce negative patient outcomes [5]. One hospital reports a 30% reduction in medical errors and an 88% decrease in the number of patient falls after implementing TeamSTEPPS® training [6].

The simulated clinical experience provides an ideal opportunity for learners to practice and refine clinical skills, teamwork, and communication in a controlled environment under the direction of faculty seeking to achieve a set of pre-determined objectives [7]. Combining simulation and the TeamSTEPPS® curriculum is an effective teaching strategy to allow learners the opportunity to engage in experiences addressing knowledge, skill, and interpersonal interactions while practicing team strategies in a safe and reproducible environment.

### Simulation Instruments

An important aspect of determining the effectiveness of simulated experiences is through evaluation. Most instruments used to measure student performance lack reported reliability and validity [8]. The utilization of instruments that have undergone appropriate psychometric testing is necessary to support reliable and valid assessment of student performance. Howard found a large number of untested instruments in current use and suggested a moratorium on further simulation instrument development until the appropriate psychometric assessments have been completed with instruments currently available [9]. In order to advance the simulation pedagogy, performance evaluation instruments from an individual and team perspective must undergo the rigor of psychometric testing.

## The TeamSTEPPS® Performance Observation Tool

The TeamSTEPPS® Performance Observation Tool (TPOT) is a 25 item instrument used to evaluate 5 domains of team performance. The domains are: team structure, leadership, situation monitoring, mutual support, and communication (Figure 1). The TPOT uses a 5-point scale that ranges from 1 (very poor) to 5 (excellent). The maximum score possible on the TPOT is 125 points.

The AHRQ and the DOD created the TPOT in an effort to quantify team performance. The tool creators acknowledge the TPOT had not been tested for reliability or validity prior to its publication nor is a standardized user menu or scoring method available [10]. At the time of this publication, no report of reliability or validity of the use of the TPOT among nurse educators was found in the literature.

## Purpose

The purpose of this study was to assess the internal consistency reliability and convergent validity of data produced by the TPOT when used by a group of nurse educators at one university in a southeastern state for evaluation of third semester Baccalaureate nursing students' team performance during a post-partum hemorrhage simulated patient care scenario. The research question was: What is the internal consistency reliability and convergent validity of TPOT

## Methods

Convenience sampling was utilized to recruit study participants. All full-time faculty and one cohort of nursing doctoral students from one school of nursing in a southeastern state were recruited. The inclusion criteria were for participants to be over 18 years of age and currently employed as a nurse educator. Institution Review Board approval was requested and exempt status was achieved.

## Data Collection

Data were collected in individual sessions or group sessions to accommodate the schedules of participants. Group session participants were instructed to avoid engaging in verbal and non-verbal communication to avoid scoring bias. Demographic information of participants was obtained. participants viewed a 10-minute pre-recorded clinical simulation scenario of third semester Baccalaureate nursing students caring for a patient experiencing a post-partum hemorrhage. Participants viewed the scenario two consecutive times. The first viewing was to observe the overall scenario content. After the initial viewing and prior to the second scenario viewing participants reviewed the TPOT instrument and received scripted scoring instructions. The second viewing occurred immediately after the first to allow scoring of the TPOT. Participants were granted no more than 10 minutes of additional time at the end of the second viewing to complete TPOT scoring.

## Data Analysis

Data were analyzed using PASW® Statistics GradPack 18 for Mac® and the SAS V9.3 system. Univariate analysis was used to examine the demographic nature of the sample. Internal consistency is the reliability estimate of a test based on a single administration [11]. To provide an estimate of internal consistency reliability, Cronbach's alpha coefficient was used along with split-half analysis. The split-half correlation is an additional method of analysis to further suggest the reliability of data as the TPOT was administered to participants on one occasion [12]. Convergent validity was assessed using 1-way analysis of covariance (ANCOVA) to detect possible differences in TPOT total scores among two distinct groups: those who teach undergraduate vs. graduate nursing courses while controlling for number of years of experience (Table 1). The TPOT total scores should ideally reflect only the quality of the scenario being evaluated and minimize subjectivity from the rater. Therefore, to establish convergent validity it was hypothesized that no systematic differences would exist among raters based on years of experience and level of teaching responsibilities. In other words, it was hypothesized that everyone in this sample would possess similar skills to evaluate the scenario at hand and therefore the number of years of experience and the level of teaching responsibilities would not systematically impact their TPOT total scores.

## Results

### Sample

Thirty-one participants were enrolled in the study (Table 2). Education preparation of the group approached equal balance between faculty with doctoral degrees (52%) and faculty with Master's degrees (48%). Teaching responsibilities among the group were equally distributed between baccalaureate (52%) and graduate (48%) degree levels. More than half of participants had completed five or more education courses at the graduate level (55%). The majority of the group had been teaching five or more years (68%). The group was nearly balanced between those currently responsible for performance based testing (48%), and those with no experience or no current experience with performance based testing (52%). A small percentage of participants indicated active teaching of the TeamSTEPPS® curriculum or of being a certified TeamSTEPPS® trainer

### Reliability

As a measure of internal consistency, Cronbach's alpha coefficient was 0.965. Split-half analysis of the TPOT was 0.943 (13 items) and 0.952 (12 items). The overall mean score of the TPOT was 70.77 (SD=21.42) (Table 1). Given all of these pieces of evidence, we find the internal consistency reliability of the TPOT to be strong.

### Validity

Instrument validity refers to how well an instrument actually measures what it is supposed to measure (Field, 2009). As a measure of convergent validity (one type of instrument validity), TPOT total scores were not found to differ significantly based on level of teaching responsibility and years of experience, $F_{(1,29)} = 0.26$, $p = .6107$, $\omega2 = 0.04$. Once again, these results were expected as no systematic differences here suggest that raters are in fact evaluating the same latent construct regardless of the raters' years of experience and level of teaching responsibilities. Graduate faculty total TPOT scores were somewhat lower (M=64.07, SD=19.0) than undergraduate faculty

(M=77.06, SD=22.21), however, these differences were not found to be statistically significant (Table 2). Subsequent ANCOVA analyses were performed on the 25 individual items of the TPOT as well. Results showed no statistical significance at the α = .05 level.

Figure 1: Team Performance observation Tool.

| Variable | Category | N (%) |
|---|---|---|
| Type of program taught | Baccalaureate | 16 (52%) |
| | Graduate | 15 (48%) |
| Number of years as nursing faculty | <1 | 1 (3%) |
| | 1-3 year | 6 (19%) |
| | 4-5 years | 3 (10%) |
| | 6-10 years | 4 (13%) |
| | >10 years | 17 (55%) |
| Highest degree completed | Master's Degree | 15 (48%) |
| | Doctoral Degree | 16 (52%) |
| Number of education courses completed at the graduate level | 0 | 4 (13%) |
| | 1 | 1 (3%) |
| | 2 | 4 (13%) |
| | 3 | 1 (3%) |
| | 4 | 4 (13%) |
| | 5 | 2 (7%) |
| | >5 | 15 (48%) |
| Experience with clinical simulation | No experience | 7 (23%) |
| | Participated as a learner in a simulated clinical environment | 5 (16%) |
| | Facilitated learning in a clinical environment | 17 (55%) |
| | Attended a simulation workshop | 1 (3%) |
| | Took a simulation elective course | 1 (3%) |
| Experience with evaluating students in a performance based assessment | No experience | 4 (13%) |
| | Some experience but none currently | 12 (39%) |
| | Responsible for evaluating performance based learning this semester | 15 (48%) |
| Indicate your experience with team work and the TeamSTEPPS curriculum | Experience with teamwork concepts, not TeamSTEPPS | 15 (48%) |
| | Familiar with TeamSTEPPS curriculum | 13 (42%) |
| | Teach TeamSTEPPS | 1 (3%) |
| | A certified TeamSTEPPS trainer | 2 (7%) |

Table 1: Participants Demographics (N=31)

| Attribute/ Group | N | Mean | Median | Std Dev | Minimum | Maximum | Lower 95% Confidence Limit | Upper 95% Confidence Limit |
|---|---|---|---|---|---|---|---|---|
| Years of Experience | 31 | 3.97 | 5.00 | 1.33 | 1.00 | 5.00 | 3.48 | 4.46 |
| TPOT Total Score | 31 | 70.77 | 66.00 | 21.42 | 28.00 | 119.00 | 62.92 | 78.63 |
| TPOT Total Score by Group | | | | | | | | |
| Undergraduate | 16 | 77.06 | 73.50 | 22.21 | 43 | 119 | 65.23 | 88.90 |
| Graduate | 15 | 64.07 | 63.00 | 19.00 | 28 | 97 | 53.55 | 74.59 |

Table 2 : TPOT Question Scores for Undergraduate and Graduate Faculty 1-way ANOVA (Undergraduate N=16 Graduate N=15)

## Discussion

This study serves to establish psychometric properties related to reliability and validity of TPOT pilot data when used to evaluate team skills of undergraduate nursing students. The findings of this study suggest the TPOT is a reliable instrument to utilize in the evaluation of team performance among undergraduate nursing students. Furthermore, this study provides the beginnings of a validity study through presenting initial evidence of convergent validity. Specifically, findings suggest that convergent validity is acceptable with no statistical differences detected among teaching responsibility groups while controlling for years of experience. T

The results of TPOT data can yield worthwhile data to healthcare teams seeking to evaluate team performance. Nurse educators may find the TPOT an effective tool to utilize in the simulated clinical environment to provide formative and/or summative assessment of team performance. Data from TPOT scoring can also provide information to educators as to the effectiveness of leadership and communication within a curriculum.

## Limitations

Several limitations of this study must be noted. First, variability occurred in how data was collected. Some participants completed the TPOT in one-on-one sessions and others completed the TPOT in small group sessions all led by the principle investigator. These small group sessions may have resulted in verbal and non-verbal communication among participants that influenced participants' TPOT score however, an attempt was made to control and minimize any such bias. Second, the scenario reviewed was a performance of novice practitioners. Various skill imperfections were present and may have distracted participants from the overall team performance. Third, the sample size was small, not randomized, and limited to one institution. Additional testing is required with a larger sample size to complete a factor analysis and compare findings among multiple institutions. While all faculty were experienced with broad concepts of teamwork, not all faculty members were actively teaching TeamSTEPPS® curriculum nor were they certified TeamSTEPPS® trainers. Unfamiliarity with the TeamSTEPPS® curriculum may have accounted for the variability in scoring. Thus, it is recommended future studies mandate certification in TeamSTEPPS® as part of the inclusive criteria for participants.

## Conclusion

Clinical simulation provides an ideal setting for providing reliable and valid assessment of student performance across multiple domains. Recommendations for further studies include repeated measures of TPOT scoring among groups to evaluate the stability of the instrument and utilizing the TPOT with simulation scenarios that differ in level of team performance to determine if the tool can detect varying abilities' of team performance. Increasing the sample size of participants will strengthen the precision of psychometric indicators of the TPOT. Research is in progress on a national scale to replicate this study with other schools of nursing faculty to determine the reliability and validity of TPOT data among a larger sample

Refined instruments for the evaluation of teams will help to standardize assessment of team performance in the simulated clinical environment and ultimately the clinical practice setting. The improved performance of healthcare teams in clinical practice will help to mitigate human factors and result in reduction of medical errors.

## References

1. Institute of Medicine (1999) To err is human: Building a safer health system.

2. Medical errors in the USA: Human or systemic (2011) The Lancet.

3. Agency for Healthcare Research and Quality (2013) TeamSTEPPS: National implementation.

4. American Institutes for Research (2010) TeamSTEPPS Teamwork Perception Questionnaire (TTPQ)

5. Courtright SH, Steward GL, Ward MM (2012) Applying research to save lives: Learning from team training approaches in aviation and health care. Organizational Dynamics, 41: 291-301.

6. Nailberk D (2012) Hospital cuts med errors 30%, falls 88% with TeamSTEPPS. Healthcare Risk Management, August, 90-91.

7. Clapper TC, Kong M(2012) TeamSTEPPS: The patient safety tool that needs to be implemented. Clinical Simulation in Nursing 8:e3670-e373.

8. Kardong-Edgren S, Adamson KA, Fitzgerald C (2010) A review of currently published evaluation instruments for human patient simulation. Clinical Simulation in Nursing, 6: e25-e35

9. Howard V (2012, December) Simulation evaluation. Webinar cosponsored by the American Association of Colleges of Nursing and the International Nursing Association for Clinical Simulation and Learning.

10. Almeida S (2009) Designing evaluation systems for TeamSTEPPS. Webinar sponsored by the American Institute for Research Designing Evaluation Systems for TeamSTEPPS.

11. Haertel EH (2006) Reliability in Brennan, R.L. (Ed.). Educational Measurement (4th ed.). National Council on Measurement in Education, American Council on Education. Westport, CT: Praeger Publishers.

12. Field A (2009) Discovering statistics using SPSS. Thousand Oaks, CA: Sage.

# 19

# Sheltering Aboriginal Women with Mental Illness in Ontario, Canada: Being "Kicked" and Nurtured

**Phyllis Montgomery[1*], Sarah Benbow[2], Laura Hall[3], Denise Newton-Mathur[1], Cheryl Forchuk[4] and Sharolyn Mossey[1]**

[1]School of Nursing, Ramsey Lake Road, Laurentian University, Sudbury, Ontario, Canada

[2]Faculty of Health Sciences, Arthur Labatt Family School of Nursing, Western University, London, Ontario, Canada

[3]York University, 4700 Keele St., Toronto, Ontario, Canada

[4]Arthur Labatt Family School of Nursing, Lawson Health Research Institute, 1151, Richmond Street, Western University, London, Ontario, Canada

*Corresponding author : Phyllis Montgomery, Professor, School of Nursing, Ramsey Lake Road, Laurentian University, Sudbury, Ontario, Canada,
E-mail: pmontgomery@laurentian.ca

## Abstract

**Objective:** For individuals living with mental health challenges, the provision of homeless shelters can offer a temporary respite in overwhelming life circumstances. There is, however, limited evidence regarding the subjective experiences associated with shelter services by Aboriginal women in Canada. The purpose of this study was to develop an understanding of the day-to-day experiences of Aboriginal women as they seek and provide safety, comfort, health, and healing in the context of mental illness and insecure housing.

**Methods:** The study design was a secondary qualitative analysis of data collected in a primary mixed method study involving persons faced with mental health and housing challenges in southern Ontario, Canada. Narrative analysis was used to identify common experiences among 11 shelter service users and 10 shelter service providers, all of whom where Aboriginal women.

**Results:** Regardless of whether the women received or provided shelter services, they consistently described experiences about being "kicked" and nurtured. Their stories about being "kicked" described experiences associated with compounding losses. Juxtaposed to this reality, were accounts about being nurtured or "lifting each other up." Nurturing relations were essential to address the pervasive health and social disparities experienced by the women. Relationships within homeless shelters were directed towards supporting the health and well-being of individual women and their broader community.

**Conclusion:** This study's findings extend the community mental health body of nursing literature regarding Aboriginal women living with mental illness and homelessness. Despite the protective and restorative components of nurturing within shelter services, cooperative networks need to be developed to build communities that eradicate the pervasive losses experienced by Aboriginal women who continue to be "kicked."

**Keywords:** Aboriginal women; Mental health; Homelessness; Shelters; Qualitative

## Introduction

In Canada, the health and well-being of Aboriginal women is particularly compromised in comparison to their non-Aboriginal female counterparts. The individual and collective vulnerabilities of Aboriginal women are represented by multiple intersecting "realities of everyday life in which Aboriginality, female gender, racism, sexism and poverty are lived and experienced simultaneously, not sequentially" [1]. It has been well documented that Canadian Aboriginal women have a significantly lower life expectancy [2] and higher prevalence of depression, addictions, and self-injury [3,4]. Further, Aboriginal women are reported to have higher social surveillance, incarceration rates, incidences of violence, transgenerational trauma, discrimination and lower income levels; all of which impact health [4-8]. As a group, Aboriginal women are more often homeless compared to both non-Aboriginal women and Aboriginal men [9], which has further compromised their overall well-being inclusive of mental health.

Impacted by entrenched historical and contemporary health and social inequities [6, 10] Aboriginal women often enter homeless shelter services to seek refuge [11,12]. For insecurely housed Canadians, such as Aboriginal women, the use of adult shelter services has been fundamental to sustaining day-to-day survival in the midst of entrenched health and social disparities. In this way, homeless services focus predominantly on fulfilling immediate basic needs [13,14]. Shelters offer services that are intended to transition vulnerable women from homelessness to stable housing through the concurrent provision of necessary health and social services. The coordination and timeliness of appropriate services to break the cyclic nature of homelessness is challenging given the variability and complexity of needs that threaten well-being [11,15].

In general, Canadian women have described their homeless shelter experiences as disempowering, un-dignifying and regimented [7,16]. Liebow's ethnographic study [17] suggested that racial divisiveness is a pervasive within shelter life. In particular for women with mental illness who may be subjected to overt and covert hostility associated with racial tensions, self-imposed isolation was a protective strategy that further undermines their mental health [17]. Other authors reported that the need to balance individual and collective security is a complex undertaking for community workers navigating cultural tensions and advocating for broader social justice [14,18,19]. Further, social disparities impede exit from the shelter circuit keeping Aboriginal women dependent on services which may not be culturally sensitive [20].

Several authors have identified the need for focused research that explores the well-being of Aboriginal women when their capacity to fulfil family and community responsibilities is disrupted [8,14,21]. The purpose of this study therefore, was to develop an understanding of the day-to-day experiences of Aboriginal women as they seek safety, comfort, health, and healing in the context of mental illness and insecure housing. More specifically, this study revealed the accounts of receiving and providing shelter services as told by Aboriginal women. Green [10] identified that individual and collective experiences of Aboriginal women are reflective of social realities that warrant acknowledgement and intervention by psychiatric mental health nurses. The results of this study have the potential to sensitize psychiatric mental health nurses to the complexity of Aboriginal women's quest to achieve wellness of body, mind and spirit as described by the First Nations and Inuit Mental Wellness Advisory Committee [22], an underdeveloped area of psychiatric mental health nursing research.

## Methods

### Design

This study`s design was a supplementary secondary qualitative approach to examine a data subset not fully addressed in a primary study [23]. The five-year primary study used a mixed methods participatory action approach to examine housing issues and solutions for individuals with mental illness [24]. It generated an extensive repository of data, approved for secondary analyses. The dataset, particular to Aboriginal women who used or provided shelter services, was accessed for this supplementary study to elicit a focused description of their knowledge about and experiences of shelter care. This secondary analysis was important to search for new knowledge that is informed by the voices of Aboriginal women [12,25,26].

Access to the ethically approved dataset and its security was maintained by an author who was also the academic lead of the original study. To uphold the ethical principle of beneficence, the anonymity and uniqueness of each woman was safeguarded through data extraction, secure storage, and representation in the findings. This was particularly salient given that participant data could reveal their identity to members of their small communities. Cultural sensitivity throughout the research process was guided by the Aboriginal research team members.

### Sample and sample

The original study recruited individuals from a variety of mental health, housing and social services in southern Ontario all of who were involved in either service use or service provision [24]. For this study, data was extracted from group interviews specific to 21 English-speaking women who self-identified as Aboriginal, including First Nation, Métis, or Inuit. It is acknowledged that each of these three

groups of Aboriginal peoples is a distinct nation with unique heritages, languages, cultural practices, and spiritual beliefs as described by the Government of Canada [27]. Of this sample, 11 self-identified as having a history of mental illness and insecure housing that required use of homeless shelter services. The remaining 10 Aboriginal women in the dataset were employed in the provision of homeless shelter services.

### Data collection and analysis

Data particular to the 21 Aboriginal women were extracted from the eight primary study tape-recorded verbatim focus group transcripts, which were anonymized. Evident across the transcripts were stories co-constructed during participation in the focus groups. Stories, the unit of analysis in this study, are told to communicate internal understanding of life experiences and situations [28,29].

Data analysis involved a structural narrative approach to systematically identify and group stories based on shared structure, meaning, and function [30]. The structure refers to how stories are constructed by participants [31]. The story meaning represents the participants' intended message [32]. Finally, the function of a story denotes the implications of what is being told to the researcher [30]. This approach necessitated the research team members to engage in serial open conversations leading to shared interpretations of the structure, meaning and function of each story grouping with the intent of honouring the voices of the participants. This interactive and iterative approach was supported by the work of Peat [33].

To preserve each Aboriginal woman's anonymity, entire stories are not presented. Rather, one or two sentences were extracted from the accounts of several women to illustrate story structure, meaning, and function while indicating auditability, analytic logic and credibility [29]. Within these extractions textual clarifications were added within square brackets. The use of quotations was to note the precise lexicon of participants not attributable to or tidied by the researchers.

## Results

The women told 124 stories, describing daily experiences involving tenacious efforts to secure a "good life" for themselves and others in the context of mental illness and insecure housing. The experiences described by shelter service users and providers were similar. Their stories, reflecting a cohesive account of sheltering while vulnerable, were labelled being "kicked" and being nurtured. To varying degrees, these two groups of contrasting stories occurred in the lives of all participants. Below is a sequential presentation of the structure, meaning, and function of each of the two story groups.

### Being "Kicked" Stories

Within this first group of stories, service users and providers described a legacy of historical oppression with which they live on a day-to-day basis. Largely influenced by negativity, the women shared experiences likened to being perpetually "kicked," and thus the labelling of this group of stories. For some service users, being "kicked" was attributed to not only having a mental illness and insecure housing but also the "colour of my skin." For some service users, being "kicked" was related to generalization of Aboriginal women as "untrustworthy."

## Structure

The common structural element across all of the "kicked" stories was that of multiple, diverse, compounding and often unresolved loss. Service users and providers detailed removal from or denial of resources such as personal possessions, relationships, autonomy, community influence, service and land often entrenched in racial discrimination. The following excerpts illustrate the element of loss within the "kicked" stories.

Service user 3: My grandfather makes [a special artefact] and he is 87 years old. He gaveme one. I had it in the apartment. I lost the apartment and I lost my treasure. He [landlord] threw everything in the dump.

Service user 5: I'm in a shelter because I lost my boyfriend and I lost our place.

Service user 9: We are actually told we [Aboriginal women] are no good for nothing and there is no way around that.

Service provider 2: And out here all we have is our skin.

Service provider 5: Our women have no property rights. When we leave [our reserve] we leave our land our home what we have built our whole life. As an Aboriginal woman I understand our reality, our issues, the Indian Act.

Service provider 6: We know what it is like to deal with people who don't care. We    know what it is like to be assumed that you are guilty even before you have a chance to explain. We know what that feeling is as it is also our experience. It is also our sisters' and brothers' experience. It happened to our parents, our cousins, our boyfriends, our girlfriends. It is there and it is bad.

The presence of repeated losses, reinforced women's perception of exclusion, objectification and deprivation, which was characteristic of the experience of being "kicked." Service users who were "kicked" out of places and service providers, who were excluded or "kicked" out of processes, witnessed the accumulation of their losses. Ultimately, this created an entrenchment of their respective needs as "virtually invisible" and unmet. Being kicked distanced them from where "they want[ed] to be and how they need[ed] to be." From a service user perspective, "always having doors slammed in your face" further threatened mental well-being. Service providers recognized that in the presence of loss and absence of stable mental health and secure housing, shelters users would remain "broken," "out of place" and preoccupied with just trying to "survive day-to-day."

## Meaning and function

The women told "kicked" stories to convey cumulative losses of that which was perceived as essential to health and well-being. Persistent discrimination and social inequities became commonplace in the lives of shelter service users and providers. Both shelter users and providers gave testimony to the contextual aggression and deprivation within their life- and work-circumstances. The participants acknowledged that an "unsupportive society" heightened suffering and perpetuated their sense of loss. With each repetitive and forceful kick, both shelter users and providers came to live in a sustained state of vulnerability. As described by a service provider, "their [shelter users'] crust starts to form," and "then their mental illness really kicks in." Succinctly stated by one shelter user, her life in disadvantage was "a constant audition" for a more meaningful and healthy existence. Overall, being kicked restricted women's capacities and opportunities for "peace."

These stories function to provide insight into the insidious nature of loss that pervades the life experiences of both shelter service users and providers in this study. Although experienced to varying degrees, each woman was affected, directly or vicariously, by society's ineffectual response to eradicate homelessness and promote mental well-being. Further, this group of stories identifies the need for mental health nurses, as members of the broader community mental health network, to provide culturally appropriate individualized assessments and cooperative interventions relative to trauma that could be experienced by some Aboriginal women using and providing homeless shelter services. A failure to consider the possibility of such trauma risks "further and further and further and further and further" omissions in the comprehensive and coordinated service provision for Aboriginal women living with mental illness and insecure housing.

## Being Nurtured Stories

Within the second group of stories, service users and providers both described the need for and practices of gently "lifting each other up" in the context of the life circumstances described in the being "kicked" stories. Most nurturing stories described providers' attempts to "contribute good things" through nurturing of self, "our sisters," and "our people as a whole." Nurturing involved a respectful attention to the physical, emotional, social, spiritual, and cultural aspects of one another.

## Structure

The common structural element across the being nurtured stories was partnering to address diverse needs. The presence of unmet needs necessitated respectful connections between service users, providers and external others to fulfil immediate needs. The following excerpts illustrate the impetus for partnering within one another within the nurturing stories.

Service user 2 : When I say I am sick, I am really sick. And just like other people I need    help from those [individuals who are supposed to help].

Service user 6: As a single mother with kids I feel I need to hook up with someone because I can't do this alone to make ends meet. I would love to be on my own but I can't right now.

Service user 7: At many shelters, there are certain times where we can't eat. We don't even have a place to sit at [name of a particular shelter]. At this shelter they do have good meals and fresh beds. If I don't have a place to sit I now know I can come here.

Service provider 8: We had a woman who was going to be evicted while she was in the hospital. She called us. We went to her house and packed her stuff up for her. Whatever we can do to help we try to do it.

Service provider 10: We care for some women who are so poor that they can't help their children. Not that they don't want to, not that they are bad people, not that they are not worthy. They simply can't do it alone

Service provider 5: The Indian Act has to be interpreted. It is huge for our people in terms of where we can live, what are our rights, all those things that significantly impact on Aboriginal women.

Nurturing involved "providing for" and "being available to" one another, "one woman at a time." The acts were to foster in the service users a sense of being "cared for" and feeling "cared about." Efforts to counter the described losses in the "kicked" stories and establish a support network required service providers to be "pretty sophisticated in social politics." Their nurturing practices were guided by reasonable actions that addressed a woman's needs rather than rigid compliance with "institutionalized routines." For example, providers recognized the need to "let some women sleep" and "take the time they needed" to initiate restoration of "body, mind and spirit." Cultural sensitivity was described as a welcome component of nurturing interactions. Simple actions such as speaking "our own languages" and sharing foods that "not only sustained us physically, but provided cultural nourishment" was described as means of connecting with and nurturing one another.

## Meaning and function

Participants told being nurtured stories to illustrate the potential of positive and authentic connectedness in overcoming unmet needs both to promote individual "balance" and a create a community of healthy Aboriginal women. This group of stories portray optimism for a future in which Aboriginal women's identity as "beautiful, strong, caring and kind" women is unmasked. These stories function to demonstrate that authentic nurturing focused on the individualized fulfilment of needs has the potential to extend "servicing" to "healing" for Aboriginal women. Nurturing and healing work that is initiated by service users and providers within homeless shelters, complements community mental health nurses' overall efforts for optimized well-being.

## Discussion

This study's findings extend the community mental health body of nursing literature regarding Aboriginal women living with mental illness and homelessness. In juxtaposition to being "kicked", being nurtured stories present a simultaneous reality characterized by genuine concern and person-centred actions between and among Aboriginal women. In concert, the two types of stories illustrate the importance of validating the historical and contemporary contextual reality of Aboriginal women and their strategic efforts to actualize person dignity and connectedness with valued others. The being "kicked" and nurtured stories depict individual and shared efforts towards balance of body, mind, and spirit. Although the mandate of homeless shelter services is not mental health, the women's stories demonstrate that nurturing has the potential to promote individual mental well-being. Within spaces that offer safety and comfort, even if time-limited, a woman's journey for physical, emotional, mental, cultural and spiritual well-being is made possible [8]. As such, individuals who receive and provide sheltering services and the organizations in which services are structured are integral to building a community that not only espouses but enacts social justice.

Community building, as conceptualized by Walter and Hyde [34] necessitates authentic "communityness," beyond the sharing of geographic space, members are connected by activities that foster a sense of belonging through the fair and equitable distribution of community resources. The nurtured stories within this study suggest the presence of emergent communityness. In contrast, "kicked" stories emphasize the ongoing presence of health and social inequities that continue to pervade the lives of Aboriginal women, hallmarks that communityness and social justice have not yet been achieved. Community building practices involve multidimensional engagements using a range of strategies to acknowledge diverse beliefs, interests, and strengths, with the goal of building "capacity of the entire system, and all its participants, to operate as community" [34].

Mental health nurses, as established members of community are well positioned to acknowledge the strengths of those with whom they interface, inclusive of shelter users, shelter workers and organizations. Exploring ways of working together for community building necessitates affirming and acknowledging one another's legitimacy and legal entitlements, embracing diversity, identifying common goals such as health equity, engaging in creative planning, integrating multiple visions and strategies, and accepting responsibility to remain connected [34]. Shelter service user and provider partnering for fulfilment of immediate needs as represented in the nurturing stories in this study can be supported by mental health nurses' conscious, inclusionary, and community building practices for individual and population health [10,34,35]. This study's results suggest an orientation for fostering community development as opposed to a singular best practice to address the disparaging circumstances of individual women involved in shelter life. As argued by Johnstone [36], mental health nurses have a responsibility to challenge the status quo and advocate for inclusivity as strategies to subvert the normalized culture of prejudice and discrimination against vulnerable populations.

The Canadian Federation of Mental Health Nurses [37] asserts that mental health nurses must consider the impact of culture, class, ethnicity, language, stigma, and social exclusion on health and health promotion. For nurses working with Aboriginal women living with mental illness and insecure housing, this is particularly relevant given historical and contemporary losses. The loss feature of the being "kicked' stories can be perceived as a manifestation of poverty and exclusion associated with colonialism [8,26]. According to de Leeuw, Greenwood and Cameron [38], the Canadian legacy of colonialization permeates the mental health of Aboriginal peoples. Thus, nurses' mindfulness of the impact of historical processes, such as the Indian Act, and social determinants, provides a more comprehensive assessment of Aboriginal women's mental health [8,13,39]. Koptie [40] cautioned that definitions of poverty, underpinned by tenets of assimilation, negate the efforts of Aboriginal people to overcome their 'trajectory of suffering' in a colonial context.

The being nurtured stories not only pay tribute to the resilience and strength of Aboriginal women in adversity, but support the movement away from an account solely focused on abuse and pain to one of strength, hope and acknowledgment of Aboriginal experiential knowledge [41,42]. Aboriginal worldviews generally tend to emphasize responsibility for the whole of the community rather than just for individual members. Nurses' awareness of this orientation may foster a partnering with Aboriginal women in their efforts to shift practices from an emphasis on service provision to connectedness and inclusivity with sensitivity to context and culture. This 'coming-to-know' [33] requires attention to processes through further dialogue among a range of community stakeholders to understand the circumstances required for Aboriginal women to actively engage in their wellness [25]. Forging authentic relations between mental health and social service providers is imperative to ensure that individual rights and needs are met, and at a much broader level social inclusion and social action for community building can be achieved for marginalized populations [14,43,44]. To bridge the chasms that continue to exist within health and social services, mental health nurses can function in a variety of roles such as care advocate, case manager, and consultant. The roles of care manager [45] and navigator [46] to support individuals living with other chronic challenges warrant examination for feasibility with this study's population.

In conclusion, future research guided by Aboriginal methodologies, such as sharing circles [47], is recommended to extend the findings of this study. Such approaches offer the possibility of acquiring further understanding of the complex realities of mental health and housing challenges for Aboriginal women in a culturally appropriate manner beyond what was accomplished in this study. This study did reveal the juxtaposed realities experiences by Aboriginal women in homeless shelters. Despite the protective and restorative components of nurturing within shelter services, cooperative networks need to be developed to build community that eradicates the pervasive losses and mental distress experienced by Aboriginal women.

## References

1.   Culhane D (2009) Narratives of hope and despair in Downtown Eastside Vancouver. In Kirmayer LJ, Valaskakis GG, In Healing Traditions: The Mental Health of Aboriginal Peoples in Canada. 160-177. University of British Columbia Press, Vancouver BC.

2.   Smylie J (2009) The health of aboriginal peoples. In Raphael D, Social determinants of health: Canadian perspectives (2nd edn p. 280–301). Canadian Scholars Press, Toronto, ON.

3.   Donner L, Isfeld H, Haworth-Brockman M, Forsey C (2008) A profile of women's health in Manitoba. Prairie Women's Health Centre of Excellence, Manitoba, Winnipeg.

4.   Reading CL, Wein F (2009) Health inequalities and social determinants of Aboriginal Peoples' health. National Collaborating Centre for Aboriginal Health, Prince George, British Columbia.

5.   Haskell L, Randall M (2009) Disrupted attachments: A social context complex trauma framework and the lives of aboriginal peoples in Canada. Journal of Aboriginal Health 5: 48- 99.

6.   Native Women's Association of Canada (2004). Aboriginal women and housing: For the Canada-Aboriginal Peoples roundtable sectoral follow-up session on housing. Native Women's Association of Canada, Ottawa, Ontario.

7.   Scott S (2007) All our sisters: Stories of homeless women in Canada. Broadview Press, Peterborough, Ontario.

8.   Stout R (2010) Urban Aboriginal women and mental health (Project #215). Prairie Women's Health Centre of Excellence, Winnipeg, Manitoba.

9.   Native Women's Association of Canada (2007) Aboriginal women and homelessness: An issue paper. Author, Corner Brook, Newfoundland.

10.  Green BL (2010) Applying interdisciplinary theory in the care of Aboriginal women's mental health. J Psychiatr Ment Health Nurs 17: 797-803.

11.  Richter MS, Chaw-Kant J (2008) A case study: Retrospective analysis of homeless women in a Canadian city. Women's Health & Urban Life 7: 7-19.

12.  Ruttan L, LaBoucane-Benson P, Munro B (2008) "A story I never heard before": Aboriginal young women, homelessness, and restoring connections. Pimatziwin: A Journal of Aboriginal and Indigenous Community Health 6: 31-54.

13.  Benbow S, Forchuk C, Ray SL (2011) Mothers with mental illness experiencing homelessness: a critical analysis. J Psychiatr Ment Health Nurs 18: 687-695.

14.  Berman H, Mulcahy GA, Forchuk C, Edmunds KA, Haldenby A, et al. (2009) Uprooted and displaced: a critical narrative study of homeless, Aboriginal, and newcomer girls in Canada. Issues Ment Health Nurs 30: 418-430.

15.  Young MG, Moses JM (2013) Noeliberalism and homelessness in the western Canadian arctic. Canadian Journal of Nonprofit and Social Economy Research 4: 7-22.

16.  Novac S (1996) A place to call one's own: New voices of dislocation and dispossession. Status of Women Canada, Ottawa, Ontario.

17.  Liebow E (1993) Tell them who I am: The lives of homeless women. Penguin Books, New York, New York.

18.  Krausz RM, Clarkson AF, Strehlau V, Torchalla I, Li K, et al. (2013) Mental disorder, service use, and barriers to care among 500 homeless people in 3 different urban settings. Soc Psychiatry Psychiatr Epidemiol 48: 1235-1243.

19.  Lyon-Callo V (2004) Inequality, poverty, and neoliberal governance: Activist ethnography in the homeless sheltering industry. Broadview Press, Peterborough, Ontario.

20.  Thurston WE, Oelke ND, Turner D, Bird C (2011) Final report: Improving housing outcomes for Aboriginal people in Western Canada: National, regional, community and individual perspectives on changing the future of homelessness. Department of Community Health Services, University of Calgary, Alberta.

21.  Ruttan L, LaBoucane-Benson P, Munro B (2010) "Home and Native Land": Aboriginal young women and homelessness in the city. First Peoples Child & Family Review 5: 67-77.

22.  First Nations and Inuit Mental Wellness Advisory Committee (2007) Draft Strategic Action Plan for First Nations and Inuit Mental Wellness. Author, Ottawa, Ontario.

23.  Heaton J (2008) Secondary analysis of qualitative data. In Alasuutari P, Bickman L, Brannen J (eds.) The SAGE handbook of social research methods (p. 506-519). SAGE Publications, London, England.

24.  Forchuk C, Csiernik R, Jensen E (2011) Homelessness, housing and the experiences of mental health consumer-survivors: Finding truths creating change. Canadian Scholars Press, Toronto, Ontario.

25.  Kenny C (2006) When the women heal: Aboriginal women speak about policies to improve the quality of life. American Behavioral Scientist: 50: 550-561.

26.  Smith LT (1999) Decolonizing Methodologies: Research and Indigenous Peoples. Zed Books, New York, New York.

27.  Government of Canada (2012) Aboriginal Affairs and Northern Development Canada: Terminology.

28.  Holloway I, Freshwater D (2007) Narrative research in nursing. Blackwell Publishing, Oxford, England.

29.  Riessman CK (2008) Narrative methods for the human sciences. SAGE Publishers, Los Angeles, California.

30.  Bailey PH, Montgomery P, Mossey S (2013) Narrative Inquiry. In Beck CT (ed.) Routledge international handbook of qualitative nursing research (p.268-281). Routledge, Abingdon, Oxon.

31.  Labov W, Waletzky J (1972) Narrative analysis: Oral versions of personal experience. In Helms J (ed.) Essays on the verbal and visual arts (p. 12-44). University of Washington Press, Washington, Seattle.

32.  Agar M, Hobbs JR (1983) Natural plans: Using AI planning in the analysis of ethnographic interviews. Ethos: 11, 33-48.

33.  Peat FD (2002) Blackfoot Physics: A journey into the Native American Worldview. Planes Press, Grand Rapids.

34.  Walter CL, Hyde CA (2012) Community building practice: An expanded conceptual framework. In Minkler M. (ed.) Community organizing and community building for health and welfare (p. 78-94). Rutgers University Press, New Brunswick.

35.  Benbow S (2009) Societal abuse in the lives of individuals with mental illness. Canadian Nurse 105: 30-32.

36.  Johnstone MJ (2001) Stigma, social justice and the rights of the mentally ill: challenging the status quo. Aust N Z J Ment Health Nurs 10: 200-209.

37.  Canadian Federation for Mental Health Nurses (2006) Canadian standards for psychiatric-mental health nursing.

38.  De Leeuw S, Greenwood M, Cameron E (2009) Deviant constructions: How governments preserve colonial narratives of addictions and poor mental health to intervene into the lives of Indigenous children and families in Canada. International Journal of Mental Health and Addictions 8: 282-295.

39.  Browne A, Smye V, Varcoe C (2005) The relevance of postcolonial theoretical perspectives to research in Aboriginal health. Canadian

Journal of Nursing Research 37: 16-37. http://www.ncbi.nlm.nih.gov/pubmed/16541817.

40. Koptie S (2010) Inferiorizing Indigenous communities and intentional colonial poverty. First Peoples Child and Family Review 5: 96-106.

41. Brascoupé S, Waters C (2009) Exploring the applicability of the concept of cultural safety to Aboriginal health and community wellness. Journal of Aboriginal Health 5: 6-41.

42. McKegney S (2007). "We have been silent too long." In Magic weapons: Aboriginal writers remaking community after Residential School (pp. 59-99). University of Manitoba Press, Winnipeg, Manitoba.

43. Canadian Nurses Association (2010) Social justice: A means to an end, an end in itself.

44. Labonte R (2012) Community, community development, and the forming of authentic partnerships: Some critical reflections. In Minkler M (ed.) Community organizing and community building for health and welfare (p. 95-109). Rutgers University Press, New Brunswick.

45. Ciccone MM, Aquilino A, Cortese F, Scicchitano P, Sassara M, et al. (2010) Feasibility and effectiveness of a disease and care management model in the primary health care system for patients with heart failure and diabetes (Project Leonardo). Vasc Health Risk Manag 6: 297-305.

46. Wells KJ, Battaglia TA, Dudley DJ, Garcia R, Greene A, et al. (2008) Patient navigation: state of the art or is it science? Cancer 113: 1999-2010.

47. Lavalle LF (2009) Practical application of an Indigenous research framework and two qualitative indigenous research methods: Sharing circles and Anishnaabe symbol-based reflection. International Institute for Qualitative Methodology 8: 21-40

# 20

# Skilled Versus Unskilled Assistance in Home Delivery: Maternal Complications, Stillbirth and Neonatal Death in Indonesia

**Fase Badriah**[1*]**, Takeru Abe**[2]**, Baequni**[1,3] **and Akihito Hagihara**[3]

[1]*Syarif Hidayatullah Islamic State University, Faculty of Medicine and Health Sciences, Department of Public Health, Indonesia*

[2]*Waseda University, Faculty of Human Sciences, Department of Health Sciences and Social Welfare, Saitama, Japan*

[3]*Osaka University, School of Human Science, Department of International Collaboration, Osaka, Japan*

[4]*Kyushu University, Graduate School of Medicine, Department of Health Services, Management and Policy, Fukuoka, Japan.*

**\*Corresponding author:** Fase Badriah, Department of Public Health, Faculty of Medicine and Health Sciences, Syarief Hidayatullah State Islamic University (UIN) Jalan Kertamukti nomor 9, Pisangan, Ciputat, Jakarta, Indonesia, 15419; E-mail: fase_bzm@uinjkt.ac.id

## Abstract

The purpose of this study was to compare adverse intra-partum and post-partum outcomes for home deliveries with skilled and unskilled birth assistance. A cross-sectional study examined Indonesia Demographic Health Survey (IDHS 2007) data for 3,811 ever-married women who had had home deliveries in 2006 and 2007. A logistic regression analysis was used to examine associations between type of assistance at delivery and outcomes. This study found that there was a significantly higher probability of adverse outcomes with skilled assistance than with unskilled assistance for complications at birth and for complications after giving birth. Home deliveries with skilled assistance are not free from the risks of maternal morbidity and neonatal death. This finding raises doubts about the impact of skilled birth assistance. These results call for appropriate training to manage complications during and after childbirth by home delivery using skilled birth assistance. Further research is required.

**Keywords:** Indonesia; Maternal complications; Stillbirth; Home delivery; Assistance at delivery

## Introduction

Unskilled health workers, or "traditional birth attendants" (TBAs), have been suggested as a cause of maternal mortality and undesired neonatal outcomes in home deliveries. In response to the high proportion of home deliveries without skilled assistance and to improve access to professional care at birth as a means of reducing child and maternal mortality, the Indonesian Ministry of Health began placing midwives in villages [1]. In addition, apart from enhancing the awareness, understanding, and appreciation of Millennium Development Goal (MDG) 5 in Indonesia, by 1996 more than 50,000 village midwives had been placed in villages around the country to support progress towards achieving the MDGs related to improving maternal and child health.

This intervention increased the proportion of deliveries attended by skilled assistants from 43% in 1997 [2] to 79% in 2007 [3]. However, previous research on local healthcare in rural villages has reported on the quality of care provided by skilled assistants [3,4] and has found that increasing the rate of skilled assistance at delivery did not reduce the maternal mortality rate or maternal morbidity [4,5].

Other studies reported that skilled delivery was not associated with reduced neonatal-maternal mortality overall, but there were interaction effects with geographic region [6-8]. Very few studies have reported associations between type of assistance and outcomes for home delivery after increasing the proportion of skilled assistants. The aim of the present study was to compare outcomes for home deliveries using skilled birth assistance (midwives) with outcomes using

unskilled birth assistance (UBA). The outcomes included complications at birth, stillbirths and neonatal outcomes.

## Methods

### Data

We used data from the 2007 Indonesia Demographic and Health Survey (IDHS), a survey conducted periodically to evaluate demographic and health situations in Indonesia. The survey is designed to provide nationally representative information on demographics and maternal and child health in Indonesia. It has been administered as part of the global MEASURE DHS (Demographic and Health Surveys) program [9]. The IDHS recode consisted of IDBR51SV (Birth Recode), IDCR51SV (Couple's Recode), IDHR51SV (Household Recode), IDKR51SV (Children's Recode), IDMR51SV (Male Recode), and IDPR52SV (Household Member Recode). This program was implemented by ICF International in Calverton, Maryland, in partnership with the Johns Hopkins Bloomberg School of Public Health [9].

### Study design and sample

This research was a cross-sectional study examining the type of delivery assistance (skilled or unskilled). **The data set has one record for every child ever born to an interviewed woman. It** contains the full history of all women interviewed, including information on pregnancy, postnatal care, immunization, and healthcare for every child born in the last 5 years. To minimize recall bias, we selected sample data on all babies born within 2 years of the survey (2006 and 2007) and their mothers. The total number of babies was 7,509.

We excluded babies born at health facilities (3,305) because this study aimed to examine home delivery. We excluded twin births (68 babies, 1.6%), babies who required medical doctors for delivery assistance (18 babies, 0.4%), babies who required nurses for delivery assistance (73 babies or 1.7%), and records with missing values (235 babies, 5.6%). The study excluded medical doctors as delivery assistants because generally in Indonesia most mothers who use medical doctors for home deliveries have a known higher risk at birth, and medical doctors are generally recommended for births at health facilities. This study excluded nurses used as delivery assistance because the number was small (1.7%) and because this study was focused on evaluating Indonesia's policy of placing midwives in villages around the country to increase the proportion of health professionals as delivery assistants. We also excluded twin births because these births might involve higher risks for low birth weight and a higher infant mortality rate [10]. Finally, 3,811 home deliveries were analyzed further (Figure 1).

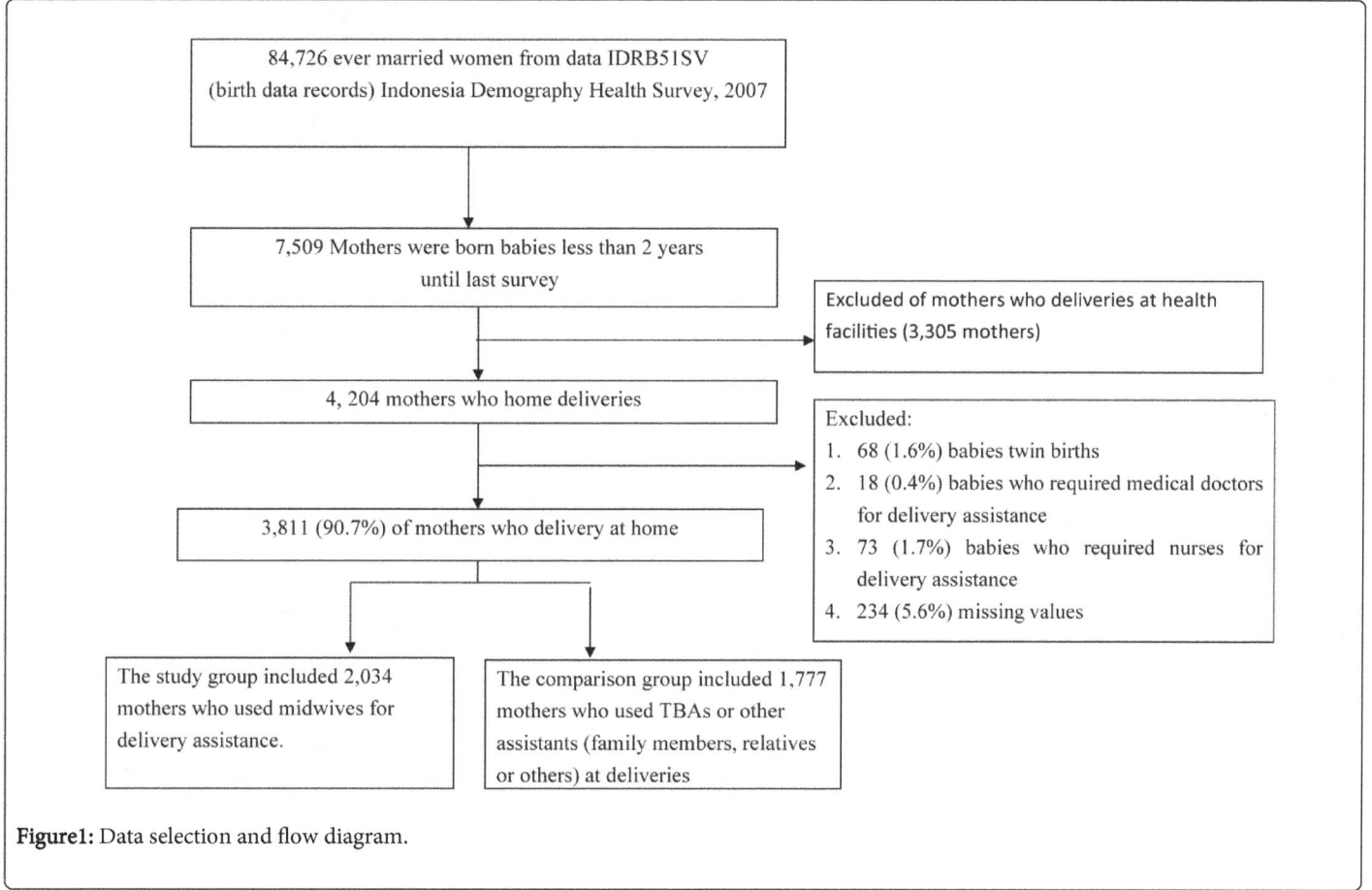

**Figure1:** Data selection and flow diagram.

## Study variables

The independent variable was the categorical variable type of delivery assistance (skilled assistance or UBA). Skilled assistance included delivery assistance by a village midwife, a local midwife, or any midwife. UBA included delivery assistance by a TBA, a relative, or a family member.

Mothers' characteristics and prenatal healthcare services during pregnancy were confounding variables for maternal and neonatal outcomes. They were included in the analysis as independent variables. Independent variables included socio-demographic factors (wealth index, which originally had five categories that were then reduced to three for the analysis; type of residence, categorized into urban and rural; and mother's education level), mothers' characteristics (the mother's age at the time of the infant's birth; parity; and complications during pregnancy, such as vaginal bleeding, fever, and convulsions; prenatal healthcare during pregnancy; and tetanus vaccine injection before birth [9].

Maternal outcomes included complications at the time of birth and complications after birth (Figure 2). The variable covering delivery complications was based on four types of obstetric complications reported by mothers: prolonged labor (referring to strong and regular contractions lasting more than 1 day and 1 night), excessive vaginal bleeding that soaked more than three pieces of cloth, high fever and foul-smelling vaginal discharge, and convulsions with loss of consciousness [9,11]. Most maternal morbidity and mortality is due to direct obstetric complications that occur during labor and after birth [12]. Stillbirths and neonatal deaths were used because the WHO reported an association between birth attendants and stillbirth and neonatal death [13-15]. Stillbirth is the birth of a baby that shows no sign of life at birth (fetal death). We used two variables for neonatal death: neonatal death (death occurring 1–28 days after live birth) and early neonatal death (death during the first 7 days of life) [16].

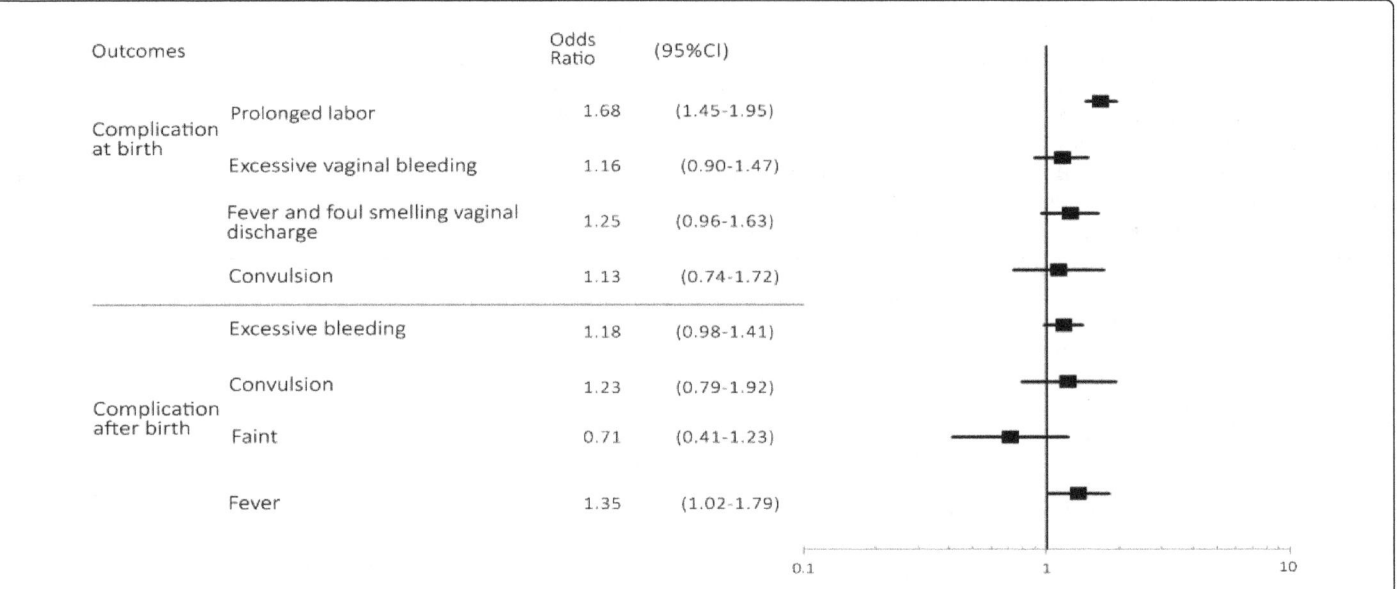

**Figure 2:** Parameter estimate (odds ratio and 95% CI) of conditional logistic regression analyses complication at birth and after birth comparing skilled versus unskilled delivery assistants.

## Statistical methods

To describe the characteristics of the mothers and prenatal care during pregnancy, we performed an analysis of frequency tabulations of all variables. We used a crude odds ratio (OR) and an adjusted odds ratio with a 95% confidence interval (CI) to investigate the estimated associations [17]. First, we used a crude model that considered how the independent variable (type of assistance at delivery) influenced all outcomes. Second, we used an adjusted model that considered how all independent variables influenced these outcomes.

We used logistic regression analyses to determine whether there was any significant association between the outcomes and the independent variable. All p-values reported are two-sided. A p-value less than 0.05 was considered to indicate statistical significance. Data analysis was conducted using SPSS software (ver. 18.0 for Windows; SPSS, Inc., Chicago, IL, USA).

## Results

Almost half of all mothers used skilled birth assistance (53.4%), and the other half used UBA (46.6%) for home deliveries. Characteristics and maternal health care differed significantly between mothers using skilled assistance and UBA, except for complications during pregnancy (p=0.713) and sex of the baby (p=0.599) (Table 1). These results did not support the assumption that a person with a risk of complications during pregnancy would benefit from skilled assistance rather than UBA.

| Variables | Skilled (n=2,034) | Unskilled assistance (n=1,777) | P value |
|---|---|---|---|
| **Mother's Characteristic** | | | |
| Wealth index | | | P<0.001 |
| Poorer | 1,165(30.57) | 1,416(37.15) | |
| Middle to richer | 869(22.80) | 361(9.47) | |
| Residence | | | P<0.001 |
| Urban | 531(13.93) | 274(7.18) | |
| Rural | 1,503(39.43) | 1,503(39.44) | |
| Mother's education | | | P<0.001 |
| Primary or less | 826(21.67) | 1,183(31.04) | |
| secondary or higher | 1,208(31.69) | 594(15.59) | |

| | | | |
|---|---|---|---|
| Mother's age at child birth | | | P<0.001 |
| Older (more than 35 year-old) | 191(5.01) | 234(6.14) | |
| Adult ( 25–35 year-old) | 1,057(27.73) | 842(22.09) | |
| Young mother (< 25 year-old) | 786(20.62) | 701(18.39) | |
| Birth-order number | | | P<0.001 |
| First born | 676(17.73) | 425(11.15) | |
| 2nd–3rd born | 969(25.42) | 775(20.33) | |
| ≥4th born | 389(25.42) | 577(15.14) | |
| Parity | | | P<0.001 |
| High, ≥4 times | 199(5.22) | 368(9.65) | |
| Low, < 4 times | 1,835(48.15) | 1,409(36.97) | |
| **Maternal health care and condition** | | | |
| Tetanus injection before birth | | | P<0.001 |
| Yes | 1,489 (39.07) | 1,007(26.42) | |
| No | 545(14.30) | 770(20.20) | |
| Prenatal care | | | P <0.001 |
| No | 1,057(27.73) | 1,095(28.73) | |
| Yes, professional health | 977(25.63) | 682(17.89) | |
| Complications during pregnancy | | | 0.713 |
| Yes | 175(4.59) | 147(3.86) | |
| No | 1859(48.7) | 1630(42.77) | |
| Child Gender | | | 0.599 |
| Female | 951(24.95) | 846(22.20) | |
| Male | 1,083(28.42) | 931(24.43) | |

**Table 1:** Mother's characteristics and maternal health care.

In terms of maternal outcomes, the mothers who used skilled assistance during delivery experienced more complications at the time of the birth (48.8%) compared with mothers who used UBA (36.3%). Compared with UBA, skilled delivery was associated with a 75% increase (adjusted OR=1.75) in the probability of complications at birth after controlling for other confounding variables. More complications after birth were also found among women who had skilled assistance (15.9%) compared with mothers who had UBA (9.83%). In addition, compared with UBA, skilled assistance was associated with a 59% increase (adjusted OR=1.59) in the probability of complications after birth after controlling for other confounding variables (Table 2).

| End point | | | | Odds ratio/ 95% CI | |
|---|---|---|---|---|---|
| | Total sample | Skilled | Unskilled assistance | Crude | Adjusted[*] |
| Maternal complication | | | | | |
| Complications at birth | 43.0 (/3811) | 48.8(994/ 2,034) | 36.3 (646/1,777) | 1.67(1.47 to 1.91)[*] | 1.75 (1.52 to 2.02)[*] |
| Complications after birth | 25.8 (2497/3811) | 15.9 (608/2,034) | 9.83 (375/1,777) | 1.73 (1.50 to 1.99)[*] | 1.59 (1.37 to 1.85)[*] |
| Neonatal outcomes | | | | | |

| | | | | | |
|---|---|---|---|---|---|
| Stillbirths | 0,7 (27/3811) | 0.4 (17/2,034) | 0.3 (10/1,777) | 1.49 (0.68 to 3.26) | 2.17 (0.92 to 5.09) |
| Neonatal death (excluding stillbirths) | | | | | |
| 1- 7 days | 1.0 (39/3811) | 0.4 (15/2,034) | 0.6 (24/1,777) | 0.54 (0.28 to 1.04) | 0.73 (0.36 to 1.47) |
| 1-28 days | 1.3 (82/3811) | 0.5 (21/2,034) | 0.7 (28/1,777) | 0.65 (0.37 to 1.15) | 0.93 (0.50 to 1.74) |

**Table 2:** Numbers and percentages of maternal-neonatal outcomes and parameter estimate (crude-adjusted odds ratios 95 % confidence interval) of regression logistic analyses. * Analyses were adjusted for variable in table 1; ** P value < 0.00.

Among complications at birth, compared with UBA, skilled assistance was associated with a 68% increase (adjusted OR=1.68) in the probability of prolonged labor after controlling for other confounding variables. Among complications after birth, compared with UBA, skilled assistance was associated with a 35% increase (adjusted OR=1.35) in the probability of fever after controlling for other confounding variables (Figure 2).

There was no significant difference between skilled assistance and UBA in terms of stillbirth. In addition, there were no statistically different outcomes in terms of neonatal death between mothers who used midwives and those who used UBA (Table 2).

These findings do not align with the general belief that skilled birth assistance can mitigate adverse outcomes. Compared with UBA, skilled delivery was associated with an increase in the probability of complications at birth (prolonged labor) and after birth (fever). Moreover, compared with UBA, skilled assistance yielded no significantly different outcomes for stillbirth and neonatal death.

## Discussion

Our findings for complications at birth and after birth raise doubts about the impact of skilled birth assistance (alone) on maternal outcomes at delivery. These findings may be attributable to the fact that the skilled assistants were placed in the community rather recently, and were thus well-educated but less experienced at managing prolonged labor at birth and fever after birth by home delivery.

Our results may have several causes. The first is the competency of skilled birth assistants for normal birth assistance. The WHO defines a skilled birth assistant as someone "trained to proficiency in the skills needed to manage normal (uncomplicated) pregnancies, childbirth and the immediate postnatal period, and in the identification, management and referral of complications in women and newborns" [18]. The skilled assistants might not have been ready to provide assistance because they lacked tool kits for home delivery. Most midwives might have spent less time in the village compared with those who provided UBA, who were more experienced and lived permanently in the village [3,19].

Home deliveries that use skilled assistance are not free from the risk of death. Mothers and babies are especially vulnerable to death; a woman with postpartum hemorrhage or a baby with birth asphyxia, sepsis, or complications from preterm birth can die within hours or even minutes if the appropriate care is not provided. Complications during childbirth are often unexpected.

We found significant differences between the two groups in parity and birth number. There were more first-time births and mothers with parity >4 among skilled assistance deliveries. This suggests that

maternal parity might also have had an impact on the adverse outcomes. Specifically, it might have triggered prolonged labor for women with first-time births and excessive bleeding for mothers with parity >4. We found that mothers with high parity were more likely to choose skilled assistance. This finding calls for appropriate training of skilled assistants to recognize when a birth is high risk and not normal, a plan for timely transfer, emergency skills to reduce hemorrhage and excessive bleeding, and emergency skills to manage prolonged labor.

This study found a higher percentage of stillbirths among mothers who used skilled assistance (0.4%) compared with mothers who used UBA (0.3%; Table 2). This might be related to childbirth complications, the first of the five major causes of stillbirth [20,21]. A high number of maternal complications at the time of birth may cause a high incidence of stillbirths among mothers who use skilled assistance at delivery.

This study found a higher proportion of neonatal deaths among mothers using UBA compared with those using skilled assistants at delivery. Similar findings have been reported in previous studies [22,23]. Neonatal infections account for about half of all neonatal deaths, and the leading causes of death are preterm birth complications, birth asphyxia, and poor obstetric care provided by unskilled birth assistants at delivery [23,24]. Although, there was no statistically significant association between type of assistance and neonatal death, the low proportion of deaths in newborn babies delivered by midwives showed better newborn care by midwives compared with unskilled birth assistants.

A previous study found that most midwives perform many tasks (including providing nutrition and immunizations) and attend few births, so their capacity to manage complications during childbirth and to recognize the need for referrals may be compromised because they encounter these situations infrequently [4]. Additionally, midwifery training focuses on normal births, which may restrict the midwife's capacity to manage complications during and after births. More importantly, there are substantial barriers to life-saving emergency obstetric care for home deliveries even when a midwife is present.

### Strengths and limitations of the study

To our knowledge, this is the first reported study to evaluate the association between type of assistance at delivery and immediate outcomes for newborn babies and mothers following home delivery. Our findings raise doubts about the impact of skilled birth assistants, because there are substantial barriers to life-saving emergency obstetric care for home deliveries even when a midwife is present.

This study has some limitations. First, we used the IDBR51SV data from the DHS, which lacks information on maternal deaths during childbirth. Second, the exclusion of mothers who required medical doctors or nurses for delivery assistance might affect the generalizability of this study. However, the number of cases excluded was relatively small (0.5% for medical doctors and 0.5% for nurses). Thus, our findings might be little affected by those exclusions. Third, the use of secondary data might have affected the validity of the findings because the data were primarily self-reported. However, the data have previously been used for research on a range of topics, and the quality of the data set had been maintained by ICF International [11]. Fourth, unknown confounding variables that were not assessed due to a lack of data, such as gestational age and birth weight of babies delivered at home, might explain why there was no statistically significant difference in neonatal mortality between mothers who used skilled assistants and those who received UBA. This might affect the generalizability of our findings to other countries.

## Conclusions

This study confirmed that skilled birth assistants cannot mitigate adverse outcomes for home deliveries. The results suggest the need to monitor and assess the quality of care provided by midwives who assist with home deliveries. We suggest a comprehensive approach to improving the performance of midwives, such as clinical training using limited tool kits and a standard operating procedure (SOP) for managing complications during and after birth for home delivery assistants before midwives are placed in a village or rural area [25,26]. The skills of midwives included management of women and newborns with complications and referral to health facilities.

Acknowledging that midwives lack experience (compared with unskilled birth assistants) may be helpful. A subsequent study investigating maternal outcomes for recently graduated skilled birth assistants compared with those who have been practicing for longer might provide some insight as to how competency assessment influences outcomes.

## References:

1. Ministry of Health, Government of Indonesia (1989) Directorate of Community Health.

2. Goverment of Indonesia, Ministary of Health (1998) The Indonesian translation of Central Agency on Statistics (BPS), & National Family Planning Coordinating Board, Ministry of Health, ORC Macro. Indonesia Demographic and Health Survey 1997. Calverton, Maryland: BPS and ORC Macro.

3. Makowiecka K, Achadi E, Izati Y, Ronsmans C (2008) Midwifery provision in two districts in Indonesia: how well are rural areas served? Health Policy Plan 23: 67-75.

4. Ronsmans C, Scott S, Qomariyah SN, Achadi E, Braunholtz D, et al. (2009) Professional assistance during birth and maternal mortality in two Indonesian districts. Bull World Health Organ 87: 416-423.

5. Graham W, Bell J, Bullough C (2001) Can skilled attendance at delivery reduce maternal mortality in developing countries? Safe motherhood strategies: a review of the evidence. Studies in Health Services Organization and Policy 17: ITG Press: 97-130.

6. Singh K, Brodish P, Suchindran C (2014) A regional multilevel analysis: can skilled birth attendants uniformly decrease neonatal mortality? Matern Child Health J 18: 242-249.

7. Anand S, Bärnighausen T (2004) Human resources and health outcomes: cross-country econometric study. Lancet 364: 1603-1609.

8. McClure EM, Goldenberg RL, Bann CM (2007) Maternal mortality, stillbirth and measures of obstetric care in developing and developed countries. Int J Gynaecol Obstet 96: 139-146.

9. http://legacy.measuredhs.com/

10. Blondel B, Kogan MD, Alexander GR, Dattani N, Kramer MS, et al. (2002) The impact of the increasing number of multiple births on the rates of preterm birth and low birthweight: an international study. Am J Public Health 92: 1323-1330.

11. ICF International (2011) Demographic and Health Surveys Methodology - Questionnaires: Household, Woman's, and Man's. MEASURE DHS Phase III: Calverton, Maryland, USA.

12. Ronsmans C1, Graham WJ; Lancet Maternal Survival Series steering group (2006) Maternal mortality: who, when, where, and why. Lancet 368: 1189-1200.

13. 2012 World Health Organization, Newborn Care at Births.

14. Yakoob MY1, Lawn JE, Darmstadt GL, Bhutta ZA (2010) Stillbirths: epidemiology, evidence, and priorities for action. Semin Perinatol 34: 387-394.

15. Yakoob MY, Ali MA, Ali MU, Imdad A, Lawn JE, et al. (2011) The effect of providing skilled birth attendance and emergency obstetric care in preventing stillbirths. BMC Public Health 11 Suppl 3: S7.

16. Tinker A, ten Hoope-Bender P, Azfar S, Bustreo F, Bell R (2005) A continuum of care to save newborn lives. Lancet 365: 822-825.

17. Rothman KJ, Greenland S, Lash L Timothy (2008) Modern Epidemiology. Philadelphia, PA: Lippincott-Raven :51-69.

18. WHO (2004) Making pregnancy safer: the critical role of the skilled attendant: a joint statement by WHO, ICM and FIGO.

19. Heywood P, Harahap NP, Ratminah, M (2010) Current situation of midwives in Indonesia: Evidence from 3 districts in West Java Province. BMC Research Notes 3: 287.

20. Stillbirth Collaborative Research Network Writing Group1 (2011) Association between stillbirth and risk factors known at pregnancy confirmation. JAMA 306: 2469-2479.

21. Stillbirths-TheLancet.com (2011) An Executive Summary for The Lancet's Series. The lancet series.

22. Black RE, Cousens S, Johnson HL, Lawn JE, Rudan I, et al. (2010) Global, regional, and national causes of child mortality in 2008: a systematic analysis. Lancet 375: 1969-1987.

23. Hatt L, Stanton C, Makowiecka K, Adisasmita A, Achadi E, et al. (2007) Did the strategy of skilled attendance at birth reach the poor in Indonesia? Bull World Health Organ 85: 774-782.

24. Hatt L, Stanton C, Ronsmans C, Makowiecka K, Adisasmita A (2009) Did professional attendance at home births improve early neonatal survival in Indonesia? Health Policy Plan 24: 270-278.

25. Koblinsky M, Matthews Z, Hussein J, Mavalankar D, Mridha MK, et al. (2006) Going to scale with professional skilled care. Lancet 368: 1377-1386.

26. Darmstadt GL, Walker N, Lawn JE, Bhutta ZA, Haws RA, et al. (2008) Saving newborn lives in Asia and Africa: cost and impact of phased scale-up of interventions within the continuum of care. Health Policy Plan 23: 101-117.

# 21

# Specific Nursing Care Rendered in Hepatic Encephalopathy: Contemporary Review and New Clinical Insights

Zeljko Vlaisavljević * and Ivan Rankovic

*University of Mississippi Clinical Centre of Serbia, Clinic for Gastroenterolgy and Hepatology, Street of Dr Koste Todorovica 2, 11 000 Belgrade, Serbia*

**\*Corresponding author:** Zeljko Vlaisavljević, Clinical Centre of Serbia, Clinic for Gastroenterolgy and Hepatology, Street of Dr Koste Todorovica 2, 11 000 Belgrade, Serbia, E-mail: kcszeljko@gmail.com

## Abstract

**Introduction:** Hepatic Encephalopathy (HE) is neuropsychiatric deterioration syndrome due to hepatic insufficiency. HE symptoms appear gradually ranging from altered mental status to deep coma and manifest as disorders of orientation, memory, perception, reasoning, focusing, rigor, and generalized convulsions. Four levels of HE exist with different symptoms.

**Aim of the paper:** To observe Specific Nursing Care rendered to hepatic encephalopathy patients and determining the significance of nurse education and employment length in HE patient healthcare.

**Methodology:** This is a cross-sectional study of 70 nurses in (Clinical Center of Serbia, Clinic for Gastroenterology and Hepatology) Between May1 to December15, 2011. The questionnaire was divided into two parts with 18 questions in total. The first part consisted of general questions (sex, professional education, working experience, working hours), while the second part had 13 questions assessing knowledge of nurses about the specificities of HE healthcare

**Results:** The most common cause of hepatic encephalopathy is ethylic cirrhosis with 69.2%, while 30.8% of patients with cirrhosis and HE died in period from 1.5.-15.12.2011. Nurses (N=70) declared that 91.4% of them had no adequate conditions to provide necessary HE patient healthcare. Out of N=70, 78.6% knew how to recognize first symptoms of HE while 64.3% nurses made no difference between HE and other diseases.

**Conclusion:** Specificity of HE patient healthcare encompassess nursing interventions and diagnosis. Through continuous education, respecting previous knowledge, it is necessary to focus on specific diseases such as hepatic encephalopathy with the aim of providing healthcare excellence.

**Keywords:** Healthcare; Hepatic encephalopathy; Nurse

## Abbreviation

HE: Hepatic Encephalopathy; CVC: Central Venous Catheter; HCC: Hepatocellular Carcinoma; SDD: Selective Digestive Decontamination; HRS: Hepatorenal Syndrome; DALY: The Disability-Adjusted Life Year; C: College; U: Univeryitet

## Introduction

Hepatic encephalopathy (HE) [1] represents potentially reversible reduction of neuropsychiatric functions due to acute and/or chronic liver disease. It occurs most often inpatients with portal hypertension. The beginning is usually insidious, and is characterized by subtle and sometimes periodical changes in memory, cognition, associative higher intellectual functions, as well as altered personality. The liver plays a central role in the regulation of other organ systems through the spectrum of its functions related to energetic metabolism, hormonal and electrolite balance, immunologic and immunomodulatory status. As a consequence, chronic liver disease causes a number of systemic manifestations that can dominate the clinical course. Some of these complications stem from the reduction in number of functional hepatocytes and the resulting loss of synthetic and metabolic functional capacity. Others consequences are from portal pressure, leading to portal vascular collaterals opening and shunting with bypassing the liver lobules. These manifestations of cirrhosis –reduced synthetic reserve and disrupted perfusion are functionally connected and can change over time depending on various pathophysiological demands. Subtle signs of hepatic encephalopathy can be observed in almost 70% of patients with liver cirrhosis and they are called the subclinical form of hepatic encephalopathy [2]. Hepatic encephalopathy can be provoked by dehydration, excessive protein intake through food and certain beverages, constipation, hypo and hyperkalemia, digestive tract haemorrhages, infections, renal failure, hypoxia, use of barbiturates and benzodiazepine, as well as changes in physical factors(climate and atmospheric disturbances). Hepatic encephalopathy is progressive in terms of its clinical prognostic character. A nurse needs to know well the symptoms of encephalopathy thus being able to react promptly and adequately in taking care of such a patient. Hepatic encephalopathy can manifest itself acutely with a rapid deterioration of mental functions leading to coma, with no previous symptomatology [3]. Being chronic reversible in patients with pronounced portal hypertension, it is caused by certain precipitating factors (constipation, bleeding, and diuretics) which can be identified and removed in most cases. The development of hepatic encephalopathy is a poor prognostic sign and is related to less than 32% of survival rate during first year. The most significant cause of this disease in the developed countries is alcohol abuse [4,5]. In Asia and Africa the most common cause of liver cirrhosis is hepatitis B virus (with or without delta antigens) [6]. The cause of cirrhosis of the liver can also be hepatitis C virus, hepatocellular carcinoma with intraparenchymatous dissemination(the so-called HCC satellite induced HE), various intoxications with heavy metals and poisonous gases, Wilson's disease (hepatolenticular degeneration), metabolic diseases (alpha-1 antitrypsin deficiency, as well as so-called storage diseases, such as hemochromatosis),while other half comprises autoimmune liver disease such as autoimmune hepatitis and primary biliary cirrhosis. HE has four grades of classification, on the basis of West-Haven Classification System [7] (Table1). HE diagnosis is established on the basis of physical clinical examination and biochemical panel. As far as biochemical markers are concerned, blood is taken for a complete blood workup which can indicate the presence of hyperammonemia usually with levels above 50mmol/l, elevated serum transaminases and bilirubin, hypokalemia, hyponatremia and azotemia. Analyses such as metabolic tests of glycaemia, serum osmolality, liver function enzymes, can point out to disorders in metabolism which are indicative for liver cirrhosis. Also urea, creatinine, eGFR, and cystatin C give away the functional capacity of kidneys whose function is also specifically altered in liver cirrhosis. If positive, hemoculture indicates the presence of pathogenic organisms, and administration of adequate antibiotics is mandatory. Coagulation status points to the presence of coagulopathy and low levels of coagulation factors predominantly factor V (with plasma half-life of 3-6h) and factor VII(also referred to as proaccelerin or labile factor) [8]. The biochemical examination of abdominal fluid, ascites (Rivalta test), bacteriological and cytomorphological examination (presence of malignant hyperchromatic cells) can also help determine the etiologic factor of liver lesion. Chest X-ray, ECG, ultrasound with portal system doppler examination and EEG are all basic diagnostic procedures that can be supplemented according to the state of the patient. The assessment of psychological status is conducted using a standardized algorithm preferably number connection test as well as using Glasgow Coma Scale when having severe HE form. Also, we must underline West-Haven criterias which are diagnostic hallmarks. Treatment is conducted through reduction of serum ammonia levels (restriction of animal proteins), administration of oral lactulose, oral or IV antibiotics, giving parenteral solutions with branched-chain amino acids, enemas, transfusions of blood and it's components, and general healthcare [9]. The final and ultimately complete treatment for liver cirrhosis with hepatic encephalopathy is liver transplantation. Transplantation is an incremental factor incuring patients with liver cirrhosis [10,11]. To accurately establish the diagnosis of hepatic encephalopathy it is necessary to determine the severity of liver disease, exclude cerebraltrauma, intracranial vascular and expansive lesions, metabolic disorders, as well as systemic hemodynamic distortions (checking continuously if cardiovascular and renal function is intact) [12]. As stated above, the approach to care differs depending on the level of encephalopathy in patients. It is necessary to establish adequate nursing diagnosis, upon which the planning goals for patient healthcare are defined. How does a patient with second (II) or third (III) grade hepatic encephalopathy clinically present? They speak incomprehensibly, they are often two or three dimensionally disoriented, with clinically pronounced abdomen due to ascites, their skin is sticky, colored from yellow too range. Their odor is sweet, as well as breath, obstipation to diarrhoea is present usually with bimodal

incontinence and oliguria. Nutrition in comatose patients is parenteral: using infusions, with nasogastric or nasojejunal tubes, or with PEG tube in most severe cases with coexisting disorders. Due to altered state of consciousness patients can be aggressive, agitated, and they can try to get out of bed and hurt themselves, therefore, they have to be placed in intensive care units under a 24-hour observation in beds with side rails.

| Grade 0 HE | **HE represents the minimal hepatic encephalopathy, known as subclinical, with minimal changes in personality and concentration.** |
|---|---|
| Grade I HE | Is characterized by trivial lack of consciousness, shortened attention span, insomnia, sleep inversion, euphoria or depression, irritability, decreased intellectual function with altered short term memory which rarely manifests |
| Grade II HE | clinically features the occurrence of lethargy, apathy, temporal disorientation, incomprehensible speech, inappropriate behavior and somnolence. |
| Grade III HE | Is characterized by somnolence, disorientation both in time and space, confusion or amnesia. |
| Grade IV | Represents coma. |

Table 1: West-Haven Classification System

## Research Material and Methods

Survey data was collected using the self-administration method to ensure the confidentiality and anonymity with a previous oral approval of nurses being questioned. The analysis of medical documentation and official protocols in the Clinic of Gastroenterology and Hepatology of the Clinical Centre of Serbia was also conducted for the time during the study period May 1. to December 15., 2011. Sample size is selected based on criteria that are nurses employed at the Clinic for Gastroenterology and Hepatology - Clinical Center of Serbia, as well as nurses who are working with patients of HE. Employed nurses that are included in the study - 70 of 98. Data processing The SPSS program for Windows, version 17.0, was used for data processing. The comparison of numerical markers between two groups (working experience and level of education) was made using the chi-square (X2) test. Values p<0.05 were taken as statistically significant. Ethical considerations This study was approved by the chief nursing educator, head-chief nurse, and department chief nurses of our clinic where the research was carried out, as well as by the head of the Department of Scientific and Research Work, Education Activity and Human Resources of the Clinic of Gastroenterology, the Director of the Clinic of Gastroenterology, and the Director of the Centre for Scientific Research Work, Education and Teaching Activities and Human Resources of the Clinical Centre of Serbia.

## General sample characteristics

Out of the total number of nurses (N=70), 62 of them (88.6%) had only secondary medical school completed, while 8 had college or university degrees (11.4%). According to the length of working experience, 30 respondents had less than 20 years of experience (42.9%), while 40 respondents had over 20 years of working experience (57.1%). The average working experience was 17.3 years. There were 6 male nurses (8.6%) and 64 female nurses (91.4%). 37 respondents worked in shifts (52.9%), while 33 of them worked only in the morning. In the hepatology ward within the Clinic of

Gastroenterohepatology, there were 30 grade I and II HE patients and 13 grade III and IV HE patients in the period between May 1 and December 15, 2011. The causes for grade III and IV patients were, results: The findings of this study revealed that the most common cause of hepatic encephalopathy is ethylic cirrhosis with 69.2%, toxic liver disease induced HE with 15.4%, autoimmune liver disease HE with 7.7%, and hepatitis C virus (HCV) HE with 7.7%. Four patients died, or 30.8% of the total number of patients with Grade III and IV HE. 38.5% suffered from portal vein thrombosis, while 66.7% had esophageal varices. Sex distribution consisted of 73.3% of male patients and 13.3% of female patients. Each one of the patients was diagnosed with hepatic encephalopathy (100%) using West-Haven criteria and adjunctive number connection test.

## Research results (Table 2)

Participants with 20 years of employment status knew that HE is disturbance of consciousness (96,7%), while those with more than 20 years of professional experience gave correct answer in 62,5%, (p=, 001), and there wasn't any statistical significance relating to the educational level between two groups. On question if they would know to recognise symptoms of HE, first group (one up to 20 years of employment) said that they would recognise (90%), and those over 20 years of experience gave positive answer in 70% (p=,044), while interpreting the educational status, there wasn't any significant statistical difference. Participants up to 20 years would know how to read blood tests (83%) and those over 20 years of employment status answered positively in 50% (p=,004).

| Question | N | C% | W% | According to working experience | | | | | According to education | | | | |
|---|---|---|---|---|---|---|---|---|---|---|---|---|---|
| | | | | Less than 20 y. C% | More than 20 y. C% | Less than 20 y. W% | More than 20 y. W% | P | SS C% | C & U C % | SS W% | C & U W % | P |
| Hepatic encephalopathy is a disorder of consciousness | 70 | 77.1 | 22.9 | 96.7 | 62.5 | 3.3 | 37.5 | 0.001 | 74.2 | 100 | 25.8 | 0 | NS |
| I know how to recognize first signs and symptoms of HE | 70 | 78.6 | 21.4 | 90 | 70 | 10 | 30 | 0.044 | 75.8 | 100 | 24 | 0 | NS |
| Can you interpret blood results# of patients with HE | 70 | 64.3 | 35.7 | 83.3 | 50 | 16.7 | 50 | 0.004 | 61.3 | 87.5 | 38.7 | 12.5 | NS |
| HE is a chronic disease | 70 | 31.4 | 68.6 | 26.7 | 35 | 73.3 | 65 | NS | 27.4 | 62.5 | 72.6 | 37.5 | 0.044 |
| Do you work in adequate conditions for HE patients care | 70 | 8.6 | 91.4 | 10 | 7.5 | 90 | 92.5 | NS | 4.8 | 37.5 | 95.2 | 62.5 | 0.002 |
| Are there procedural standards for providing health care to HE patients | 70 | 5.7 | 94.3 | 3.3 | 7.5 | 96.7 | 92.5 | NS | 3.2 | 25 | 96.8 | 75 | 0.013 |

**Table 2:** Knowledge and attitude of nurses toward hepatic encephalopathy Knowledge and attitude of nurses toward hepatic encephalopathy, N – total, C – correct answer, W – wrong answer, SS – Secondary medical school, C – College, U – University, NS-not significant, #Blood results: urea, creatinine, hepatic transaminases

The fact that HE is chronical disease nurses with higher education (C* i U*) knew in 62, 5%, while nurses that just graduated from high school didn't know that (72,6%) (p=,044). Up to 91, 4% of nurses said that they don't have adequate conditions for taking care of HE patients i.e. nurses with high school (95,2%) and those with higher education (62,5%) (p=,044). On question are there standards in healthcare procedures, 94,3% of all replied negatively, and influence of education for this question gave statistically significant result in those with high school in 96,8%, and in those with higher education in 75% ( p=,013).

## Discussion

Liver cirrhosis represents around 1% of overall global disease burden expressed in DALY (The disability-adjusted life year). The share of cirrhosis in global structure of dying is 1.4% [13]. In line with this non-negligible percentage, the prevention of this disease is of great importance. And if disease does appear, high-quality healthcare is

crucial in the clinical management process. Liver diseases comprised 1.0% of the total mortality rate in central Serbia and Vojvodina in 2000 [14]. Accessing the medical documentation, one can observe that share of cirrhosis in the structure of dying is correlating with prevailing alcohol intake as the primary etiological factor. Regardless of etiology, patients with hepatic encephalopathy have multiple specificities of health care. This paper aims to present the specificities of health care through nursing interventions in the purpose of providing better excellence in healthcare. Adequate care is of utmost importance in all phases of HE [12]. The specificity of health care for such patients would reflect in: Low-protein diet (meat and meat products), mushy and/or liquid food (due to accompanying esophagogastric varices). Diet regulates protein catabolism and allows the ammonia levels nivelating in blood, simultaneously leading to adequate passage through intestines which prevents the occurrence of constipation. The limited intake of proteins is an important part of therapy, since it enables the correction of nitrogenous substances balance in the organism [12]. The intake of probiotics regulates the gut flora and bowel movement, on the one hand, while it reduces the risk of bacterial translocation and subsequent septicemia as a common secondary complication in HE patients, on the other. The reduction in the possibility of sepsis development improves the prognosis of patients with hepatic dysfunction, thus the intake of yoghurt with added probiotics is recommended as an adjuvant nutritional therapy [15].

The intake of lactulose, a non-absorbable disaccharide which reduces the level of serum ammonia concentration, as well as its absorption, is the cornerstone therapy in the overall strategy of HE treatment [4,16,17]. A patient should not be administered any oral therapy two hours before and after the intake of lactulose to achieve full therapeutic effect of administered drug. The optimal intake of liquid is of great importance due to ascites, with special attention on avoiding the over diuresis syndrome. The effective diuresis larger than 600-800/24h must not be provoked because it leads to prerenal azotemia, which further deteriorates cerebral perfusion, increasing the severity of HE. Every infection can lead to or deteriorate the condition of patients into encephalopathy, thus, for the purpose of monitoring the transaminases in blood, bilirubin, proteins and other biochemical factors, a nurse has to perform venepuncture almost daily. Therefore, placing a CVC is recommended, naturally, only if the coagulation status of the patient allows such an intervention. Infections increase the mortality of HE cirrhotic patients, especially pneumonia, sometimes with the main cause of death in such patients [18]. Special attention should be focused on decubital ulcers which may appear due to prolonged bed lying. The risk of cellulitis also increases because of poor skin integrity and development of peripheral edema [8]. Inadequately treated cellulitis can lead to fasciitis and a potentially lethal phlegmon – Vibrio vulnificus cellulitis. Urinary catheter insertion. Everyday care of catheter should be overall clinical strategy hallmark. Continuous diuresis monitoring with the measurement of urine outputshould be an important parameter which pinpoints the beginning of hepatorenal syndrome (HRS). Time span development of low urine output is the differentiation stigmata between type I and type II of HRS. Type I HRS is the prognostic omen sign of the primary liver disease [19].Rinsing the bladder and clearing or other undesirable contents is beneficial thus preventing post renal insufficiency or azotaemia [20].Treatment of mouth cavity, where candida may appear due to overzealous antibiotic administration should also be considered as the mainstay of therapy. These patients have ascites and large abdominal girth, their skin should be treated with hydrating creams, especially in abdominal region, since there skin is stretched and the feeling of pain and tension is highly pronounced. Positive reciprocal correlation and associated with both hepatic encephalopathy and асцитес as a risk factor for these complications and for death [21]. Abdominal therapeutic and diagnostic puncture and centhesis should be performed rationally and moderately. The use of diuretics and abdominal centhesis leads to positive response in 90% of patients, with the decrease in total body weight being the best indicator of diuretic, nutritional-dietetic and interventional therapy. However, the decrease in total bodyweight must not exceed 10% during a weekly period [22]. The hepatorenal syndrome (HRS) may insidiously overcome compensatory mechanisms and administered therapy and is characterized by acute renal failure with decrease in total urine output. It occurs in approximately 10% of patients with disease progression [23]. Using diuretics, nutrition and interventional techniques should be cautious respecting hemodynamically over-sensed nephrons. In some patients, progressive oliguria appears with rapid increase in serum concentration of creatinine, and this is type I of hepatorenal syndrome. Type II HRS appears more frequently and it is characterized by increase in serum concentration of creatinine and urea with chronic to moderate progression which usually takes place in the time period of six or over six weeks from the disease starting point (pathological black point).Care of IV cannulas. Every intravenous route is a potential place of infection entry [8]. Bacterial infections are present in about 15% -47% of patients with cirrhosis of the liver, especially in relation to gram-negative bacteria. The most common spontaneous bacterial peritonitis (SBP), urinary tract infection, pneumonia, pleural empyema and sepsis[24].The patient receives infusions through one or preferably more IV routes, most often glucose or 0.9% NaCl with added potassium, magnesium sulfate or concentrated 3%NaCl [25]. Here the nurses role is pivotal giving the therapy strategy cornerstones of not only maintaining IV routes but also recognizing complications early e.g. thrombophlebitis, deep vein thrombosis or apparent hemorrhagic cutaneous or mucosal syndrome. Patients with acute liver failure, with grade III or more importantly grade IV HE, need to be intubated and put on mechanical ventilation following gas analyses every8 hours. This should be standard of nursing monitoring care surveilling respiratory insufficiency (most frequently etiological factor is hepatopulmonary syndrome).Mechanical ventilation should be with sedating agents like fentanyl aiming the protection of respiratory system and/or phenobarbital which is a neurocerebral modulatory agent for early treatment of cerebral edema by decreasing intracranial pressure as well as maintaining sedation [3]. Central nursing fields of intensive treatment should encompass knowing all the principal pharmacodynamics and pharmacokinetics of neuromodulatory agents which have effect on respiratory function. Nurses should be able to recognize overdosing of these agents since they are pulmonary function depressants when used in higher doses. Bleeding in the digestive tract complicates further HE patients treatment since proteins from blood contribute to high levels of serum ammonia. Therefore, intestines should be decontaminated and cleared of its content. This maneuver is called selective digestive decontamination (SDD). Also bleeding induced infections can occur, so proper use of antibiotic prophylaxis should be given respecting pharmacokinetic profiles of given antibiotics. One old and good technique which is in use for decadesis SDD through deep enemas with or without lactulose. Therefore, nurses need to independently perform an intervention of giving deep enemas as an overall therapeutic modality. In the case of hematemesis doctor inserts the Sengstaken-Blakemoor tube with the necessity to provide drainage and skin care around the nostrils. A nurse has to prepare both the adequate material and the patient, and she or he has to assist actively in passing the tube. Blood vomiting usually occurs due to the varicosity in the upper portions of the digestive tract. Esophageal varices are present in 30% of patients with liver cirrhosis and 60% of patients with decompensated liver cirrhosis. Every episode of repeated bleeding carries 20%mortality rate [8,26].The oxygen therapy is necessary in patients with altered consciousness. Oxygen should be administered through a nasal catheter, best using a mask. The continuous assessment of the respiratory status, including the respiratory rate, and oxygen saturation, should be performed through constant gas analyses. Passing an arterial cannula in Gr IV HE patients with acute liver failure should be particularly emphasized, since it allows for a continuous monitoring not only of blood oxygen saturation, but also of lactate and bicarbonate blood levels. The arterial cannulation gives as a clear-cut, always accessible arterial blood pH, without repeated punctures of arteries [22]. When noticing that pH curve is shifting it should alarm the nursing staff that with it hemoglobin oxygen saturation curve shifts as well prompting doctors evaluation and therapeutic intervention. Regular monitoring of total body weight and abdominal girth. Receiving therapy and abdomen ascites centhesis leads to change in abdominal girth and total body weight. Patient should loose from 0.3 to 0.5kg per day, however, if weight loss is greater it can lead to renal failure, since kidneys become more hypo perfused and sensitive to hemodynamic alterations [22]. Multimodality monitoring is tracking of multiple parameters of brain activity (monitoring intracranial pressure, EEG waves). This modern monitoring system has been used worldwide for over 20 years in neurointensive care units [27], facilitating the work of nurses and doctors, and influencing timely and accurately interventions with the improvement in patient's condition through its parameters and clinical status. Patient communication is hampered, i.e. they pronounce words with difficulty and speak incoherently, therefore it is necessary to spend enough time with them to show empathy and understanding. Communication with the patient's family is of utmost importance. Adequate communication with family members in relation to changes in the clinical status and condition offers the family an insight into the actual situation concerning prognosis and course of the disease [8,28]. In a healthcare institution, it is preferable to have a written document stating what kind of information concerning the patient's condition a nurse can convey to patient's family members. From the available medical literature, but above all from the experience of doctors with whom nurses work with, it is a well-known fact that a well educated and problem solving oriented nurse is crucial for the success of intensive care interventional procedures performed by doctors. A nurse offers psychological stability to the entire team led by a doctor, and helps the creation of positive atmosphere when highly complex procedures are performed such as insertion of a hemodialysis two lumen catheter through jugular venous system especially if low access point in the internal jugular vein is chosen or subclavian vein access point. Through their calmness and positive attitude, nurses often make the difference between success and failure of interventions performed by doctors in the intensive care units. This study examines the specificities of healthcare in patients, as well as the influence of knowledge and attitudes of nurses in providing best healthcare to patients with hepatic encephalopathy. Since knowledge is an socio-epidemiological determinant which is also related to informational level of the individual it can be concluded that respondents did not possess a substantial knowledge level of HE. Obtained research results show that correlation between the work quality factors (elaborated in more detail in the conclusion of this study) and ill-informed nurses, i.e. their lack of knowledge (44.3% stated that they did not receive any information at all), is statistically important and it carries a significant statistical relativerisk. Furthermore, the use of the Internet as an universal electronic tool for continuous medical education and self-evaluation is at a very low level, and it speaks of poor motivation of the staff for self-improvement and self-education, which is increasingly present both in contemporary literature and modern medical trends (personalized medical self-education –medline or medline plus networks and medscape internet community). Aspect of interpersonal relationships should also be mentioned, where the flow of information between doctors and head nurses, on the one hand, and ward nurses, on the other, is below the level necessary for further development and improvement of work quality (just 25.7% and 22.9%of staff personnel with secondary education received information from doctors and head nurses). Speaking of interpersonal relationships, it should be emphasized that they can have a beneficial or adverse influence on all

three factors of work quality, defined and explained in more detail in the conclusion chapter of this study. Therefore, interpersonal relationships should be highlighted due to their prospective and universal importance, which makes the man inevitable part of any future epidemiological study dealing with the same or similar medical topic. It is precisely because of the fact that an integrated approach to HE patients is needed, statistically significant percent of nurses need (72.9% of respondents) continuous medical education. Moreover, it is believed that a better organization of continuous medical education would contribute at first hand to the increase in staff interest for further tertiary education, as well as the higher quality of secondary education. Secondly, the choice of topics of continuous medical education should be closely related to the specificities of HE patient care so as to have not only scientific and theoretical, but also practical significance. Thirdly, nurses need to participate actively in education, best in the format of panel discussion which needs to be implemented into continuous medical education, which will allow interactive approach making education clearer and more efficient. Therefore, it is not only sufficient to maintain continuous medical education, but to be modified as well. Since the staff personnel awareness is at respectable level (54.3% of nurses realized the importance of adequate and specific care of HE patients), it is also necessary to introduce the regulated improved official guidelines to nursing care, which would raise the existing awareness of the staff in the HE patient care. Healthcare is part of curative, restorative-healing, invigorating and rehabilitating process. The provided nursing care is of great importance in the treatment of HE patients [29]. Recognition and treatment of encephalopathy is critical for improving survival outcome with less complications in critically ill patients [29]. Managing complications in patients with cirrhosis in intensive care settings requires knowledge of various fields of medicine for doctors [10], which should also apply to nurses. Clinical guidelines already exist for doctors in this institution, but having in mind that the majority of staff recognizes their pivotal role in the complete medical therapy, it is necessary for such guidelines to exist for the nursing staff as well making the roles of doctors and nurses mutually complementary. Furthermore, this would ensure better interpersonal relationships, since it would define the position or place of every nurse in the medical team. Nursing guidelines would contribute to the standardization, as well as uniformity, of educational and interventional factors of work quality. Guidelines could also be modified on the basis of recognizing the importance of adequate and specific care of HE patients thus preparing nurses for addressing adequately any clinical problem and/or complication in HE patients. Clinical nursing guidelines would also allow better medical economics, i.e. pharmacoeconomics, since they would avoid the problems of nursing polypragmasia or economic dispersion in interventional procedures. In addition, such guidelines would define when and which signs, symptoms, i.e. complications, in HE patients call for an alarming situation and establish the list of priorities that would eventually lead to great cost savings. In severe liver diseases, where there is no possibility of curative treatment, it is necessary to provide palliative care. Nurses and doctors are best aware of the symptoms which cause significant quality of patient's life impairment. Their task should be that as a team ensure a general sense of well-being of the patient and a dignified passing if it occurs. It is of great importance to alleviate the final moments of life when it is needed [8], which implies comprehensive engagement of health staff with the provision of organized palliative care. Based on the conducted research in our center, we believe that there are three principal factors that would improve the work of the medical staff with HE patients: economical, educational, and interventional. Hospitals are not only institutions where medical help is provided, but also institutions of social and economic character.

## Economical factor

The lack of equipment and working conditions which hinder adequate treatment of HE patients, but also impair further education of the staff with secondary education.

## Educational factor

A statistically relevant number of questioned staff with secondary education knows how to recognize the manifestations of HE in patients with liver cirrhosis thus accurately establishing appropriate nursing diagnosis, leading to temporal optimization of therapy commencement. The continuous education and improvement of nurses is of significance when it comes to new medical apprehension and technologies being implemented into practice. Educational factor would ensure that quality of provided care is both effective and efficient. In our research, nurses expressed a good will for continuous education, which should be made possible for them.

## Interventional factor

The results show that majority of respondents don't know the difference between the nursing treatment of HE patients and other patients, which results in a poor interventional skills and therapeutic procedures during the course of the treatment.

## Conclusion

The specificity of health care in patients with hepatic encephalopathy is of multilevel nature clinically speaking and of great importance in the overall treatment process. Nurses should have the necessary work conditions and continuous education thus enabling effective and efficient care through nursing interventions. The above mentioned three principal factors (economic, educational, and interventional) lead to work improvement of the secondary staff education and better therapeutic modality of HE patient's treatment. These three factors are universal and can be applied as parameters of quality in every health care institution, i.e. at every intensive care unit regardless of the specific clinical pathology. Therefore, this paper has a universal meaning that should help the secondary staff education no matter in which medical institution or ward they are currently employed. The mentioned factors are in a direct correlation with each other and they can be only observed as a whole, where the failure to meet one of the factors is sufficient to make the algorithm of HE patient healthcare unsuccessful. It can be concluded that, apart from the substantial level of staff education, further education process has to improve the other two factors of quality of work, which are: the interventional - therapeutic skills of nursing staff and the upgrade of equipment and improvement of general working conditions.

## References

1. Salgado M, Cortes Y (2013) Hepatic encephalopathy: diagnosis and treatment. Compend Contin Educ Vet. 35: E1-E10.

2. Ferenci P (2003) Hepatic encephalopathy. In: Bockus Gastroenterology, Haubrich WS, Schaffner F, Berk JE (eds.,), WB Saunders, Philadelphia, Pa.

3. Kappus MR, Bajaj JS (2012) Covert hepatic encephalopathy: not as minimal as you might think. Clin Gastroenterol Hepatol 10: 1208-1219.

4. Findlay JY, Fix OK, Paugam-Burtz C, Liu L, Sood P, et al. (2011) Critical care of the end-stage liver disease patient awaiting liver transplantation. Liver Transpl 17: 496-510.

5. Singh GK, Hoyert D (2000) Social epidemiology of chronic liver disease end cirrhosis mortality in the United States, 1935-1997: trends end differentials by ethnicity, socioeconomic status end alcohol consumption, Hum Biol. 72: 801-20.

6. Dusheiko G. Hoofnagle JH (1991) Viral hepatitis In: Oxford textbook of clinical hepatology, N. Maclntyre, JP Benhamou, J Bircher, M. Rizzetto, J. Rodes (ed.,) Oxford University Press. 1: 371-92.

7. Kalaitzakis E, Josefsson A, Björnsson E (2008) Type and etiology of liver cirrhosis are not related to the presence of hepatic encephalopathy or health-related quality of life: a cross-sectional study. BMC Gastroenterol 8: 46.

8. Perumalswami PV, Schiano TD (2011) The management of hospitalized patients with cirrhosis: the Mount Sinai experience and a guide for hospitalists. Dig Dis Sci 56: 1266-1281.

9. Mohammad RA, Regal RE, Alaniz C (2012) Combination therapy for the treatment and prevention of hepatic encephalopathy. Ann Pharmacother 46: 1559-1563.

10. Bajaj JS1 (2010) Review article: the modern management of hepatic encephalopathy. Aliment Pharmacol Ther 31: 537-547.

11. Al-Khafaji A, Huang DT (2011) Critical care management of patients with end-stage liver disease. Crit Care Med 39: 1157-1166.

12. Blei AT1, Córdoba J; Practice Parameters Committee of the American College of Gastroenterology (2001) Hepatic Encephalopathy. Am J Gastroenterol 96: 1968-1976.

13. WHO: (2002) World Health Report, Geneva, World Health Organisation.

14. Federal Statistical Office: (2002) Demographic statistics 2000, the Federal Bureau of Statistics. Belgrade. 8-48.

15. Chadalavada R, Sappati Biyyani RS, Maxwell J, Mullen K (2010) Nutrition in hepatic encephalopathy. Nutr Clin Pract 25: 257-264.

16. Jia JD (2012) Lactulose in the treatment of hepatic encephalopathy: new evidence for an old modality. J Gastroenterol Hepatol 27: 1262-1263.

17. Prakash R, Mullen KD (2010) Mechanisms, diagnosis and management of hepatic encephalopathy. Nat Rev Gastroenterol Hepatol 7: 515-525.

18. Hung TH, Lay CJ, Chang CM, Tsai JJ, Tsai CC, et al. (2013) The effect of infections on the mortality of cirrhotic patients with hepatic encephalopathy. Epidemiol Infect 141: 2671-2678.

19. Bruner end Suddarths (2009) Textbook of medical Surgical Nursing. Smeltzer C.S.Bare B.G.Hinkle JL. Cheever KH (ed.,).

20. Martinesen TE (2004) Procedure, Guidance for nurses. Association of Nurses of Serbia. Beograd. 331-333.

21. Almeida JR, Araújo RC1, Castilho GV1, Stahelin L1, Pandolfi Ldos R1, et al. (2015) Usefulness of a new prognostic index for alcoholic hepatitis. Arq Gastroenterol 52: 22-26.

22. Sargent S (2006) Management of patients with advanced liver cirrhosis. Nurs Stand 21: 48-56.

23. Ginès P, Cárdenas A, Arroyo V, Rodés J (2004) Management of cirrhosis and ascites. N Engl J Med 350: 1646-1654.

24. Garcovich M, Zocco MA, Roccarina D, Ponziani FR, Gasbarrini A (2012) Prevention and treatment of hepatic encephalopathy: focusing on gut microbiota. World J Gastroenterol 18: 6693-6700.

25. McCormick PA, O'Keefe C (2001) Improving prognosis following a first variceal haemorrhage over four decades. Gut 49: 682-685.

26. Rankovic I. Stojkovic MLj, Mijac D, Culafic D, Vlaisavljevic Z, Jovicic I.et al. (2012) New therapeutic aspects of acute hepatic insufficiency: early correction of hyponatremia and its consequences.Medicinskicasopis sup. 46: 25-26

27. Wijman CA, Smirnakis SM, Vespa P, Szigeti K, Ziai WC, et al. (2012) Research and technology in neurocritical care. Neurocrit Care 16: 42-54.

28. Olson JC, Wendon JA, Kramer DJ, Arroyo V, Jalan R, et al. (2011) Intensive care of the patient with cirrhosis. Hepatology 54: 1864-1872.

29. Li – Hung Tsai (2008) Nursing Care for Patients with Hepatic Encephalopathy. TzuChi Nursing Journal. 7: 73-79.

# 22

# Steps towards Updating the Curriculum and Teaching Methods in Obstetrics, Gynaecology and Neonatology in Mongolia

**Annette Burgess**[1*], **Heather Jeffery**[2], **Shinetugs Bayanbileg**[3], **Erdenekhuu Nansalmaa**[4] and **Kirsten Black**[5]

[1]*Education Office, Sydney Medical School, The University of Sydney, Sydney, NSW, Australia*

[2]*School of Public Health, Sydney Medical School, The University of Sydney, Sydney, NSW, Australia*

[3]*United Nations Population Fund, Mongolia*

[4]*Education, Policy and Management, Mongolian National University of Medical Sciences, Mongolia*

[5]*Sydney Medical School – Central, The University of Sydney, Sydney, NSW, Australia*

*\*Corresponding author:* Annette Burgess, Education Office, Sydney Medical School, The University of Sydney, Room 205, Edward Ford Building A27, Missenden Road, Camperdown, New South Wales 2050, Australia, E-mail: annette.burgess@sydney.edu.au

## Abstract

**Background:** Medical education in Mongolia faces many challenges in terms of staff capacity, large student numbers, and limited access to clinical experience. The Government of Mongolia has placed a high priority on reducing maternal and infant mortality, necessitating improvements to the quality of medical training, ensuring a highly skilled health workforce is produced and maintained. In 2014, a team of academic staff from Sydney Medical School were appointed by United Nations Population Fund (UNFPA) to assist in reviewing and updating the medical student curriculum in obstetrics, gynaecology and neonatology in accordance with international best practice. The first phase involved a visit from a senior delegation from Mongolia, including representatives from the Mongolian National University of Medical Sciences (MNUMS), UNFPA and the Mongolian Ministry of Health to Sydney. The week long programme was designed to demonstrate best practice in obstetrics, gynaecology and neonatology undergraduate medical education; and display modern teaching practices.

**Methods:** Course design included demonstration and participation in a four station Structured, Clinical, Objective, Reference, problem-oriented, Integrated, and Organised (SCORPIO); observation of a Clinical Reasoning Session (CRS); demonstration and participation in a four station OSCE, and teaching of best practice in writing single-best answer multiple choice questions. Participants also took part in a teacher training session. The programme was implemented at a large teaching hospital in Sydney, Australia. We employed mixed-methods to evaluate the programme, using pre- and post-questionnaires and a focus group.

**Results:** The programme increased participants' perceived understanding and ability to apply educational principles, plan learning activities, and provide feedback. In particular, participants perceived that their understanding how to implement SCORPIO, CRS and OSCE had increased. However, participants would have liked greater opportunity to observe bedside teaching. Participants foresaw challenges to the implementation of educational changes in Mongolia, including the anticipated difficulty of engaging hospital staff in teaching; implementing a student-centred approach to teaching; and providing a large number of students with adequate clinical experience.

**Conclusion:** Changes in educational strategy in Mongolia may assist medical schools to produce clinically competent graduates. Our programme provided an effective means to introduce Mongolian leaders in health and education to modern student-centred medical education teaching and assessment methods; and to highlight the importance of teacher training and evaluation as a strategy to engage both university and hospital staff in medical education. Additionally, programme outcomes assisted in subsequent phases of the project, including in-country needs assessment, curriculum development and delivery.

**Keywords:** Obstetrics; Gynaecology; Neonatology; Undergraduate teaching; Curriculum medical education OSCE Objective Structured Clinical Examination; CRS: Clinical Reasoning Session

## Abbreviations

SCORPIO: Structured, Clinical, Objective, Referenced, Problem-oriented, Integrated and Organised; PT: Peer Teaching; SMP: Sydney Medical Programme; PPH: Post-Partum Haemorrhage; ISBAR: Identity, Situation, Background, Assessment and Recommendation;

## Background

Medical education in Mongolia faces many challenges in terms of staff capacity, the large number of public and private medical schools and students' limited access to clinical experience. The Government of Mongolia has placed a high priority on reducing maternal and infant mortality, and has made significant progress since 2001 [1]. The major focus of maternal health has resulted in 81% of women attending at least four antenatal visits and 98% of women being delivered by skilled birth attendants (98.0%), along with government efforts to build capacity of doctors, introducing universal standards and guidelines for services needed for delivery [2]. However, care of new-borns is lagging with new-born deaths accounting for 56.7% of all incidents of under 5 mortality in Mongolia; levels that have remained stagnant during the last decade. Despite advances in maternity care, the Maternal Mortality Rate of 68 per 100 000 live births in 2010, is relatively high compared to countries with similar service coverage and large disparities exist between urban and rural residents and between women of different socio-economic backgrounds. An assessment of Basic Emergency Obstetric and New-born Care needs conducted by the United Nations Children's Fund (UNICEF) and the Ministry of Health in 2010 found very few staff was properly managing deliveries (13%) and there was a lack of skills in new-born care, particularly in performing neonatal resuscitation [3]. Interviews with clients revealed counselling of mothers was insufficient in urban hospitals with only 10% of clients prepared for possible complications during childbirth. Improvements are needed in the quality and standards of care, clinical protocols, and guideline development.

Mongolia has experienced significant health sector reform. The Mongolian Health Sector Strategic Master Plan (2006-2015), a long-term policy framework – was approved in 2005 [4]. The objectives of the plan include increased life expectancy, a reduction in the infant, child and maternal mortality rates, improved nutritional status, particularly micronutrient status among children and women, reduced household health expenditure, especially among the poor, a more effective, efficient and decentralised health system, and an increase in the number of client-centred and user-friendly health facilities and institutions. Improving the quality of care is a key objective and a requirement for achieving the plan. This will necessitate quality training and a highly skilled health workforce.

For a long time medical education in Mongolia followed the former Soviet school of medicine. Although evidence-based international clinical guidelines are now available, the management of common complications of pregnancy, childbirth and the postpartum period for mother and baby, as taught in the medical student curriculum, has been slow to incorporate these ideas. The recommended textbooks are from the Russian language and are outdated. A survey among graduates of the medical schools in Mongolia revealed that training was heavily biased towards the basic sciences and that there was a lack of exposure to common clinical conditions.

The Mongolian National University of Medical Sciences (MNUMS) is the main state funded university providing training to medical students and over the six year programme, has approximately 450 students per year. Obstetrics and Gynaecology has been taught in year four and six of the programme, with limited teaching in neonatology during the paediatric term. MNUMS falls under the Ministry of Education and Sciences, but the hospitals responsible for providing clinical experience, including the First Maternity Hospital, fall under the Ministry of Health. These teaching hospitals have become overcrowded with undergraduate and graduate students and this

problem, combined with a lack of clinical skill laboratories, means that many graduates emerge from the course lacking in basic skills in managing normal pregnancy and common new-born/neonatal problems. In collaboration with the Government of Mongolia, the UNFPA 5th Country Programme (2012-2016) plans to upgrade graduate and residency curricula of the NMUMS in obstetrics and midwifery training according to the international guidelines [5]. To achieve this, UNFPA sought consultancy from Sydney Medical School. Although no mention was made in the Country Programme (2012-2016) report regarding inclusion of neonatology within the curricula, it is important to note that this forms an essential component.

In 2014, a team of academic staff from Sydney Medical School, The University of Sydney responded to a tender by UNFPA to review and update the Obstetrics and Gynaecology and Neonatology curriculum for the Mongolian National University of Medical Sciences (MNUMS). The team comprised an Obstetrician and Gynaecology, a Neonatologist, and an Educationalist. The purpose of the project was aligned with the aims and objectives identified in Mongolia's Health Sector Strategy (2006-2015) [4]: to review and update the obstetrics, gynaecology and neonatology curriculum for undergraduate medical students in accordance with international best practice, and in accordance with the institutional mission of the MNUMS. The project was undertaken in three phases. Phase 1 involved a visit from a delegation from Mongolia to the Sydney Medical School. Phase 2 involved a needs assessment visit from the Sydney Medical School staff. Phase 3 involved a return visit to Mongolia to deliver the curriculum.

Phase 1 of the consultancy involved a week long programme that formed part of the initial process towards the development of the O&G curriculum in Mongolia. The programme was designed to both emphasise and demonstrate best practice in undergraduate medical education within obstetrics, gynaecology and neonatology and to introduce and demonstrate modern teaching methodologies. The purpose of our study was to evaluate Phase 1 of the project.

## Methods

### Course design

Course design included demonstration and participation in a four station Structured, Clinical, Objective, Reference, Problem-oriented, Integrated and Organised (SCORPIO) [6,7]; observation of a Clinical Reasoning Session (CRS) [8]; demonstration and participation in a four station Objective Structured Clinical Examination (OSCE) [9]; teaching of the ISBAR method of handover (Identity of patient, Situation, Background, Assessment and action, Response and rationale) [10]; teaching of best practice in writing single-best answer multiple choice questions; and a half day attendance at a Hospital conference designed to provide update of current relevant topics in Obstetrics, Gynaecology and Neonatology. Participants also took part in a half day teacher training session. Topics within the programme are outlined in Figure 1.

- An introduction to the Sydney Medical Programme (SMP)

- An overview of the SMP Obstetrics, Gynaecology and Neonatology curriculum

- Teaching in professionalism

- Introduction to SCORPIO and practical application as a candidate in the SCORPIO (Structured, Clinical, Objective, Referenced, Problem –based, Integrated and Organised) [5,6]. Stations included Post-Partum Haemorrhage (PPH), Normal Vaginal Delivery, Newborn Anthropometry, and Resuscitation of the Neonate.

- Introduction to Teaching skills training (Bedside teaching, small group teaching, giving feedback)

- Introduction to ISBAR teaching (Identity, Situation, Background, Assessment and Recommendation) [9].

- Introduction to OSCEs and practical application as a co-examiner. Stations included Respiratory distress, pap smear, caesarean) [8]

- Observation of Clinical Reasoning Sessions (CRS) [7]

- Introduction to Single Best Answer examination (SBA)

- OSCE writing session

- half day attendance at a Hospital conference designed to provide update of current relevant topics in Obstetrics, Gynaecology and Neonatology.

Figure 1: Topics covered during the week.

## Course participants

Six Mongolian delegates participated in the programme, including three females and three males. Delegates included four staff members from the MNUMS, including two obstetricians and gynaecologists and two senior academic staff; a technical adviser from Reproductive Health, UNFPA; and a senior staff member from the Mongolian Ministry for Health. No neonatologist/paediatrician was included.

## Course facilitators

Expertise was drawn from various departments within Sydney Medical School and Royal Prince Alfred Hospital. Facilitators included two neonatologists, two midwives, three obstetricians and gynaecologists, one respiratory paediatrician, one surgeon, one educationalist, and one statistician. All facilitators had previous training and experience in teaching and assessment within the medical education context.

## Study design

We employed a mixed-method study using both a structured questionnaires and a focus group to investigate participants' perceptions of the programme.

## Quantitative data

Quantitative data were collected by pre and post-programme questionnaires, reflecting on participants' perceived ability with respect to the learning outcomes of the programme. Participants were asked to respond to 11 closed questions, such as "I understand how to set up and run an OSCE", using a five-point Likert scale ranging from 'strongly disagree' (1) to 'strongly agree' (5). Data were analysed using descriptive statistics [11].

## Qualitative data

Qualitative data were collected by questionnaire and focus group. Open ended questions were included in the post questionnaire to identify participants' perceptions of the programme. Additionally, all participants were invited to attend a focus group session to explore their perspectives, attitudes and experiences of the programme in depth. The session was taped and transcribed verbatim. Thematic analysis was used to code, categorise and identify themes in the qualitative data [12].

## Results

All six delegates completed the programme. Four of the participants reported having previous teaching experience, as well as having completed a professional development programme. As shown in Figure 2, the programme increased participants' perceived understanding and ability to apply educational principles, plan learning activities, and provide feedback. In particular, participants perceived that their understanding of a CRS, OSCE and SCORPIO had increased.

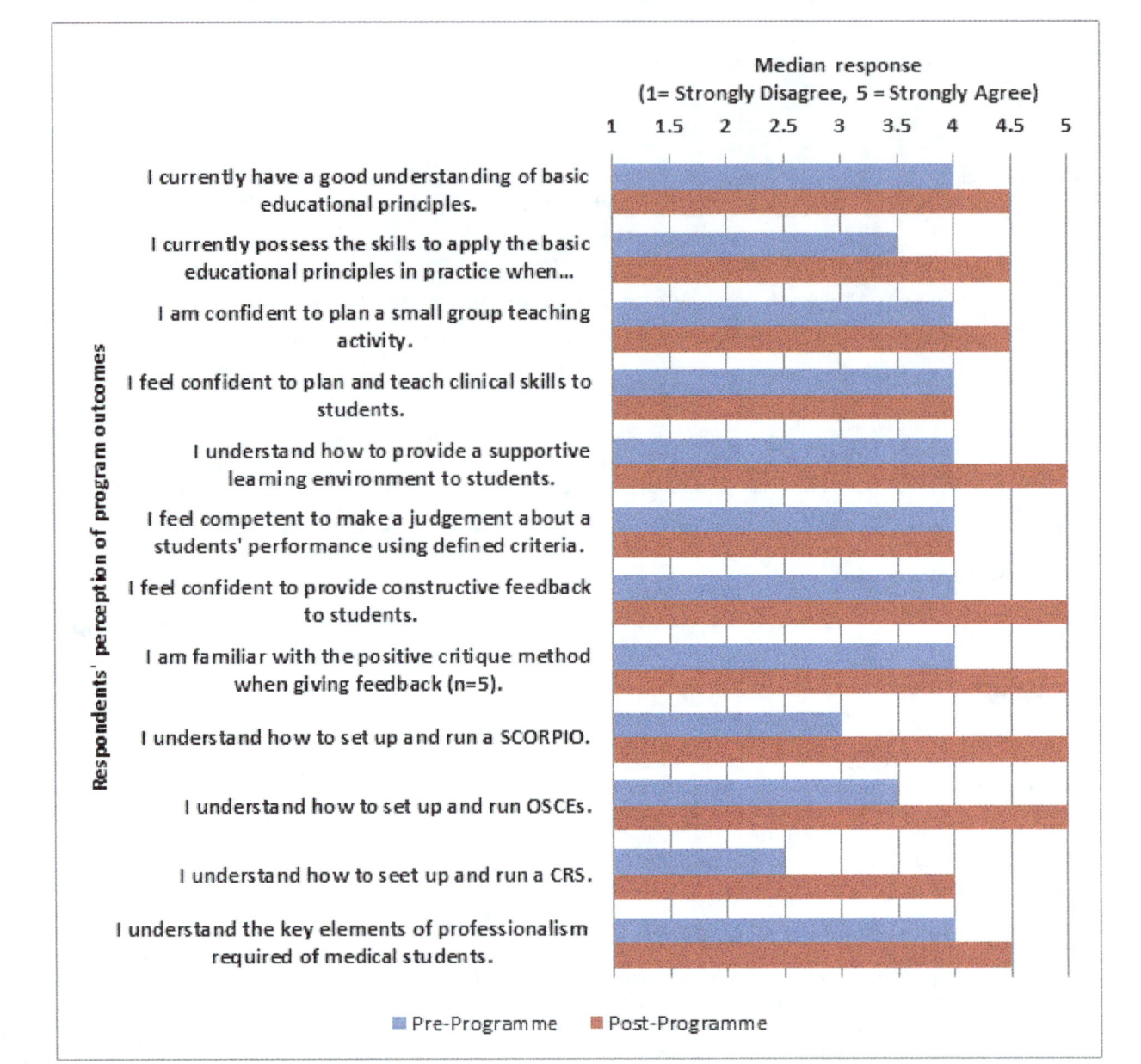

**Figure 2:** Comparison of Mongolian delegates' (N=6) Pre- and Post-programme median responses regarding perception of intended programme outcomes.

Qualitative responses by participants gave an indication of their attitudes to different aspects of the programme. These are categorised as: 1) most useful aspects of the course, 2) needs for improvement and 3) anticipated challenges for change implementation.

## Most Useful Aspects of the Course

When asked "What were the most useful aspects of the course?" participants particularly valued learning about modern teaching and assessment methods with learner centred approaches to teaching. These teaching methods included SCORPIO, Clinical Reasoning Sessions (CRS), ISBAR and OSCE, as presented below.

## SCORPIO

Participants felt that during the SCORPIO, learning was driven not only by active participation, but also by formative assessment and feedback from teachers.

*"The best training for the clinicians happens during the SCORPIO event. They were also assessed during this."*

Participants felt that the SCORPIO allowed evaluation of the teaching.

*"We were doing the SCORPIO, but the clinician who was presenting the case, was actually scored by the professors, so I think this was the*

*best way to train clinicians and also get them very interested in this type of training."*

## Clinical Reasoning Session (CRS)

On observation of the CRS, Mongolian delegates were impressed by the quality and commitment to teaching by a non-university (hospital employed), junior registrar, who had facilitated the session.

*"It was very impressive....the quality of the discussion...the capacity of this registrar, who is not university staff, dealing with each of the students, trying not to leave anything out, giving clear answers."*

Teaching in Mongolia takes place in much larger groups of 10-20, working on different cases, with multiple groups facilitated simultaneously by one tutor, and with less active participation by students.

*"I was very impressed with the capacity of the students to respond and to discuss, what not an easy case was at all. However, they were always having something to say. It's very different in Mongolia, we have 10 in one group, here are 6 or 7. Teachers have three to four small groups and different problems are used for each group."*

## ISBAR

Participants felt the use of ISBAR in both undergraduate and postgraduate medical education may provide a useful teaching method for communication skills.

*"The ISBAR was very good. We lose a lot of time when we are communicating. Sometimes we don't understand what they are stating, and we're very confused. So this was very concise. I think the best thing for this, for example, when we train student to give the student presenting the case. We can teach them to be concise and precise. Otherwise sometimes the student does not really know how to express themselves. There is a lack of communication skills. This is also needed for our teachers."*

## Teacher Training Course

Participants felt that teacher training would help to generally focus teaching on the need for learner-centred approaches to teaching.

*"This is sometimes a missing point in Mongolia. Because the teacher are very teacher-like, and clinicians very clinician like. There are gaps, so it will be useful to train teachers".*

Further to this, participants felt that implementation of teacher training would build engagement in teaching from both hospital and university staff.

*"This will create a very good connection between hospital and university. But our side is university, so clinical is clinical, so there's a very big gap here."*

## OSCE

Participants felt that although they already have OSCEs in within the medical curriculum, improvements would likely increase the objectivity and standardisation of this method of assessment.

*"We do OSCE already, but this should be very well standardised. Maybe we rely more on the teachers' experience, but this is more* *detailed and more objective, in this one, they use that kind of system. We can improve the process of the OSCE, it's clearer."*

## Multiple Choice Setting with Single Best Answer

Participants found it useful to be briefed on question writing and standard setting in MCQ.

*"There were some useful tips actually to improve the questions... Like more negative questions."*

## Suggested Improvements to the Programme

Participants' expectations were largely met during the week long programme. However, participants reported that they would have liked to have gained information and experience regarding the curriculum content and bedside teaching. In particular, Mongolian staff were disappointed that they were not provided with an opportunity to observe bedside teaching in Obstetrics, Gynaecology and Neonatology.

*"We wanted to see bedside teaching, curriculum content, student lectures, student log book."*

## Anticipated Changes

When asked how they felt changes might be implemented in Mongolia following the week long program, participants felt motivated to introduce SCORPIO and ISBAR, and introduce more interactive, student-centred approaches to teaching. They viewed formative assessment with feedback to be integral to improving students' learning outcomes.

*"We will change our teaching environments...we will use interactive teaching. But we begin by introducing SCORPIO and ISBAR...We will introduce formative assessment with feedback."*

*"We will use the positive critique method when giving feedback."*

## Future Challenges for Implementation

Participants identified five key challenges to the design, implementation of change in the Mongolian curriculum. These included access to the large hospitals; large number of students; lack of resources; engaging hospital staff in teaching; and ensuring collaboration between government departments.

*"One of the challenges when we return is to get more space and facilities for the teaching from bigger hospitals there. And in this case it's a trade-off I think, these facilities and this faculty also can use this methods actually to train the staff that is already working, like young doctors, midwives. And so this will be a kind of trade-off, for the hospitals to collaborate. So I think hopefully the Ministry will push on this. We'll also advocate for collaborate between the Ministry of Health and medical university and other hospitals, because it is very important".*

*"Very timely training as the MNUMS is in a time of change. Now leadership to influence the hospitals to provide facilities and staff is going to be very important."*

*"The teaching environment is poor. We will need constant training and a change in attitudes of other team. There are also logistics issues with the hospitals."*

*"Accommodating large numbers of students and lack of training manikins and instruments."*

## Discussion

The purpose of this study was to evaluate Phase 1 of the consultancy, which was designed to highlight best practice in obstetrics, gynaecology and neonatology undergraduate medical education; and demonstrate modern teaching practices. Participants identified benefits to the programme; made suggestions for improvement; and anticipated challenges to implementation of curriculum improvements and modern teaching methods in Mongolia.

The programme increased participants' perceived ability to apply basic educational principles, plan teaching activities, create supportive learning environments, and provide constructive feedback to students. Participants were introduced to student-centred, small group teaching and assessment methods, including SCORPIO [6,7], and Clinical Reasoning Sessions (CRS). They reported an improvement in confidence in being able to deliver these different teaching methods. Although the Objective Structured Clinical Examination (OSCE) is an assessment method already used widely in Mongolia, participants reported an increased understanding of this technique. There were some areas for which they sought greater exposure including a deeper understanding of the content of the Australian obstetrics, gynaecology and neonatology curriculum, and demonstration of clinical teaching through bedside tutorials. The intensive course provided the participants with ideas for improving their teaching, assessment and feedback methods. However, they recognised they faced significant barriers to implementing changes.

The shift from teacher centred approaches to education to a student centred one was recognised as the key to successful transition but the major challenge. The move to learner centred strategies which commenced in the 1990s [13] had major implications for faculty development at all levels from the institutional to the individual. Mongolia has yet to adopt a learner centred approach to medical education and has been adhering to the Soviet model of the teacher as the person who determines what, when, and how learners will learn. Didactic teaching has remained the predominant method. The delegates recognised the importance of creating an environment in which students can learn effectively and efficiently [14]. In fact, having the Mongolian delegation actively participate in SCORPIO, OSCE and ISBAR sessions, may have reinforced the benefits of these strategies [15].

The role of feedback, following observation of skills performance and formative assessment, was recognised by participants as integral to improving learning outcomes for students and enriching their learning experience. This is likely due to the repeated use of feedback within the SCORPIO and the formative OSCE, as well as the demonstration of feedback itself as a learned skill within the 'teacher training' session. Despite the important role of feedback in effective teaching and learning, skills in giving feedback are rarely taught to clinicians [16], something that participants would like to address within medical education in Mongolia.

Challenges for the future influencing the culture within the hospitals so that clinical staff understand the important role they play in educating the next generation of doctors and are able to work collaboratively with the academic staff to ensure students are exposed to a wide range of clinical experiences. Without being properly addressed, this issue may be compounded by the pending addition of new public and private hospitals, and rise in student numbers [16]. The Mongolian delegation felt that few academics or clinicians had been formally taught how to teach, assess or provide feedback to students, an issue also highlighted in developed countries [16-18]. On a positive note, participants felt that the introduction of 'teacher training' may provide an avenue to engage staff from both entities (hospital and university), in a collaborative effort to improve the quality of teaching. Indeed, in order to increase the quality of medical education, hospital medical culture needs to embrace education as a core task in health care [18].

## Limitations

The small sample size is a limitation of this study.

## Conclusion

Major problems facing medical education in Mongolia include the large number of students; limited opportunities made available for clinical experience, and restricted leadership in medical education. Changes in educational strategy will assist medical schools to produce clinically competent graduates. Our Phase 1, week long programme provided an effective means to introduce Mongolian leaders in health and education to current student-centred medical education strategies; assessment methods that ensure that competence is assessed rather than simply recalled; and to highlight the importance of teacher training and evaluation as a strategy to engage both university and hospital staff in medical education.

## Competing Interests

The authors declare that they have no competing interests.

## Authors' Contribution

AB, HJ, KB: Contributed to the study design, analysis and interpretation of data, drafting of manuscript, and critical revision for important intellectual content. SB, EN: Contributed to the critical revision of the manuscript for important intellectual content. All authors read and approved the final manuscript for important intellectual content.

## Acknowledgement

We wish to acknowledge the Mongolian delegates who generously gave their time to take part in the study.

## References

1.  Analysis of the Situation of Children in Mongolia 2014. Unicef 2014.

2.  Mongolia. Social Indicator Sample Survey (SISS) (2014) Key Findings. National Statistical Office of Mongolia.

3.  United Nations Children's Fund (UNICEF) (2013) Mongolia. Supporting health and nutrition actions.

4.  Government of Mongolia Ministry of Health (2005) Health Sector Strategic Master Plan 2006-2015, Ulaanbaatar.

5.  UNFPA Mongolia. Programme of Cooperation between the Government of Mongolia and The United Nations Population Fund. Country Programme Action Plan (CPAP) 2012-2016 Revision made in July 2014 for the period 2014-16 UNFPA Mongolia.

6.  Hill DA (1992) SCORPIO: A system of medical teaching. Med Teach 14: 37-41.

7.  Hill DA (1997) A strategy for teaching and learning in the PBL clerkship. Med Teach 19: 1.

8.  Harris A, Boyce P, Ajjawi R (2011) Clinical reasoning sessions: Back to the patient. Clin Teach 8: 13-16.

9.  Gormley G (2011) Summative OSCEs in undergraduate medical education. Ulster Med J 80: 127-132.

10. Thompson JE, Collett LW, Langbart MJ, Purcell NJ, Boyd SM (2011) Using ISBAR handover tool in Junior Medical Officer handover: A study in an Australian Teritiary Hospital. Postgrad Med J 87: 340-344.

11. Creswell J (2002) Educational research: Planning, conducting and evaluating quantitative and qualitative research, Merrill, Upper Saddle River, NJ, USA.

12. Braun V, Clarke V (2006) Using thematic analysis in psychology. Qual Res Psychol 3: 77-101.

13. Spencer JA, Jordan RK (1999) Learner centred approaches in medical education. BMJ 318: 1280-1283.

14. Irby DM (1994) What clinical teachers in medicine need to know. Acad Med 69: 333-342.

15. Schumacher DJ, Englander R, Carraccio C (2013) Developing the master learner: applying learning theory to the learner, the teacher and the learning environment. Acad Med 88: 1635-1645.

16. Burgess A, Mellis C (2015) Feedback and assessment for clinical placements: achieving the right balance. Adv Med Educ Pract 6: 373-381.

17. Sanson-Fisher RW, Rolfe IE, Williams N (2005) Competency based teaching: The need for a new approach to teaching clinical kills in the undergraduate medical education course. Med Teach 27: 29-36.

18. Gibson DR, Campbell RM (2000) Promoting effective teaching and learning: hospital consultants identify their needs. Med Educ 34: 126-130.

# 23

# Student's Academic Transition Issues: Associate Degree to Baccalaureate Nursing

**Kathleen Bradshaw LaSala[1]\*** and **Karen Gorton[2]**

[1]*University Of South Carolina, USA*

[2]*University of Colorado Anschutz Medical Campus, USA*

\***Corresponding author:** Kathleen Bradshaw LaSala , Associate Dean Academics and Professor, University Of South Carolina, College of Nursing, 1601 Greene Street, Columbi, SC 29208, United States, E-mail: LASALA@mailbox.sc.edu

### Abstract

Health care requires increasing the number and quality of registered nurses to the baccalaureate level to address part of the critical nurse shortage problem and need for highly qualified professionals. Two major national initiatives examining the nursing workforce issue in the United States recommend decreasing barriers, refining academic pathways and facilitating nurses return to school for higher levels of education by streamlining nursing education between community colleges and baccalaureate programs. Nurses prepared at higher levels have demonstrated stronger patient outcomes and ability to provide safe and effective care. This study sought to define barriers, priorities and enhancement/motivational factors, as identified by students, during transition from associate degree to baccalaureate nursing degree completion programs. Additionally, demographic data was compared to barriers and enhancement factors to determine if any associations between these exist. Students were provided with an electronic survey tool that allowed easy access and return. The outcome data from this pilot study provides nursing educators and professional practice leaders a better understanding the barrier factors, allowing leaders to design programs, delivery models, advising, and address needed areas of additional support or elimination to promote student success. At the same time, identified enhancement factors can be increased, streamlined for students.

**Keywords:** Academic transition; Barriers; Motivators; Enhancements; Priorities; Nursing education

## Introduction

The Institute of Medicine [1] and Carnegie Foundation for the Advancement of Teaching [2] recommend decreasing barriers by improving academic pathways to promote seamless progression from community colleges and baccalaureate programs to promote earlier, more efficient, access and cost-effective completion of a baccalaureate programs. In response to these key recommendations to the nursing profession, the authors designed a study to explore the transition issues as defined by the students, to guide nursing education and practice responses.

## Background/Review of Literature

The Institute of Medicine's [1] Future of Nursing: Leading Change, Advancing Health outlines eight recommendations to improve health care in the United States (U.S.) via nursing changes. Recommendations for nursing address the need to increase the U.S. proportion of nurses with baccalaureate degree to 80 percent by 2020. The IOM report elaborates on the need to decrease barriers by defining academic pathways that promote seamless progression and access for nurses to higher levels of education; promotion and support (financial) by health care agencies; salary differential for employed nurses with higher degrees; expanding baccalaureate programs through increased funding, scholarships and loan programs; early and continuous intra-professional collaboration with other disciplines; and recruitment of diverse student populations [1]. The Carnegie Foundation for the Advancement of Teaching: Preparation for the

Professions report Educating Nurses: A Call for Radical Transformation recommends an immediate need to streamline nursing education between community colleges and baccalaureate programs, "to allow for early completion of a baccalaureate program that are feasible, fair, and affordable for all nursing students" [2]. Health care practice requires increasing the quantity and quality of registered nurses to the baccalaureate level to address part of the critical nurse shortage problem and need for highly qualified professionals [1].

Experts on U.S. workforce issues predict a major shortage of nurses of up to million by 2020, related to the following factors: increased numbers of newly insured under the Affordable Health Care Act; increased numbers in the population; increased numbers of older individuals; an aging of the nursing workforce; and expanded areas of health care service [3]. The shortage is based on a supply-demand model that indicates a growing demand for nurses related to an increased general population, increase in those older than 65 years of age, and increase in the number of people gaining access to health care as a result of the Affordable Care Act [4]. The supply of nurses remains a challenge due to a high portion of nurses approaching retirement age and limitations on enrollment rate in schools of nursing due to the faculty shortage and clinical placements [5]. The current U.S. percentage of nurses prepared at the Associate Degree (ADN) level is 45.5% and Baccalaureate degree (BS/BSN) level is 33.7% [4].

The Institute of Medicine's report [1] states health care will need more nurses to address the predicted shortage. Additionally, these nurses should have higher levels of preparation to address improved patient outcomes. Evidence supports the IOM recommendation, indicating nurses with baccalaureate degrees are linked to lower rates of mortality [6,7]; are better prepared to provide safe and effective care than associate degree nurses [8]; and demonstrate better communication skills, knowledge, problem solving, patient-teaching and psychosocial skills [9]. More nurses will be needed with advanced education and skill to meet the demands of the future [1]. Meeting this need will require streamlining programs to produce increase the number nurses prepared at the baccalaureate, or higher level of education.

The U.S. Tri-Council for nursing [10] endorsed a position statement on the need to enhance the educational advancement of registered nurses. In response, many academic nursing programs continued to develop articulation partnerships spelling out the necessary coursework for degree transition from community college to baccalaureate education. Presently, students still find many challenges that influence their decision to pursue and attain advanced education. Researchers have explored personal characteristics, work attributes and work attitudes to predict if a nurse with an associate or bachelor's degree would enroll or complete a higher educational level [11], finding predictors of obtaining the BSN degree include: being black, living in a rural area, non-nursing work experience, higher work motivation, working in the intensive care units and working day shifts.

There is limited current data on barriers and enhancing factors related to transition from the associate to baccalaureate nursing degrees offered through Registered Nurse to Baccalaureate (RN-BS/BSN) programs, although there is rich anecdotal data. Students report complicated admissions requirements, including pre-requisite nursing courses and liberal arts and sciences classes that vary from one institution to another; financial barriers; conflicting responsibilities of work or family; and lack of guidance [12]. Only two older qualitative studies [13,14] explored the transition issues, revealing several barrier themes, including: a variation of expectations, tentative beginnings, limited time, lack of confidence/fear, insufficient recognition for past educational and life experiences, insufficient differentiation in roles of different registered nurses (RNs) prepared at different educational levels, and lack of basic academic support. Students in these studies identified several factors (enhancement/motivational) that facilitated advancing their education, including: it was the right time and place in life to go to school, looking forward/continuing job opportunities, achieving a personal goal, and obtaining support and encouragement to return to school identification of cornerstone courses that led to significant change [13,14]. Nurse educators and clinical leaders have actively pursued measures to ease the transition in RN-BSN programs, including articulation models, joint enrollment projects, cohort admission programs with clinical agencies and various other measures. However, most of the measures are relatively new and have not been analyzed for impact. In order to best understand the issue and develop solutions, the current study explored students' perceptions of barriers and enhancement factors in academic transition in this decade.

## Purpose of the Study/Aim

The purpose of the study was twofold; 1) define barriers, priorities and enhancement/motivational factors perceived by students as they transition from associate (ADN) to baccalaureate (BS/BSN) nursing programs and 2) explore associations of barriers and enhancing factors with demographics to better understand student issues. Barriers were defined as factors that interfered or made pursuing education more difficult; whereas enhancement/motivating factors were identified as factors that helped facilitate or made pursuit of education easier. The

study is designed to gather current data from nurses in this decade, knowledge that is missing from the literature.

## Methods

### Research Design:

The research was undertaken with an exploratory approach as there is limited current data noted in the literature related to academic transitions of the RN to BS/BSN student. A descriptive survey method, using an electronic Qualtrics survey tool was used (http://www.qualtrics.com).

### Research Questions

The research questions related to barriers, priorities and enhancement/motivation factors to obtaining a bachelor's degree and factors which assisted in pursuing this degree among students with an associate degree or diploma in nursing. In a descriptive survey, nursing students were given options/choices to select, and an open-ended "other" selection. Actual subset questions are listed in tables 1 and 2. The research questions were as follows:

- What are the barriers in obtaining a BS/BSN degree?
- What are the enhancement/motivating factors in obtaining a BS/BSN degree?
- Is there a relationship between students' demographic factors and barriers and enhancement factors in obtaining a BS/BSN degree?
- What priority factors are related to the selection of the RN-BS/BSN program?
- What priority factors made going back to school for a BS/BSN degree easier?

### Research Instrument:

The survey instrument was developed by the investigators based on research findings in qualitative studies of Kovner et al., [11], Delany &Piscopo [13], Megginson [14]. In addition, questions reflected anecdotal information and suggestions obtained from Deans/Directors who have worked with RN-BSN students in the state surveyed. Once developed, the instrument was peer-reviewed by a panel of ten Deans/Directors for content validity and readability, then revised appropriately prior to use. The survey collected demographic data, 41 items multiple-choice selections for questions related to barriers, priorities and enhancement factors, and open-ended "other" area for comments.

### Procedure/Sample/Data Collection/Analysis:

After receiving institutional review board approval for the study, an electronic letter was sent to ten Nursing Deans/Directors of national nursing accredited programs in the selected state with RN-BS/BSN programs introducing the leaders to the survey. The letter discussed the survey, shared the institutional review board (IRB) approval and explained that informed consent would be documented by willingness to participate in survey. The Dean/Director was then asked to forward an attachment letter with a link to the survey to their RN-BS/BSN students. The letter to the students also included the information on IRB approval and the assumed consent by participation explanation. Based upon an estimated number of 520 RN-BS/BSN students enrolled in the state programs in 2014, the return rate was approximately 10% (N=52).

Data was analyzed using frequency, distributions and correlations using the Statistical Package for Social Sciences [15] (with a significance level of $p<0.05$). Since written comments were limited, all were included in the findings. All demographic data was reported in aggregate format and grouped into meaningful categories, then re-analyzed and determined to meet normalcy distribution of data.

## Results

### Demographic Findings

Respondents were 100% female; primarily white/Caucasian (96%), with 18% (20-29 years old), 32% (30-39 years old), 32% (40-49 years old) and 28% greater than 50 years old. Most of the subjects were married (71%), with 16% separated or divorced, 10% single and 4% with domestic partners. A small percentage (12%) were not working, while 6% were working part time between 12-25 hours, and 82% were working 25 or more hours a week. Although the RN-BS/BSN programs were located in one state, 44% (n= 23) of the students were from other states as a result of the distance offerings. Students were from a variety of regional locations; with 35% from rural and 65% from urban areas. Although this demographic data is close to the demographic data of the state surveyed, the gender and race demographics of the U.S. are more diverse.

The students had completed previous degrees, primarily at ADN (92%), and 8% Diploma graduates and 65% with bachelor's degrees in another field. The students had completed all their previous degrees at various ages, with 48% completing by age 30; 38% by age 40, and 14% after the age of 40. Most (81%) completed their previous nursing degree/diploma in less than four years. The number of years between completing the previous degree and starting the RN-BSN program varied, with 20% starting within the first year, 12% from year 1-3, with equal number (8%) between 3-5 years, 5-7 years, 7-9 years, 9-11 years, and 11-13 years, 2% at 13-15 years and 27% completing after 15 or more years. When asked how long they thought the RN-BSN program would take them to complete, 10% reported less than a year, 45% reported 1-2 years, 35% 2-3 years and 10% thought it would take more than 3 years. Most respondents calculated it would take them at least two years to complete the nursing courses (79%), as well as taking them two years to complete the non-nursing requirements (93%).

### Barriers for Students Pursuing a RN-BS/BSN Degree

Respondents identified barriers they faced while pursuing additional education at the BS/BSN level (Table 1). Major barriers included issues with educational and work issues, family and personal responsibilities and financial restraints. In the area of "other", participants entered free text noting such factors as additional lack of/cost of childcare, professional employment dedication, work responsibilities, learning disability and time constraints were added.

| Barriers for Students Pursuing a RN-BSN degree | N | Percentage |
|---|---|---|
| Cost (tuition and fees) | 40 | 82% |
| Family responsibilities | 25 | 51% |
| Obtaining pre-requisite coursework for admissions | 10 | 20% |
| Lack of employer support | 9 | 18% |
| Lack of motivation | 8 | 16% |
| Lack of family/significant others' support | 8 | 16% |
| Other (see discussion section for specific responses) | 6 | 12% |
| Lack of Childcare | 4 | 8% |
| Time away from employment | 3 | 6% |
| Lack of RN-BSN program in my area | 2 | 4% |
| None | 2 | 4% |
| Long acceptance time into BSN programs | 1 | 2% |

Table 1: Barriers for Students Pursuing a RN-BSN Degree.

### Enhancements/Motivational Factors for Students Pursuing a RN to BS/BSN Degree

Factors that motivated students to return to school for their BS/BSN degree completions (Table 2) included internally motivating factors such as desire for continued education/professional development and support of one's family and significant others. External factors included financial and family/employer support, and increased opportunities at the baccalaureate degree level. Educational incentives included having a choice of a number of programs, ease of completing pre-requisite courses and a short acceptance time for admissions. However, employer mandates were a very low motivating factor. When describing the "other" factors, individual nurses wrote that multiple factors encouraged them including the desire to pursue graduate school, scholarship and tuition support, availability of online programs, limitations for opportunity at the ADN level, promotion options and being a role model for one's own children.

| Enhancements/Motivational Factors for Students Pursuing the RN-BSN Degree | N | Percentage |
|---|---|---|
| Personal motivation for increased education/professional development | 35 | 73% |
| Short acceptance time into BSN program | 27 | 56% |
| Family/significant other support | 24 | 50% |
| Tuition support | 23 | 48% |
| Other (see discussion section for specific responses) | 15 | 31% |
| Increased job opportunities at the BSN level | 13 | 27% |
| Many RN-BSN programs to choose from | 13 | 27% |
| Ease of completing pre-requisites | 11 | 23% |
| Employer encouraged | 10 | 21% |
| Employer support | 9 | 19% |
| Employer provides release time for coursework that is paid time | 4 | 8% |
| Employer mandate (required to keep one's job) | 3 | 6% |
| None | 1 | 2% |
| Provision of childcare | 0 | 0% |
| Increased pay level for BSN | 0 | 0% |

Table 2: Enhancements/Motivational Factors for Students Pursuing the RN-BSN degree.

## Relationship of Demographic Data and Barriers and Enhancement Factors

Analysis of age and family/significant other support was found to be statistically significant (0.005). Analysis between age and incentives (employer mandate to keep my job) demonstrated a statistically significant relationship (0.005).

An association between partner status and a variety of barriers were noted to be statistically significant, including: the relationship between partner status and barriers (tuition and fees) (0.01); the relationship between partner status and the barrier of family responsibilities (0.05); the relationship between partner status and the barriers of family responsibilities (0.05) and partner status and lack of family/significant others support (0.011); and the relationship between partner status and lack of RN to BSN programs in my area (0.016). However, partner status and motivational factors for returning for the RN –BS/BSN degree were not found to be statistically significant.

## Priority Factors Related to Selection of RN-BSN Program

Analysis of factors related to selection of RN-BS/BSN program revealed participants reported receiving their initial information about the RN-BS/BSN program from a website (58%), program advisors (44%) and from College Network (15%), with some indicating more than one source. Information about non-nursing required courses was received from the similar sources and most (94%) believed the

information was easy to understand and helped motivate them to move forward with their educational program. The majority (73%) of students received individual advising prior to admission and most (84%) only applied to one program. All of the RN-BS/BSN programs that these students attended were either totally online or hybrid programs. Participants were asked to rank the most important priority factors in selection of an RN-BS/BSN program (Table 3). In addition to the responses provided, individual nursing students identified the following factors in the "other" selection: A quick enrollment and admissions process; accredited program; ability to self-pace; discounts provided through employer; assistance with disability; and desiring a program with graduate programs.

| Priority Factors Related to Selection of RN-BSN program | # 1 Priority | #2 Priority | #3 Priority |
|---|---|---|---|
| Online program delivery | 55% (N=27) | 22% (N=11) | 8% (N=4) |
| Reputation of the school | 20% (N=10) | 31% (N=15) | 18% (N=9) |
| Scholarship/financial assistance | 8% (N=4) | 12% (N=6) | 2% (N=1) |
| Pre-requisite and/or non-nursing course requirements | 6% (N=3) | 18% (N=9) | 29% (N=14) |
| Other (see discussion section for specific responses) | 6% (N=3) | 10% (N=5) | 10% (N=5) |
| Location, onsite program delivery | 2% (N=1) | 0% (N=0) | 6% (N=3) |

Table 3: Priority Factors Related to Selection of RN-BSN program

## Factors that Made Going Back to School Easier

Students identified factors that made going back to school easier in rank order:

- Personal motivation
- Online/distance program availability
- Financial support
- Family/significant other's support
- Employer support
- Strong academic advising
- Well-planned curriculum with ease of transition
- Onsite delivery method

## Positive Impact Factors the BSN Would have on Nursing Career

When reporting positive impact factors they felt the BSN would have on their nursing career, the students rank ordered:

- Increase opportunity to pursue graduate education
- Increase my career mobility
- Provide additional knowledge and skills as closely related impacts

In the open-ended section that included "other" option, one student nurse wrote the BSN degree would increase respect from my colleagues and another individual wrote the BSN would qualify them to teach at a community college.

## Factors Delaying Progression in the RN-BSN Program

Major factors identified as delaying progression in the RN-BSN were costs and life events. Some of the nurses (24%) expected to work in the same area following graduation, but others (76%) saw future opportunities as possibilities. Over half (67%) of the survey respondents expected to attend graduate school within the next five years. In response to "other" option, two students indicated some concern with general education and pre-requisite courses taken as part of the ADN programs that did not translate into accepted credits at the BSN level. Several of the nurses found it difficult to arrange their own clinical experiences as required by their program. One non-clinical nurse also found assignments directly relating to clinical/service learning activities difficult to complete. In addition, one student reported academic advising was not available to them prior to admission to the RN-BS/BSN program, which set up barriers of additional coursework that could have been avoided. Another student wrote the costs and current economic instability made a difficult and unpredictable time to assume student loans. Lastly, three students were disappointed that the nursing profession has not focused more attention on the baccalaureate level of education until now.

## Discussion

This study provided new preliminary findings on RN-BSN educational issues and confirmed some existing, but limited data in the literature. The findings confirm some commonly held beliefs based on anecdotal information about this student population that had not been previously identified in research. On a positive side, personal motivation was rated by most as the greatest incentive to return for the BS/BSN, including opportunities for continued education, professional development and future employment choices. This finding was not reported in the previous literature and reflects a change in enhancement/motivating factors. In addition, new educational factors that helped motivate students included short acceptance time into a program. Family and employer support was found in earlier studies and continues to be a strong motivational factor. A new finding revealed age and employer incentives were demonstrated to have a statistically significant relationship, indicating the influence the employer can have on individuals pursuing higher education at different stages of their career. Additionally, as health care agencies attain/maintain Magnet status, increased BS/BSN leaders will help advance the initiative. Nurses who are early or mid-career are finding the longevity need for a BS/BSN more predominant than their predecessors. The clear message for higher education is being better delivered through both education and practice leaders.

Priorities for education have shifted, reflected in the top two priorities for program selection being the online/distance delivery model and reputation of the school. These are new findings and reflect the current student's need for flexibility and quality through distance education, shifting away from onsite/local education demands. Students identified pre-requisite and non-nursing course requirements as a lower priority, which did not confirm the anecdotal data supplied by students and some deans/directors in the study's region.

Multiple barriers associated with the RN-BS/BSN academic transition are identified. Supporting the existing literature, costs and financial issues and family responsibilities remain highly ranked issues, while new data reflected the barriers of obtaining pre-requisite coursework and support of employers and family were added to the list of primary barriers to pursuing a BS/BSN degree. It is clear that employers and family support can be both a positive and negative factor in continuing one's education, Lack of educational opportunities is clearly not an issue for most students completing this study, which may or may not differ from the general population of students.

The students indicated that online and hybrid programs as their number one priority, reflecting need for flexibility and choice. The widespread access to distance education programs helped the students deal with juggling the demands of work and family responsibilities; however these responsibilities continue to serve as major barriers. Working full time and/or carrying for others left little time for focus and study in school. Concurrently, students' reported employer support with both encouragement and tuition assistance as an enhancement to success.

## Limitations and Strengths of Study

As a pilot study, the findings are limited due to the small number of participants, regional limitations and response rate. A reminder notice was sent out for a second response opportunity, but generated little additional participation. However, the procedural and study findings help guide broader national or international study that can be helpful in guiding education and practice. In addition the pilot study helped identify changes/shifts in the priorities and issues students perceive related to advancing their education.

## Conclusion

In addressing the purpose of the study, the barriers, priorities and enhancement/motivational factors associated with RN-BS/BSN academic transition were well defined. The primary enhancement/ motivator finding that most students are self-motivated to advance their education needs to be capitalized by employers and educators, expanding awareness of opportunities higher education can provide, support students in their educational process through resources (e.g., financial, time), and providing quality online academic experiences. The barriers identified indicate individuals pursuing additional education sometimes have barriers outside of their control: cost, time, family responsibilities, work demands and time constraints; therefore development and implementation of flexible educational programs, with online delivery methods are overwhelming preferred and allow nurses prepared at the associate degree level pursue their baccalaureate degree. Even with the online method, educators and employers need to continue to demonstrate flexibility with scheduling in both the work place and academic arenas. For education, this may mean the development of adaptable course delivery models, schedules and academic advising. For employers, this may mean the development of work schedules that plan for school participation.

To address the barriers to seamless education and costs, educators need to adequately guide students to obtain correct non-nursing courses and pre-requisites and prevent unnecessary duplication of nursing courses to help defer additional costs. The pre-requisite coursework requirements were not identified as a priority by students, yet they were listed as barriers. Further investigation is needed in this area, as it also has an impact on cost and time. Early advising and degree audits in the associate degree programs can aid in this issue, but due to the variety of BS/BSN programs available it is not always easy to predict where a student will chose to attend. Nursing educators have a clear impact on streamlining pre-requisite (non-nursing) courses required and improving communication with associate degree programs; however, less control exists in non-nursing college/ university requirements for graduation and the school students choose to attend. In addition, educational institutions need to continue to provide online education programs and pursue scholarships and grants for students, and share funding opportunities with students at all stages of their academic careers. Since choice of programs was identified as an incentive, advisors at the associate degree level will need to become more versed in BS/BSN programs available and requirements.

The identification of support by family and significant others as both a barrier and enhancement factor was interesting. This leads the researchers to extrapolate that the level of support identified by the student may be a key to how it was viewed by the student. Returning to school puts a stress on time, money, childcare, eldercare responsibilities and work commitments for the students; therefore, program advisors and practice partners to support the student with stress management and time management skills. The use of "step-out options" for students that do not result in significant delay in their plan of study should also be considered. Both partners need to focus on connecting school with work, and perhaps, even connecting family with school by including the family in the orientation process. Students in the study indicated a desire to serve as a role model for their children in pursuit of higher education; therefore, involving the family could be a positive factor.

By better understanding the barriers factors influencing academic transition, decision-makers can begin to design programs, delivery models, advising and other areas of support to help decrease or eliminate these distractions from success, while strengthening motivational factors. Understandably, there may be regional differences in barriers to students and this study provided information on the experience of nurses from one region, unique student profiles may exist in various regions of the U.S. and globally. This study supports existing findings and provides new knowledge related to barriers and enhancing factors to nurses pursuing an RN-BS/BSN degree. A partnership between educators, practice leaders, families/ significant others and students is essential for the success of the student goals.

## References

1.  Institute of Medicine (IOM) (2011) The future of nursing: Leading change, advancing health. Washington, DC: The National Academies Press.

2.  Benner P, Stuphen Leonard, Day (2010) Educating nurses: A call for radical transformation. San Francisco: Jossey-Bass.

3.  Buerhaus PI, Auerbach DI, Staiger DO (2009) The recent surge in nurse employment: causes and implications. Health Aff (Millwood) 28: w657-668.

4.  Health Resources and Services Administration (2010) The registered nurse population: Initial findings in the 2008 national sample survey of registered nurses. U.S. Department of Health and Human Services Resources and Services Administration. Washington DC.

5.  American Association of Colleges of Nursing (AACN) (2014)2013-14 Enrollment and graduations in baccalaureate and graduate programs in nursing. Washington DC.

6.  Kutney-Lee A, Sloane DM, Aiken LH (2013) An increase in the number of nurses with baccalaureate degrees is linked to lower rates of postsurgery mortality. Health Aff (Millwood) 32: 579-586.

7.  Aiken LH, Clarke SP, Cheung RB, Sloane DM, Silber JH (2003) Educational levels of hospital nurses and surgical patient mortality. Journal of the American Medical Association, 290, 1617-1623.

8.  Berkow S, Virkstis K, Stewart J, Conway L (2009) Assessing new graduate nurse performance. Nurse Educ 34: 17-22.

9.  Friese CR, Lake ET, Aiken LH, Sibler JH and Sochalski J (2008) Hospital nurse practice environments and outcomes for surgical oncology patients. Health Services Research, 43, 1145-1163.

10.  Tri-Council for Nursing (2010) Educational advancement of registered nurses: A consensus position.

11.  Kovner CT1, Brewer C, Katigbak C, Djukic M, Fatehi F (2012) Charting the course for nurses' achievement of higher education levels. J Prof Nurs 28: 333-343.

12.  Personal Communication (2014) Personal communication with Deans and Directors of all RN-BSN programs in state XXX.

13.  Delaney C1, Piscopo B (2007) There really is a difference: nurses' experiences with transitioning from RNs to BSNs.J Prof Nurs 23: 167-173.

14.  Megginson LA1 (2008) RN-BSN education: 21st century barriers and incentives. J NursManag 16: 47-55.

15.  SPSS Version 22 (2014)IMB SPSS Version 22 Statistical Package for Social Sciences. International Business Machines.

# 24

# Ethical Model - A Synthesis between Caring Sciences and Nursing Administration

**Frilund Marianne**[1*] and **Lisbeth Maria Fagerstrom**[2]

[1]*Faculty of Medicine and Health Sciences, NTNU University, Aalesund, Norway*

[2]*Department of Nursing Science, Drammen, Norway*

[*]**Corresponding author:** Frilund Marianne, Associate Professor, Faculty of Medicine and Health Sciences, NTNU University, Aalesund, Norway, E-mail: mafr@ntnu.no

**Abstract**

We want more than we have realistically possibilities to do. Caregivers are aware about how they have to act in the daily work in patient settings. Still we have to stat that we don´t can guarantee ethically good care of patients.

**Aim:** Aim of the study is to describe and explain the relationship between the ethos of caring and nursing intensity, based on a theory model developed by a hermeneutic approach.

**Method:** The study is a theoretically study with a hermeneutic approach and a hypothetic-deductive design. Materials are results from four sub-studies published between 2009 and 2013.

**Findings:** The model includes for corn stones and sex interoperations patters witch keep the corn stones together in a process of moving.

**Conclusion:** The theoretical model explained in this paper has opportunities to guide the caregivers in their daily work for providing ethically good care to older people.

**Keywords:** Caregivers; Nursing

## Background

Everyday work for nurses includes lot of ethical challenges and in the future ethical dilemmas and problem will increase because of the changes in the public healthcare. Today politicians and the financially responsible ask for efficiency, productivity and high quality standards of service from health care. They want the care providers to do the job cost-effectively and ethically [1-3]. In the public health-care, we have much more needs to meet then we have professional caregivers available. People over 65 years-old increase. They have more complex care needs and they know much more about their rights and benefits in case of illness and desire. Still the patient, now days, want to make their own decisions in relation to their own life's [4,5]. The nursing intensity will be higher, problems more complex and money less [6]. This is the reality and we have to find out how to manage these challenges and make the good ethical care possibly in the future.

This paper is based on thesis by Frilund in the field of Caring science and Nursing administration. The synthesis between ethos and nursing intensity evolves thought a hermeneutic moment between understanding and interpretation, in a dialectic tension between thesis and antithesis [7], i.e., the ethos of caring and nursing intensity [8]. The thesis had three main aims, the first aim was to deepen the understanding of caring ethos, the second aim was to deepen the understanding of the nursing intensity within the care of older people and the third aim was to create a theoretical model describing the synthesis between the caring ethos and nursing intensity. A theoretical model was developed by four sub-studies [9-12]. Propose of clinical

caring-science is to form the ethical ideals and to implement the ideals into the reality [13,14]. These kinds of knowledge expansion and theoretical formation described in the study had a hypothetic-deductive design, [15] in accordance with a humanistic tradition [16].

The synthesis between the ethos of caring and nursing intensity highlight new knowledge formation in a theoretical model, and took place in a process of creativity [4]. Propose of the model was to start a discussion about ethic and ethical manners in praxis. Good care is in constant movement and tension between the ethical and the unethical. The caregivers are aware about the ethics in the daily work but they lack realistic possibilities to act in an ethical manner in their daily work. Good Care is always at risk of changing into more or less unethical care, despite good intension of the caregivers [17,18].

Based on earlier research we can state that basic ethical values can be summered into four values: dignity [19,20], autonomy [21,22], safety [23] and caring community [24]. The caregivers most often accept these values, but they not necessary guide the nurses in their daily work. Researches stat that still the care of older people are stereotypic and based on routines. Patient's autonomy and integrity safeguarded in an unsatisfactory manner [18,19] Research shows that especially in care of older people the risk of being carried of tiered and stressed caregivers increase. Nursing today will be a job with lot of stress and impossibilities to provide a care in accordions with the ideals of the caregivers. The everyday work don´t take account the older persons individual needs and don't planning patient's care from this point of view [8].

Most of the nurses' will everyday meet ethical dilemmas and challenges. Ethical discussions and problem-solving are necessary, and it is the leader how have the responsibility to start the process and make good ethical care possible [8,9].

The caring ethos, ethical values or caritativ caring ethics are used as synonyms in the study, and they have to be understood from a caring science perspective. The concept "nursing intensity" will be an administrative concept witch refers to the patients 'needs and how well the nurses experience they have had possibilities to meet the needs [25]. For to guarantee the patient an ethical good care it will be important that the patients 'needs will be in balance with available resources [26]. It will be one of the nursing leaders' main task to make "good ethical care" possibly by relevant resource allocation, recruitment and the development of the staff to provide good care [1,11,27].

The propos of this paper is to describe the theoretical model called a synthesis between ethical values and nursing intensity. The model was developed thought a hermeneutic movement between understanding and interpretation, in a dialectic tension between thesis (ethos of caring) and antithesis (nursing intensity) [28].

## Aim

Aim of the study is to describe and explain the relationship between the ethos of caring and nursing intensity, based on a theory model developed by a hermeneutic approach.

## Research Questions

What central entities does a theoretical model consist of when the aim is to support the ethos of caring as well as ethical manners?

How can we describe the relationship between ethos and nursing intensity?

## Methods

The sub-studies had a hypothetical- deductive design. Previous research, theoretical standpoints of relevance for the study has provided the interpretive framework. Data for building the model was four sub-studies, Frilund et al. [9-12]. The authors interpreted and analyzed findings from the studies and by a hermeneutic process the model was formed. The model that describes the synthesis between caring ethos and nursing intensity consist of four cornerstones and sex interpretation patterns The concept used in the model has been chosen in line with the theory of caritative. The model has to be understood from a caring and nursing management perspective. That constituted for the researcher new pre-understanding for further interpretation.

The model for to describe ethical values and nursing intensity was formed by a logical deductive process and with a hermeneutic approach [29] based on Ghadames's philosophy. The synthesis between ethos of caring and nursing intensity took place in a process of creativity and logical deduction. The analyze process, was done in three steps.

The first step of the analyze process was based on result from the four sub studies mined above. The sub studies was early published and thereby been reviewed. Conclusion from the analyze process was explained as theoretical patterns of interpretation. In the second step a new logical deductive process was done and the results of this process results in four corn stones for the model. The meaning for the model

was given by using concepts that liked together the cornerstones as well as the interpretation patterns. The final model formation was the third phases in the inquiry of the process. Corn-stones and patters of interpretation form the model and the model will be understood by the concepts and relations between the concepts from clinical nursing science and nursing administration point of wave. The model has been reviewed by researches from different countries and the model has been found logical and reliable. The process of review was taken place before my dissertation.

## Findings

A theoretical model showing the synthesis between ethos of caring and nursing intensity grew up and started with six patterns of interpretation, i.e. new horizon of interpretation in accidence with a hermeneutic approach. The "patterns of interpretation" was named: the ethical ideals, ethical wishes and expectations, ethical manners, the older persons caring needs and optimal level of nursing intensity, ethical dilemmas and challengers and finally ethical leadership [8-11,13]. The corner stones was named; ethical values as ideals, ethical wishes' and expectations in relation to nursing intensity, ethically possibilities, and ethically leadership [3].

First, we want to explain the six interpretative patterns that step forward in the analysis and interpretation of results.

The ethical ideals Good ethical care starts with ethical values. The sub study two [10] show four ethical values of relevancy to provide good ethical care for older people; autonomy (integrity), safety, dignity and caring community. This values where accepted by the participants based on the findings in the study two [10] at a high level of agreement, but not good enough for guarantee patient good quality care, regardless of caregivers [8-10].

Ethical wishes and exceptions: Interpretation process indicate that ethical awareness and consensus needs to be done in the team of caregivers. Good ethical care also indicates that the patients' needs, wishes and expectations have to been met. Without ethical awareness you cannot be award ethical expectations and wishes of the patient.

For to meet the needs, expectations and wishes of the patient the nursing intensity at the unit has to be in balance. That means a balance between needs and available resources [26,28]. For to state the level of optimal nursing intensity the caregivers needs methods for assess the nursing intensity level, and well defined criteria's what good ethical care means at the unit in case. Caregivers have opportunities to assess this by using tools for nursing intensity measurement in relation to the criteria's of good care made by the staff at the unit. Based on study four we can state that RAFAELA system is a valid and reliable system to measure Nursing Intensity [12-31]. The optimal nursing intensity level describe a level there resources and the patients' needs will be in balance, a level for the unit in case [11]. The study three shows that RAFAELA- system has the opportunities to determine the optimal nursing intensity in care of older people.

Optimal Nursing Intensity level is a determining factor for the patient's possibilities to got good ethical care. The sub study two show a remarkable result. Opportunities to provide ethical good care varies significantly. Based on early research one reason might be the unbalance between patients' needs and resources [30]. Good ethical care will thereby be in in a constant tension between the ethical and the unethical. Despite of good intensions good ethical care is always at risk of changing into more or less unethical care [9,10]. In order to guarantee the older person an ethical care based on dignity, a caring community, safety and integrity in caring, in the future, the caregivers need for an awareness of and responsibility for those entities from witch good care are grooving up (ethical values and ethos), otherwise ethical problems and dilemmas hidden the good intention of ethical care [8,9]. The caregivers have to be awereness of ethical dilemma and together make ethical consensus about how to act in the daily work. The point is, everybody has to take responsibility for good ethical care.

Caring with dignity as ideal longs for a care where compassion and mercy prevails. Other ideals as autonomy take account the older person´s free will to act (autonomy) and decide in cases that belongs to her care. To assert that the patient has received good care according to the department has established criteria for good care, both needs and wishes has to be met [8,11,13].

From the "patters of interpretation" four cornerstones was drawing out; such as ethics as ideals, wishes ethical manners and ethical leadership. Good care based on the values dignity, a caring community, safety and integrity, receive their legitimacy thought ethical awareness and consent among caregivers. The ethical awareness deepens the understanding of wishes and expectations that may arise as a result of ethical openness (Figure 1).

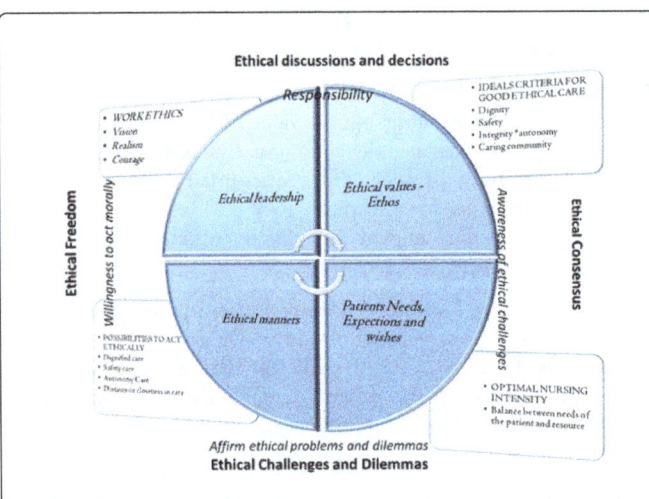

**Figure 1:** Syntheses between ethical values and nursing intensity.

Good care requires an awareness of balance between the patient´s care needs and optimal level of nursing intensity. An ethical leader considers a work situation where optimal nursing intensity and optimal resource allocation makes good care possible, i.e., the caregiver have the opportunity to meet the patients 'needs, wishes and expectation in an optimal level. When ethical wishes and expectations can be met, we have an optimal nursing intensity with possibilities for ethical manners. The nursing process has to be supported by good leadership. An ethical aware leader proposes ethical discussions and ethical decision-making in the daily work. The ethical freedom is a task for the leader. He or she has to form a culture were goodness has a possibility to grow and caregivers has courage and willingness to do good for the patients.

The theoretical model presented is an ideal typical reasoning. The model can be used as a thought structure to develop an ethical transparency and in creating ethical consensus decision between caregivers. Ethical values creates ethical desires and expectations, and

only when ethical aspirations, expectations and needs can be met, the patient can guarantee good care, the department is at an optimal nursing intensity level. An optimal Nursing Intensity level makes good ethical manners possibly. Based on early research can we state that caregivers know and want to act ethically, but they do not always have possibilities to act in accordance with their wishes.

## Discussion

Ethical good care requires affirmed ethical values among caregivers and consent when the team of caregivers make a common decision about ethical values for to guide them I their daily care of patients. The caregivers need courage to see wishes and expectations of the patients, but they also need support of their nursing manager [1]. They need to know that their attitudes and manners make difference for the organization. Whiteout support and supervising the caregivers' don´t see their own responsibility for good ethical care in the caring team. To do well the caregivers have to feel there will be balance between expectations and the realistic possibilities to provide "good ethical care". Based on my study we can state that a prerequisite for meeting this needs are balance between available resources and caring needs [8,26]. The theoretical model show above have opportunities to guide the manager in here task to promote good care for older people. He or she can step by step, lead and supervise the caregivers in their professional development. Ethical values, nursing intensity, ethical manners would continuously be discussed. By interpretation of the entities in the model, the understanding of the possibilities of ethics in daily work deepens. Previous research shows that caregivers almost daily, face ethical problems and challenges. The caregivers are aware about the ethics in the daily work with older people, but they feel they lack realistic possibilities to act in ethical manners they would like to [1,9].

The care of older people faces great challengers due to the increase of number of older people and the decrease in available personnel. Society glorifies economically principles, efficiency and productivity, values that are hard to combine with "good ethical care", still it will be a very important area to find out a way for common communication [31]. Economic and ethics needs a common dialog. The field of work with older people is commonly considered unattractive, knowledge is lacking and recruiting staff is becoming more and more difficult to find. Care of older people needs highly professional caregivers and status of an attractive work area. Every caregiver have her his ideal about the good care, and they want to act in accordance with this ideals. Research has found that caregivers don\t stay in the caring area if they every day have to compromises with their conscience. The caregivers have to protect themselves and they have different ways to handle, they either live the caring area or they would get burnout.

## Conclusion

Good care occurs when different professions work together develops ethical processes with ethical reflections in the daily work; the theoretically model would give the structure for this development process. Caregivers and leaders have to communicate with each other, take each caregivers experience in account and in an effective way eliminate inhibited factors for ethical good care. The entities in the model have been found reliable and logical. The model would need further research for to develop the entities and concepts. Further research is also needed for to find out how the model can support clinical praxis and ethical development. I look forward to start the process and I hope other researches would be interesting to develop the model by research.

The author takes responsibility for the article and we have now economical or other benefits of the article. I am grateful to my supervisor Lisbeth Fagerstrom, professor at the Åbo Academy University, how guided me in the research process.

## References

1. Frilund M (2015) Leadership ideals- A study with prospective nursing leaders. Open Journal of Nursing 5: 508-515.

2. Brewer GA, Kellough EJ (2016) Administrative values and public personel management: reflections on civil service reform. Public Personnel Management 45: 171-189.

3. Papastavrou E, Efstathiou G, Tsangar H, Karlou C, Patiraki E, et al. (2015) Patients' diaconal control over care: a cross-national comparison from both the patients' and nurses' points of view. Scandinavian Journal of Caring Science 1-11.

4. Aiken LH, Clarke SP, Sloane (2000) Hospital staffing, organization and quality of care. International Journal for Quality in Health Care 14: 5-13.

5. Martinsen K, Eriksson K (2009) Evidens- begrensende eller opplysende? Å se og innse om olike former for evidens Arkibe Oslo 52: 81-165.

6. Fjetland KJ, Søreide GE (2010). Etichal dilemmas; A Resource in Public Health Nurse's' everyday work. Scandinavian Journal of Caring Science 24: 75-83.

7. Fagerström L, Bergbom I (2010) The use of Hegelian dialectics in Nursing Science. Nursing Science Quarterly 23: 79-81.

8. Frilund M (2013) En vårdvetenskaplig syntes mellan vårdandets ethos och vårdintensitet. (1stedn), Åbo Akademi, Vasa.

9. Frilund M, Eriksson K, Fagerström L (2013) The caregivers 'possibilities of providing ethically good care for older people. Scandinavian Journal of Caring Science 4: 13.

10. Frilund M, Eriksson K, Fagerström L, Eklund P (2013) Assessment of ethical ideals and ethical manners in care of older people. Nursing Research and Practice 1-11 L.

11. Frilund M, Fagerström L (2009) Managing the optimal workload by the PAONCIL method- a challenge for nursing leadership in care of older people. Journal of Nursing Management 17: 426-434.

12. Frilund M, Fagerstrom, L (2009b) Validity and reliability testing of the Oulu Patient Classification: instrument within primary health care for the older people. International Journal of Older People Nursing 4: 280-287.

13. Eriksson K (2002) Caring science in a new key. Nursing Science Quarterly 15: 61-65.

14. Eriksson K (2010) Concept determination as part of the development of knowledge in caring science. Scandinavian Journal of Caring Sciences 24: 2–11.

15. Føllesdal D, Walløe L (2000) Argumentajonsteori, språk og vetenskapsfilosofi. (1stedtn), Universitets förlaget, Oslo.

16. Flemming V, Robb Y (2003). Hermeneutic rescearch in nursing; a developing a Gadamerian – based research method. Nursing Inquiry 10: 113-120.

17. Randers, Mattiasson AC (2004) Autonomy and integrity: Upholding older adult patients' dignity. Journal of Advanced Nursing 45: 63-71.

18. Randers, Mattiasson AC, Olson T (2002) Conforming older adult patients' view of who they are and would like to be. Nursing Ethics 9: 416-430.

19. Edberg M (2002) Människans värdighet ett grundbegrepp inom vårdvetenskapen. (1st edtn), Akademisk avhandling, Åbo.

20. Andenberg P, Sean P Berglund, AL, Segersten K (2007). Preserving dignity in caring for older adults: A concept analysis. Journal of Advanced Nursing 59: 635-645.

21. Boisaubin E, Chu A, Catalano J (2007) Perceptions of long-term care, Autonomy and dignity by residents, Family and Caregivers: the Houston Experience. Journal of Medicine and Philosophy 32: 447-464.

22. Davies S, Ellis L, Laker S (2000) Promoting autonomy and independence for older people within nursing practice: An observational study. Journal of Clinical Nursing 9: 127-136.

23. Melander Wikman A (2008) Safety and privacy; elderly person´s experience of a mobile safety alarm. Health and Social Care in Community 16: 337-346.

24. Eriksson K (2010). Concept determination as part of the Development of knowledge in caring science. Scandinavian Journal of Caring Sciences 11: 195-198.

25. Fagerström L (1999) The Patient´s Caring needs- to understand and measure the unmeasurable. (8thedtn), Åbo Akademis Förlag.

26. Ito C, Natsume M (2016) Ethical dilemmas facing chief nurses in Japan: A Pilot study. Nursing ethics 23: 432-441.

27. Rauhala A, Fagerström L (2004) Determining optimal nursing intensity: The RAFAELA method. Journal of Advanced Nursing 45: 351-359.

28. Fagerström L, Bergbom I (2010) The use of Hegelian dialectics in nursing science. Nursing Science Quarterly 23: 79-84.

29. Eriksson K, Lindström UA (2007) Vårdvetenskapens vetenskapsteori på hermeneutisk grund- några grunddrag. (2ndedtn) I Eriksson, Lindström, Matilainen, Lindholm. I hermeneutikens landskap. Gryning III, vårdvetenskap och hermeneutik. Enheten för vårdvetenskap, Åbo Akademi, Multiprint, Vasa.

30. Rauhala A, Fagerström L (2004) Determining optimal Nursing Intensity: The RAFAELA method. Journal of Advanced Nursing 45: 351-359.

31. Martinsen K (2009) Evidens- begrensende eller opplysende? (1stedtn). Å se og Å innse om olike former for evidens. Arkibe, Oslo.

# 25

# Strengthening of Health Locus of Control could Increase the Independence of Post Stroke Patients in Implementing the Daily Activities at Home

**Ali Hamzah\* and Sugiyanto**

*Bandung Nursing Department, Bandung Health Politechnic, Indonesia*

**\*Corresponding author**: Ali Hamzah, Bandung Nursing Department, Bandung Health Politechnic, Indonesia, E-mail: alihamzahbandung@yahoo.co.id

## Abstract

According to the data released by the Ministry of Health of Indonesia in 2009 shown that stroke was reported as the first number cause of death in patients who's hospitalized and it placed the eleventh rank of the most diseases in outpatient wards. Strokes often cause a lot of problems, especially interferes in the functioning of the body movement then prequently lead to disability, dependence on the other and inability to carry out daily activities. It is not only the healing process that takes time but also stroke treatment and rehabilitation does too gradually it leads to boredom and frustration. Furthermore, if the patient want to return to their productive phase they have to be confidence to have a self-control of their health problems (health locus of control) so that their level of independence in carrying out their daily activities can be improved. This study is aimed to determine the effect of strengthening health locus of control to the independence of post stroke patients in carrying out daily activities at home. The research method used a quasi-experimental with pre and post test without control design, and used the 31 post-stroke patients who are undergoing treatment at the Polyclinic stroke of Al Islam Hospital Bandung, Indonesia, as sample. The samples were taken by purposive sampling technique. Data analysis consisted of univariate analysis using the mean score and standard deviation as well as bivariate analysis using t-test dependent. Based on the analysis obtained that the strengthening of the Health locus of control influence was highly effectively to increase the independence of post stroke patients in carrying out his daily activities, so the nurse suggested that the strengthening health locus of control should be continued to be implemented to the post- stroke patients to continue treatment at home in order to increase their independence.

**Keywords:** Strengthening health locus of control; Independence in implementing daily actvities; Stroke

## Introduction

Based on the data taken from the Ministry of Health of Indonesia in the year 2009 shown that stroke was considered as the first cause of death to hospitalized patients and it ranked as the eleventh most diseases in outpatient wards. Meanwhile, according to report done by the Fundamental Health Research in 2007 stroke was prevailed in Indonesia was about 8.3 per 1000, in the province of West Java was 0.9%, and in Bandung city reached 1.1%.

However, the results made by Thomas and Santoso (2003) in Dr. Kariadi hospital Semarang was only 7.7% of suffer can perform their daily activities independently after they had been undergone treatment in such particular hospital [1]. While the remaining, 77.8% suffer need family assistance to be able to perform their daily activities and 22.2% was highly dependent on their family to perform daily activities. In regard, to the stroke patients who's undergone advanced treatment program requires the presence of a health locus of control/HLoC.

The health Locus Of Control is the degree of belief in one's health that his health is determined by internal factors or external factors. It means that the patient him self feels responsible for his health. Several studies related to the health locus of control had been done before; Nurina Dewi Pratita used the method of correlation studies to assess the relationship of spousal support and the health locus of control with compliance in undergoing the treatment of type 2 diabetes, the obtained results indicated that there was a high relationship (close)

between spousal support and the health locus of control with compliance in undergoing the treatment of type 2 diabetes (r=0884 p=0.0001) [2]. Similarly, another research conducted by Yunita Mandasari about the relationship health locus of control among smoker and assertive behavior in teen, the results obtained p value = 0.0005, which mean that there was a significant relationship between significant others health locus of control and assertive behavior in adolescents who smoke [3].

Referring to such metters, the importance of health locus of control in determining compliance patient post- stroke treatment program will also directly determine their independence in meeting his daily needs the further research on the influence of these factors HLoC. Hence, the purpose of this study is: "to determine the effect of strengthening of the health locus of control to independence of post-stroke patients in carrying out their daily activities at home".

## Conceptual framework

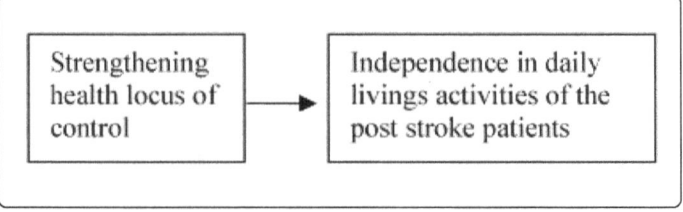

## Definition of term

Strengthening of Health Locus of Control (HLOC), an independent variabel is kind of effort done by researchers to enhance a patient's self confidence level to have a self control on health of post-stroke patients, through the approach of giving educational home visits twice a week, counseling once and motivation once a week, for at least 45 minutes.

Consequently, the independence level to carry out daily activities done by post-stroke patients that is considered as a dependent variable was performing the activities of eating, bathing, dressing ornate, defecation, urination, toileting, moving from bed to chair or conversely, move, and up or down stairs, both before and after strengthening health locus of control as measured by observation using the Barthel index. The results of a range of values that range from 0-100, the higher the value obtained patients show that the patients increasingly independent, and it is in ratio scale.

## Research Methodology

This study used a quasi experiment with pre and post test design without control. It has been implemented since September 2012 up to October 2013, using the 31 post- stroke patients who were undergone a treatment at the polyclinic stroke in Al Islam hospital Bandung. The data was obtained by using purposive sampling technique. The patients who were selected are undergoing post-stroke treatment program. It was not taken from hemoraghic stroke criteria. The condition of the patient is conscious and calm, cooperative, able to listen and speak clearly and willing to be respondent. Data collection is begun by identifying post- stroke patients who meet the inclusion criteria, then patients who met the inclusion criteria provided an informed consent and asked approval is for being the respondents. Subsequently measured respondent level of independence in performing daily activities at home before being given treatment (pre-test), and then do the strengthening health locus of control, consisting of a package modul as much as 4 times, consist of 2 times a week for education program and each education program need 45 minutes with the topic: care and stroke rehabilitation program at home and efforts to improve post- stroke patient independence in performing activities of daily living, the next was given counseling 1 times (45 minutes) and finally was given motivation to the patient 1 times (45 minutes) too, due home visit to each patient's residence. After patients completed a whole series of these treatments directly measured the level of independence in performing activities of daily living as a data post-test. Data processing was done by step: editing, coding, entrying, cleaning and processing, data. Further data analysis through univariate analysis using the mean and standard deviation as well as bivariate analysis using t-test dependent.

## Result

### Univariate analysis

#### Respondent characteristic

| | Respondent characteristic | f | % |
|---|---|---|---|
| 1. | Age: | | |
| | Adult (18-45 years old) | 1 | 3,23 |
| | Pre elderly (46-59 years old) | 6 | 19,35 |
| | Elderly (≥ 60 years old) | 24 | 77,42 |
| | Number | 31 | 100 |
| 2. | Experienced of having patient in stroke frequency: 1 times | 12 | 38,71 |
| | ≥ 2 times | 19 | 61,29 |
| | Number | 31 | 100 |
| 3. | Patient relationship with the family: | | |
| | Spouse (husband/wife) | 19 | 61,29 |
| | Children | 12 | 38,71 |
| | Number | 31 | 100 |

Table 1: Respondent Characteristic (Post Stroke patient who undergo to Polyclinic stroke of Al Islam hospital)

Referring to Table 1 it appears that patient post-stroke who are undergoing treatment at the clinic of the stroke program Al Islam Hospital Bandung majority (77.42%) categorized as elderly age (≥ 60 years), most of them also had suffered a stroke ≥ 2 times and only a small part for the first time had suffered a stroke and suffered a stroke during their general lives with her partner (husband/wife) at home.

## Mean score independence in daily activities of the post stroke patients before and after streghtening health locus of control/HLoC

| Indepedence of Post Stroke Patient | Mean | N | Sd |
|---|---|---|---|
| Before strengthening health locus of control | 62.74 | 31 | 26.23 |
| After strengthening health locus of control | 46.61 | 31 | 22.38 |

Tabel 2: Mean score of Indepedence Post Stroke Patient (before and after strengthening health locus of control)

Based on Table 2 the mean score of post-stroke patient independence in performing their daily activities at home before being given the strengthening HLOC is 46.61 with a standard deviation of 26.23 and after strengthening HLOC increased to 62.74 with a standard deviation of 22.38.

## Bivariate analysis

Results of t-dependent test analysis as shown in Table 3.

| Data | Avg Mean | Sd | Std. Error Mean | t | p- Value |
|---|---|---|---|---|---|
| Post Test - Pre Test | 16.13 | 10.54 | 1.89 | 8.517 | 0.0001 |

Tabel 3: Analysis of the average difference before and after intervention strengthening health locus of control to post-stroke patients.

Table 3 shows that the difference in average scores indepedence of the post stroke patient before and after streghtening HLoC is 16,13 with standard deviation is 10,54, a value of t = 8,517 and 0.0001 probability value ≤ 0.05. These results indicate that there is a significant effect of strengthening to the independence HLOC on improving post-stroke patients in carrying out his daily activities at home.

## Discussion

The results indicate that efforts to strengthen HLOC through 4 types implementation two times giving education, counseling and motivation by home visit. It is proven to increase on average of independence significantly. This suggests that in addition to the familiar program implemented by the health care team in the hospital such as blood pressure control, continuing treatment and medical rehabilitation programs, nurses also need to make another effort, especially in strengthening and improving the health locus of control patient in dealing with the problem at hand stroke so the patients have confidence with high motivation, strong spirit and exercise, as a result their level of dependence on others reduce or having self independence. Through strengthening this HLOC a patient has given the opportunity to convey his feeling or expressing emotions therefore the patient feel more recognized, listened to his complaint and made him aware of changes, getting solutions and motivation to pace his problem.

Referring to the opinion Wallston and Walston (2002) that "health locus of control is influenced by several factors, including the age factor, older the patient is, the higher the belief of HLoC is. In accordance to the theory many strokes patients occur in middle age above. However, in this study found a very young age of stroke patients at the age of 31 years old. When associated with research, it turns out the age factor in this study has a strengthening effect also affects HLOC, where the young age of the patient, the easier and excited in doing exercises so it's easier HLOC strengthened. Some patients at adult age categories (18 - 45 years) and pre- elderly (46 - 59 years) responded well when given training Range Of Motion (ROM) and their motivation to improve HLOC, some of them made progress, due to his productive age. This can be seen at the second and third visits generally they have increased ability to perform daily activities.

Besides the age factor, the influence of the strengthening HLOC to be independence in carrying out their daily activities to the post-stroke patients are also influenced by the experience of having patient in stroke frequency. According to the research Cadena et al. (2011), in examining the relationship of locus of control with work experience, found that "experience can change a person's belief in self-control" [4]. In this study, the majority (61.29%) of respondents had suffered a stroke the same experience or more than 2 times.

Experience of suffering a stroke more than 2 times will affect the patient's ability to accept and digest the information given by the researchers in the form of education, counseling and motivation due to the many functions of neurons that have been damaged. Smeltzer (2002) and Sylvia Anderson (2006) revealed that "more often patient having a stroke, the risk of damage to the neurons in the brain affected and the more widespread", in which it will also influence the noble functions including a memory function and motoric patient. In contrast to the small proportion of respondents (38.71%) for the first time having stroke, the risk of damage to the neurons in his brain will be fewer and smaller, so that the ability of some of its noble function,

especially memory can still have function properly when handling fast and proper [5].

In addition, the presence and involvement of people who matter to patient especially from spouse (husband/wifes) is very important in the success of this intervention HLOC strengthening the independence of post- stroke patient. Referring to Table 1, the majority (61.29%) of respondents suffered from stroke during their generally treatment by her partner (husband/wife) or if the deceased spouse was a minority (38.71%) of respondents cared for by children. Based on the observations in most patient researchers got positive support and motivation, especially attention from both families of couples (husband/wife) or their children apperently increase. Average the level of independence, otherwise the patient who has lack off support is less concerned from his family because of busy working or over protective than the patient has generally less motivated and willing to attempt to break away from dependence of the family, hence the average level of independence less likely to increase or even stagnant. Thus the stronger the family support for the patient, the faster the patients can achieve independence to carry out their daily activities.

Simirarly, the research conducted by Nurina Dewi Pratita (2012) shown that there is a relationship between spousal support and the Health Locus Of Control with compliance in undergoing the treatment of type 2 diabetes (r=0884 and p=0.0001) [2]. Likewise, the results of research conducted Yunita Mandasari (2011) of the relationship health locus of control and assertive behavior of a teen smoker, shown a significant correlation between significant others health locus of control and assertive behavior in adolescents who smoke (p=0.005 ) [3]. The results are not much different shown by Enejoh A Victor and Karick Haruna (2012) in this study of Relationship between health locus of control and sexual risk behavior concluded that there was statistically significant effect HLOC on risky sexual behavior (p ≤ 0.05).

The level of health locus of control is different for each person, this is due to differences in assessment and experiences during his life span. Some patients displayed more positive behavior, when they were motivated to maintain their life by getting the treatment and rehabilitation programs on a regular basis. So that, they feel that they are still able to perform their activities like everyone else, even a little. Here is encourage them to seek independently in carrying out their daily activities needs. However the majority of patients who have a pessimistic sense of the condition of his health, they need to be encouraged by others because they thought that he was not able to do anything else because all that has been determined by God [6].

According to these result, it is necessary to strengthen HLOC ifor patients who have chronic diseases and requires continuoustly treatment, such as: the stroke patients need to be handled by the nurse that the patient can continue to be motivated to continue treatment and rehabilitation programs that ultimately will be self-sufficient in patient health control, especially in carrying out daily activities [7-12].

## Limitation

This research study has some limitations especially on the research design that didn't use control group or another group intervention, because we had very difficult to find appropriate patients criteria and we couldn't control confounding factors such as medication program.Therefore, the result couldn't compare with the others and it will influence the conclussion [13-22].

Strengthening of Health Locus of Control could Increase the Independence of Post Stroke Patients...

137

## Conclusion

Strengthening health locus of control will effectively be increase self independence in performing daily activities at home for the post-stroke patients who were adjusted to the Polyclinic stroke of Al Islam hospital Bandung.

## Suggestions

Nurses need to continue an integration effort to strengthen the HLOC treatment for the post stroke patients in their home in order to increase their independence, by integrating these efforts with the home care program.

Nurses also must cooperate and always involve which the family in providing support to post-stroke patients who were treated at home so that patients can continue to improved their HLOC and independence of him.

## Acknowledgements

Great appreciation is given to Director of Bandung Health Polytechnic, and Chairperson of Bandung Nursing department who has supported and giving budget for this research project. We would also like to thank to the Director and the head of nurse of Bandung Al Islam hospital, in Bandung, who has given us permission to conduct research. I am gratefully indebted for all of patients and family members of the stroke patients who participated in this study.

## References

1. Santoso, Thomas A (2003) Kemandirian Aktivitas Makan, Mandi Dan Berpakaian Pada Penderita Stroke 6-24 Bulan Pasca Okupasi Terapi. Skripsi. Semarang: Universitas Diponegoro.

2. Pratita ND (2012) Hubungan Dukungan Pasangan Dan Health Locus Of Control Dengan Kepatuhan Dalam Menjalani Proses Pengobatan Pada Penderita Diabetes Mellitus Tipe-2, Jurnal Ilmiah Mahasiswa Universitas Surabaya Vol.1 No.1.

3. Mandasari Y (2011) Health Locus of Control Relationships and Assertive Behavior In smoker Teens, Gunadarma University Library.

4. David Cadena BS, Sandra B, Inez Cruz MSW, Ashok K, Robert F (2011) Correlation between locus of control and opportunities for health behaviors, The University of texas Health Science Centre at San Antonio.

5. Price, Sylvia A (2006) Patofisiologi Konsep Klinik Proses-proses Penyakit Edisi 4. Jakarta : EGC.

6. Lau RR (1982) Origins of health locus of control beliefs. J Pers Soc Psychol 42: 322-334.

7. Brenda GB, Suzanne CS (2002) Brunner & Suddarth: Text Book of Medical Surgical Nursing, W.B. Sounders. Philadelphia.

8. Depkes (2009) Badan Penelitian dan Pengembangan Kesehatan Departemen Kesehatan, Republik Indonesia.

9. Departement of Psycology and School of Public Health (1999) Does locus of control moderate the effect of tailored health education materials?, St Louis University, St Louis, MO 63108, USA.

10. Dinkes TK I Jawa Barat (2007) Profil Kesehatan Jawa Barat. Bandung : Dinkes Provinsi Jawa Barat.

11. Schlenk EA, Hart LK (1984) Relationship between health locus of control, health value, and social support and compliance of persons with diabetes mellitus. Diabetes Care 7: 566-574.

12. Mulyatsih E (2006) Stroke, Petunjuk Praktis bagi Pengasuh dan Keluarga Pasien Pasca Stroke, Jakarta: Balai Penerbit FKUI.

13. Victor EA, Haruna K (2012) Relationship between health locus of control and sexual risk behavior. Retrovirology 9: P62.

14. Ida F (2009) Mengantisipasi Stroke Petunjuk Mudah, Legkap dan Praktis Sehari-Hari. Yogyakarta: Buku biru.

15. Indriyati (2009) Hubungan Activity Daily Living (adl) Berdasarkan Indeks Barthel Dengan Tingkat Depresi Pada Pasien Stroke Di Bangsal Anggrek 1 RS Dr. Moewardi Surakarta. Skripsi. Surakarta: Universitas Muhamadiyah Surakarta.

16. Muhammad I (2010) Fisioterapi Bagi Insan Stroke. Yogyakarta:Graham Ilmu.

17. Muttaqin A (2008) Asuhan Keperawatan Klien Dengan Gangguan Sistem Persarapan. Jakarta : Salemba Medika.

18. Niven ON (2002) Psikologi Kesehatan Pengantar Untuk Perawat dan Professional Kesehatan Lainnya. Jakarta: EGC.

19. Nursalam (2008) Konsep & Penerapan Metodologi Penelitian Ilmu Keperawatan: Pedoman Skripsi, Tesis, dan Instrumen Penelitian. Jakarta; Salemba Medika.

20. Pinzon R, Laksmi A (2010) Awas Stroke! Pengertian, Gejala, Tindakan, Perawatan dan Pencegahan. Yogyakarta: Andi.

21. http://www.yastroki.or.id/read.php?id=300.

22. Health Locus of Control Scales (2002) In H. Lefcourt (Ed.) Research With The Locus of Control. New York: Academic Press.

# 26

# The Effect of Hand Hygiene Promotion in a University Hospital in China

**Li-Li Xiang**[1], **Duo-Shuang Xie**[2,3*], **Rui Li**[2], **Xiang-Yun Fu**[2], **Hui-Fang Wang**[2],**Qiao Hu**[2], **Qin-Qing Luo**[2], **Lei Wang**[4], **Rui-Ping Lai**[2] and **Han-Lin Liao**[2]

[1]*Physical examination center, Taihe Hospital, Hubei University of Medicine, Shiyan, Hubei, China*

[2]*Department of Infection Control, Taihe Hospital, Hubei University of Medicine, Shiyan, Hubei, China*

[3]*Center of Health Administration and Development studies, Hubei University of Medicine, Shiyan, Hubei, China*

[4]*Hospital Administration Office, Taihe Hospital, Hubei University of Medicine, Shiyan, Hubei, China*

**\*Corresponding author: Duo-Shuang Xie,** Department of Infection Control, Taihe Hospital, Hubei University of Medicine, No 32 Renmin Road, Shiyan, Hubei 430030, PR China, E-mail: xieds8@163.com

## Abstract

**Objective:** Implementing a multimodal campaign could be resulted in a sustained increase in hand hygiene (HH) compliance rates. However, most studies of HH campaign have been conducted in the developed countries. This study was aimed to evaluate the effectiveness of hand hygiene campaign in a university hospital in China.

**Methods:** During the period of the HH campaign, the WHO hand hygiene improvement strategy was implemented to improve hand hygiene compliance. We collected and evaluated the effect of hand hygiene campaign by the questionnaire of WHO hand hygiene observation, consumption of alcohol-based hand rub (AHR), liquid soap and gloves, and the quality of HH by adenosine triphosphate (ATP) test.

**Results:** Of the 4,177 opportunities of hand hygiene evaluated, the HH compliance improved significantly from 24.2% to 41.0% after the intervention. Health care workers in the ICU showed higher hand hygiene compliance compared with those in other departments. In general, Nurses' hand hygiene compliance was higher than those of physicians and surgeons. The consumption of AHR and the ATP pass rate increased after the intervention.

**Conclusion:** Through the intervention, medical staff hand hygiene compliance was greatly improved from 24.2% to 41.0%. The WHO Hand Hygiene Strategy was also effective in hospital of China.

**Keywords:** Hand hygiene campaign; Compliance; Healthcare associated infection; China

## Introduction

Healthcare-associated infection (HAI) accounts for one of the most common complications in hospitalized patients, and is a major contributor to prolonged hospital stay and increased healthcare costs [1,2].

In recent years, improving patient safety has received more and more attention, and the first goal of the World Health Organization (WHO) World Alliance for Patient Safety is "the Clean Care is Safer Care" [3]. Hand hygiene (HH), i.e. washing hand with soap and water, or disinfecting hands with alcohol-based hand rub (AHR), is considered to be a simple, but most effective method of preventing HAI and cutting off the spread of antimicrobial-resistant pathogens [4-6]. In 2009, the WHO has issued hand hygiene guidelines for health care workers (HCW) [2].

The efficiency of HH is well-known, however, numerous studies have shown that without any intervention the rate of HH compliance remained low [7,8].

It's been reported that implementing a multimodal campaign could resulted in a sustained increase in HH compliance rates. However, most studies of HH campaign have been conducted in the developed countries [5,8-11]. In 2009, the Ministry of Health of China (MOH)

issued a national health industry standard Hand Hygiene Norms for Medical Staff [12]. From then on, HH campaigns were conducted in a few hospitals in China. In Taihe Hospital, Hand Hygiene Campaign was conducted with those effective tools. This study was undertaken to evaluate HH behavior of HCW before and after the HH campaign in the hospital, and to add the experience of the WHO Hand Hygiene Strategy conducted in the developing countries.

## Materials and Methods

### Setting

The study was performed from January 2012 to April 2013 in Taihe Hospital. Taihe Hospital, also named the Affiliated Hospital of Hubei University of Medicine, is a tertiary hospital, founded in 1965 and located in the City of Shiyan, Hubei Province of China. There are 2900 beds for adults and children, and 1067 nurses and 707 physicians or surgeons in the hospital totally, with 99 000 admissions in 2012. The hospital included a general intensive care unit (ICU) and all medical specialties being represented. Due to the limitation of research labor power, we selected the following departments to conduct the study: internal medicine (comprising respiratory, gastroenterology, cardiology, endocrinology, hepatology, nephrology, hematology, and neurology), departments of surgery (comprising general surgery, cardiac and cerebral surgery, neurosurgery, orthopedics, urology, plastic and burn, oncology, obstetrics and gynecology), pediatrics,

ICUs, and others (comprising Chinese traditional medicine, dentistry, ENT [ears, nose and throat] medicine, ophthalmology and dermatology). This study was reviewed and approved by the Ethics and Health Research Review Committee of Taihe Hospital, Hubei University of Medicine.

## Design

The baseline HH compliance rate of HCW was established from January to August 2012. After the first observation period, comprehensive intervention was implemented in September and October, 2012 by the infection control team. We conducted this study using the WHO hand hygiene improvement strategy.

The strategy consists of 5 core elements [13]:

(1) System change, including access to AHR at the point of patient care and to liquid soap, towels, and a safe, continuous water supply. AHR bottles were installed along the passageway and the foot of every patient bed in an attempt to enable easy access by HCW to the HH products.

(2) Training and educating HCWs: All the HCW in the hospital received the theoretical and practical training which was delivered by the director or the trained nurses of the infection control team, and we tried some innovative training methods, such as hand hygiene slogan and promotional items solicitation and hand hygiene knowledge contest.

(3) Monitoring practices and providing feedback on performance. Data of HH compliance and consumption of AHR, liquid soap and gloves were provided monthly for each ward by our study team.

(4) Posting visual reminders in the workplace.

(5) Creating a safety climate within the institution with the active, visible participation of both individual HCW and senior hospital managers. Before the intervention, each wards must paid for these HH products, including AHR, liquid soap, gloves, and hand tissue. After the intervention, these items were provided by the hospital, and the consumption of related HH material didn't add any financial burden to each ward.

## Data collection

For the evaluation of these opportunities, a special assessment sheet was provided. The following parameters were recorded: (1) the name and type of the wards, (2) the type of opportunity for HH, and (3) the type of action performed (washing hands, AHR, glove, no action). The observations was performed respectively before and after the intervention at least 50 opportunities in each wards to ensure a standardized manner of observation. Compliance rates were then calculated as percentages, using direct observation by trained observers via a standardized assessment sheet designed by WHO. These opportunities were evaluated according to the standardized WHO definitions and divided it into 5 groups [14]: (1) before contact to the patient, (2) before aseptic practice, (3) after contact to potentially infectious agents, (4) after contact to the patient, and (5) after contact to patients' environment. Results of HH compliance rates were calculated separately for different category of departments, and different medical professionals.

In addition, consumption of AHR, liquid soap, and glove were recorded and evaluated monthly by our study team.

## Adenosine triphosphate monitering

Except for hand hygiene improvement strategy, adenosine triphosphate (ATP) was used to monitor and improve the quality of hand hygiene in this study. In each wards, HCW were selected at random and asked to wash their hands with liquid soap and running water. When the hands were completely dry, the investigator rubbed the swab against the tips of each finger, in between each finger and then in an S-shape along the palm of one hand. Then the swab was placed in the monitor, and in no time the results recorded automatically. An explanation of the score was given and the improvement in technique to achieve cleaner hands was discussed with HCW in the spot.

The ATP monitoring system was System SURE Plus, produced by Hygiena International, Watford, UK, 2011. The score <30 was considered pass according the manufacturer's recommendation. During the observations of hand hygiene compliance at each department, the 2-3 HCW who washed his/her hands with flowing water were chosen to be tested by ATP detection.

## Statistical analyses

Statistical analysis was performed using descriptive statistics such as frequency, percentage of HH compliance and the 95% confidence interval (CI). Statistical analysis was performed by SAS, version 8.2.,and Bartlett's Chi-squared test was used to evaluate the inequality of percentages, and P values <0.05 (two-tailed) were considered statistically significant.

## Results

### HH compliance rates

Overall, 4177 opportunities events requiring HH were observed during all phases of the study, with 1914 opportunities before the intervention and 2263 after. There were more than 700 HCW attended the hand hygiene slogan and promotional items solicitation, and hand hygiene knowledge contest. During the period of HH campaign, more than 423 HH slogans and 40 HH promotional items were created personally by HCW of Taihe Hospital.

Compliance rates of investigated groups were summarized and presented in Table 1. From January to August 2012 before the intervention, the HH compliance was 24.2%. After the intervention a significant improvement of HH compliance was assessed in the period from September 2012 to April 2013 (from overall 24.2% to 41.0%, P< . 0000).

There was significant difference in HH compliance among departments and professionals both before and after the intervention. Before the intervention, the highest rate of HH compliance was observed in ICU (30.4%), followed by the internal medicine units (27.3%) and the pediatric units (24.0%). After the intervention, the high rate were noticed in ICU (47.2%), then the surgical wards (46.7%) and others departments (42.3%). Compared with physicians and surgeons, nurses were noticed with the higher rate of HH compliance both before (30.9%) and after (44.8%) the intervention.

According to the 5 groups of opportunities defined by WHO, HH was performed more frequently after body fluid exposure risk.

| Variable | Baseline | | | Follow-up | | | P |
|---|---|---|---|---|---|---|---|
| | No. of hand hygiene actions | No. (%) of hand hygiene opportunities | Compliance, % (95% CI) | No. of hand hygiene actions | No. (%) of hand hygiene opportunities | Compliance, % (95% CI) | |
| Overall | 464 | 1914 | 24.2(22.3-26.2) | 927 | 2263 | 41.0(38.9-43.0) | 0.00 |
| Departments | | | | | | | |
| Internal medicine | 132 | 483 | 27.3(23.4-31.3) | 173 | 552 | 31.3(27.5-35.2) | 0.16 |
| Surgical | 86 | 459 | 18.7(15.2-22.3) | 398 | 852 | 46.7(43.4-50.1) | 0.00 |
| ICU | 75 | 247 | 30.4(24.6-36.1) | 137 | 290 | 47.2(41.5-53.0) | 0.00 |
| Pediatric | 82 | 342 | 24.0(19.5-28.5) | 117 | 328 | 35.7(30.5-40.9) | 0.00 |
| Others departments | 89 | 383 | 23.2(19.0-27.5) | 102 | 241 | 42.3(36.1-48.6) | 0.00 |
| Professional category | | | | | | | |
| Nurse | 311 | 1006 | 30.9(28.1-33.8) | 601 | 1342 | 44.8(42.1-47.4) | 0.00 |
| Physician | 63 | 324 | 19.4(15.1-23.8) | 120 | 350 | 34.3(29.3-39.3) | 0.00 |
| Surgeon | 90 | 584 | 15.4(12.5-18.3) | 206 | 571 | 36.1(32.1-40.0) | 0.00 |
| Indications | | | | | | | |
| Before patient contact | 131 | 579 | 22.6(19.2-26.0) | 153 | 437 | 35.0(30.5-39.5) | 0.00 |
| Before aseptic procedure | 108 | 365 | 29.6(24.9-34.3) | 186 | 376 | 49.5(44.4-54.5) | 0.00 |
| After body fluid exposure risk | 87 | 157 | 55.4(47.6-63.2) | 130 | 190 | 68.4(61.8-75.0) | 0.01 |
| After patient contact | 76 | 422 | 18.0(14.3-21.7) | 352 | 916 | 38.4(35.3-41.6) | 0.00 |
| After contact to patients environment | 62 | 391 | 15.9(12.2-19.5) | 106 | 344 | 30.8(25.9-35.7) | 0.00 |

**Table 1:** Compliance rates of investigated subgroups in a university hospital in China.

Others departments, Departments of Chinese traditional medicine, dentistry, ENT [ears, nose and throat] medicine, ophthalmology, and dermatology.

The most extensive improvement of HH compliance was recognized on our surgical ward (18.7%), which ended up reaching the higher HH compliance rates of all (46.7% after the intervention). Lowest improvement after the intervention (4.0%) was evaluated on internal medicine wards (31.3% after the intervention).

### AHR, liquid soap and glove consumption

The overall use of AHR, liquid soap and glove by HCW in different departments increased significantly. Before the Clean Hands Campaign, the highest AHR consumption rates were recorded in ICU (median: 11.8 mL per patient-day), followed by the surgical wards (3.0 mL) and the pediatric wards (1.4 mL). Meanwhile, the highest liquid soap consumption was in ICU (median: 25.3 mL per patient-day), followed by the surgical wards (8.8 mL), and the Internal medicine wards (4.3 mL). The median AHR, liquid soap and glove of all participating wards is presented in Table 2 and Figure 1.

| Departments | Period | | AHR | Liquid soap | Glove |
|---|---|---|---|---|---|
| Internal medicine | Before intervention | Jan.-Apr., 2012 | 0.2 | 2.7 | 0.3 |
| | | May-Aug., 2012 | 0.6 | 5.7 | 0.3 |
| | After intervention | Sep.-Dec., 2012 | 4.0 | 8.9 | 0.3 |
| | | Jan.-Apr., 2013 | 4.1 | 8.3 | 0.4 |
| Surgical | Before intervention | Jan.-Apr., 2012 | 2.8 | 7.1 | 0.2 |
| | | May-Aug., 2012 | 3.1 | 10.3 | 0.2 |
| | After intervention | Sep.-Dec., 2012 | 5.0 | 16.5 | 0.2 |
| | | Jan.-Apr., 2013 | 3.9 | 12.9 | 0.2 |

| | | | | | | |
|---|---|---|---|---|---|---|
| ICU | Before intervention | Jan.-Apr., 2012 | 45.2 | 26.5 | 1.6 |
| | | May-Aug., 2012 | 48.9 | 23.8 | 2.6 |
| | After intervention | Sep.-Dec., 2012 | 79.8 | 31.4 | 2.6 |
| | | Jan.-Apr., 2013 | 63.2 | 34.1 | 2.9 |
| Pediatric | Before intervention | Jan.-Apr., 2012 | 1.2 | 1.7 | 0.2 |
| | | May-Aug., 2012 | 1.5 | 2.6 | 0.1 |
| | After intervention | Sep.-Dec., 2012 | 4.5 | 4.3 | 0.2 |
| | | Jan.-Apr., 2013 | 4.0 | 6.7 | 0.1 |
| Others departments | Before intervention | Jan.-Apr., 2012 | 0.3 | 3.3 | 0.3 |
| | | May-Aug., 2012 | 0.6 | 3.5 | 0.3 |
| | After intervention | Sep.-Dec., 2012 | 2.1 | 5.0 | 0.3 |
| | | Jan.-Apr., 2013 | 1.8 | 6.0 | 0.3 |

**Table 2:** AHR, liquid soap and gloves consumption of investigated subgroups in a university hospital in China.

NOTE: Others departments, Departments of Chinese traditional medicine, dentistry, ENT [ears, nose and throat] medicine, ophthalmology, and dermatology. Values are median; milliliter per patient-day for AHR and liquid soap, pair per patient-day for glove.

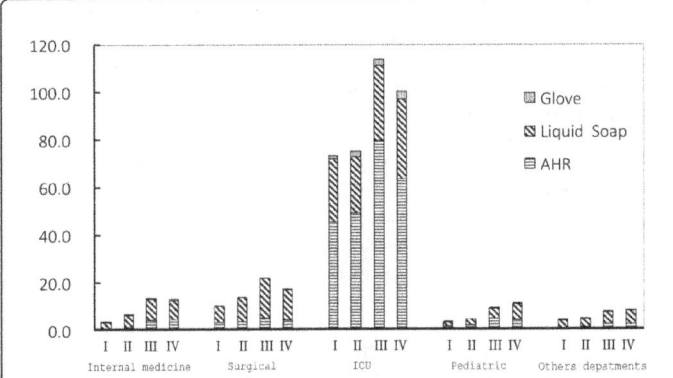

**Figure 1:** AHR, liquid soap and gloves consumption of investigated subgroups in a university hospital in China.

NOTE. AHR, alcohol-based hand rub. Others departmens, Departments of Chinese traditional medicine, dentistry, ENT [ears, nose and throat] medicine, ophthalmology, and dermatology.,Jan.-Apr. 2012;, May-Aug., 2012; , Sep.-Dec., 2012; , Jan.- Apr., 2013.

## ATP results

In the ATP test, 333 subjects were testedand the pass rate was 86.79%. The mean pass rate prior to the HH intervention was 79.75% (126of 158 HCW had scores <30). After the intervention, the rate increased to 93.14% (163of 175 HCW had scores <30)(P< 0.001).

## Discussion

HH was widely accepted as an effective measure to reduce HAI in healthcare settings. Implementation of infection control in the developing countries was complex and must take into account many factors, including costs, lack of knowledge, deficient infrastructure, and cultural issues [15].

To our knowledge, few data about HH compliance rates in China hospitals have been previously reported in international journals. In comparison with data from other institutions [9,10], compliance rates at Taihe Hospital seem to be rather low before the intervention, but enhancement was obvious after the intervention. In this hospital, enhancement was still possible and very much required.

In the health system of China, state financing only counted to about 25-30% of total costs [16]. Medical institutions must try to save costs. Before the intervention, materials of hand hygiene always were inadequate in this hospital. Beginning from September 2012, the hospital provided adequate AHR, liquid soap and hand towel for all the wards. The financial policy that each ward needn't pay for these materials encouraged the HH compliance. The WHO guidelines for hand hygiene reflected evidence that accessibility to AHR near patient locations is key to assist HCW to practice hand hygiene [2].

It is reported that training in HH should be a key element for a successful education, especially in academic professions. Intensive training and education are essential to improve compliance rates and to achieve sustained effect. In this study, we added some games such as hand hygiene slogan and promotional items solicitation, and hand hygiene knowledge contest. The use of gaming technology to provide education and assessment not only improved technique, but also increased compliance with the Five Moments for Hand Hygiene across the hospital [10].

Consistent with the previous reports [17,18], compliance with hand hygiene varied across indications, medical specialties, and HCW categories. Like other studies [9,18-21], compliance improved across all medical specialties and all professional categories after the intervention. As demonstrated by this study, the intervention had an effective influence on the overall HH compliance rate among the medical staff.

The professional status of a HCW was an influencing factor of HH compliance in several studies [7,22,23]. A systematic review published in 2010 showed that the median hand hygiene compliance was 40%, and among physicians, in intensive care units and prior to patient contact the hand hygiene compliance was lower [24].

Similarly, a difference in compliance between the professional groups in our hospital became apparent during the Campaign. All groups, including nurses, physicians, and surgeons improved with respect to HH compliance, but this effect was much more evident in the surgeons' group. The present study showed that most of the missed HH actions were after touching the patient environment and after/ before patient contact, meanwhile, the highest rate of HH compliance indication was after body fluid exposure risk. This finding is in agreement with many published studies [25,26]. The reason might be that HCW scared more for their own protection rather than their patients.

The compliance rates of HH among the medical staff of the 5 departments were different both before and after the intervention. In ICU, severely immuno-compromised patients are treated. This fact seems to enhance HCWs HH compliance. In this study, its compliance rate of HH was the highest one. This observation is concordant with other studies [17,18].

After the intervention, the surgical units showed the best improvement of HH in our institution with compliance rates ranging from 18.7% to 46.7%. A reason for this observation may be that the baseline compliance was rather low.

AHR and liquid soap consumption can reflect the real HH compliance. In China, there isn't a national reference data of AHR consumption. After the intervention, the AHR consumption in the study was 63.2-79.8 mL per patient-day in ICU, and 1.8-5.0 mL per patient-dayinnon-ICUs, while in a study conducted in Germany in 2009, in which the median AHR in 543 ICUs was 83 mL per patient-day, and the median AHR in 3339 non-ICUs was 18 mL/patient-day [27]. The AHR removes microorganisms effectively, requires less time and irritates hands less often than does hand washing with soap or other antiseptic agents and water [28]. In our study, in non-ICUs, the liquid soap consumption was more than AHR. The reason might be the difference of work habit and needs more detailed research to find out.

There are several limitations in our studies. First, our study was conducted using the direct observation method. There are concerns about the methods used for training the observers, the assessment of inter-rater reliability and the potential bias for staff members to change their behavior when they know that they are being observed [29,30]. Second, the follow-up period was short and further studies are needed to evaluate the sustainability of the intervention of HH campaign. Third, the present study was inability to identify the most effective element(s) of the intervention.

Despite these limitations, we consider the observed improvements to be very promising, because compliance was poor at baseline and this multifaceted approach was introduced for the first time in this cultural context. We recognize, however, that further progress needs to be made.

Next, further study is needed to confirm the improvements in the HAI rates and infections due to multidrug-resistant bacteria associated with the improved rate of HH compliance.

## Conclusion

In this study, we have compared compliance rates before and after the intervention of hand hygiene Campaign in a university hospital in China. In our study we found that HH campaign is feasible and effective in a healthcare setting in , similar to other countries. Otherwise, the WHO strategy and derived tools are evidence-based and ready-to-use in planning and conducting hand hygiene promotion in healthcare facilities all over the world, including China.

## Acknowledgments

Financial support. This study was no funded.

Potential conflicts of interest- All authors report no conflicts of interest relevant to this article.

## References

1.  Burke JP (2003) Infection control - a problem for patient safety. N Engl J Med 348: 651-656.

2.  Mathai E, Allegranzi B, Kilpatrick C, Pittet D (2010) Prevention and control of health care-associated infections through improved hand hygiene. Indian J Med Microbiol 28: 100-106.

3.  World Health Organization (2013)WHO programmes and activities: First Global Patient Safety Challenge - Clean Care is Safer Care

4.  Duckro AN, Blom DW, Lyle EA, Weinstein RA, Hayden MK (2005) Transfer of vancomycin-resistant enterococci via health care worker hands. Arch Intern Med 165: 302-307.

5.  Pittet D, Hugonnet S, Harbarth S, Mourouga P, Sauvan V, et al. (2000) Effectiveness of a hospital-wide programme to improve compliance with hand hygiene. Infection Control Programme. Lancet 356: 1307-1312.

6.  Pittet D, Allegranzi B, Sax H, Dharan S, Pessoa-Silva CL, et al. (2006) Evidence-based model for hand transmission during patient care and the role of improved practices. Lancet Infect Dis 6: 641-652.

7.  Erasmus V, Daha TJ, Brug H, Richardus JH, Behrendt MD, et al. (2010) Systematic review of studies on compliance with hand hygiene guidelines in hospital care. Infect Control Hosp Epidemiol 31: 283-294.

8.  Scheithauer S, Oude-Aost J, Heimann K, Haefner H, Schwanz T, et al. (2011) Hand hygiene in pediatric and neonatal intensive care unit patients: daily opportunities and indication- and profession-specific analyses of compliance. Am J Infect Control 39: 732-737.

9.  Aboumatar H, Ristaino P, Davis RO, et al. (2012) Infection Prevention Promotion Program Based on the PRECEDE Model: Improving Hand Hygiene Behaviors among Healthcare Personnel. Infect Control Hosp Epidemiol 33: 144-151.

10. Barrera L, Zingg W, Mendez F, Pittet D (2011) Effectiveness of a hand hygiene promotion strategy using alcohol-based handrub in 6 intensive care units in Colombia. Am J Infect Control 39: 633-639.

11. Helder OK, Brug J, Goudoever JB, Looman CWN, Reiss IKM, Kornelisse RF(2014) Sequential hand hygiene promotion contributes to a reduced nosocomial bloodstream infection rate among very low-birth weight infants: An interrupted time series over a 10-year period. Am J Infect Control 42: 718-722.

12. The Ministry of Health of China. Norm of hand hygiene for health care workers (in Chinese). 2009.

13. Pittet D, Allegranzi B, Storr J (2008) The WHO Clean Care is Safer Care programme: field-testing to enhance sustainability and spread of hand hygiene improvements. J Infect Public Health 1: 4-10.

14. Pittet D, Allegranzi B, Boyce J (2014) For the World Health Organization World Alliance for Patient Safety First Global Patient Safety Challenge Core Group of Experts. The World Health Organization Guidelines on Hand Hygiene in Health Care and Their Consensus Recommendations. Infect Control Hosp Epidemiol 30:611-622.

15. Raka L (2009) Lowbury Lecture 2008: infection control and limited resources--searching for the best solutions. J Hosp Infect 72: 292-298.

16. Liu X, Liu Y, Chen N (2000) The Chinese experience of hospital price regulation. Health Policy Plan 15: 157-163.

17. Mazi W, Senok AC, Al-Kahldy S, Abdullah D (2013) Implementation of the world health organization hand hygiene improvement strategy in critical care units. Antimicrob Resist Infect Control 2: 15.

18. Rosenthal VD, Pawar M, Leblebicioglu H, Navoa-Ng JA, Villamil-GÏŒmez W, et al. (2013) Impact of the International Nosocomial Infection Control Consortium (INICC) Multidimensional Hand Hygiene Approach over 13 Years in 51 Cities of 19 Limited-Resource Countries from Latin America, Asia, the Middle East, and Europe. Infect Control Hosp Epidemiol 34: 415-423.

19. Salama MF, Jamal WY, Mousa HA, Al-Abdulghani KA, Rotimi VO (2013) The effect of hand hygiene compliance on hospital-acquired

infections in an ICU setting in a Kuwaiti teaching hospital. J Infect Public Health 6: 27-34.

20. Sahay S, Panja S, Ray S, Rao BK (2010) Diurnal variation in hand hygiene compliance in a tertiary level multidisciplinary intensive care unit. Am J Infect Control 38: 535-539.

21. Scheithauer S, Haefner H, Schwanz T, Schulze-Steinen H, Schiefer J, et al. (2009) Compliance with hand hygiene on surgical, medical, and neurologic intensive care units: direct observation versus calculated disinfectant usage. Am J Infect Control 37: 835-841.

22. Chaberny IF, Möller I, Graf K (2009) Hand hygiene and campaigns. Pneumologie 63: 219-221.

23. Helms B, Dorval S, Laurent PS, Winter M (2010) Improving hand hygiene compliance: a multidisciplinary approach. J Infect Control 38: 572-574.

24. Erasmus V, Daha TJ, Brug H, Richardus JH, Behrendt MD, et al. (2010) Systematic review of studies on compliance with hand hygiene guidelines in hospital care. Infect Control Hosp Epidemiol 31: 283-294.

25. O'Boyle CA, Henly SJ, Larson E (2001) Understanding adherence to hand hygiene recommendations: the theory of planned behavior. Am J Infect Control 29: 352-360.

26. Novoa AM, Pi-Sunyer T, Sala M, Molins E, Castells X (2007) Evaluation of hand hygiene adherence in a tertiary hospital. Am J Infect Control 35: 676-683.

27. Reichardt C, KA–niger D, Bunte-SchA–nberger K, Linden P, MA–nch N, et al. (2013) Three years of national hand hygiene campaign in Germany: what are the key conclusions for clinical practice? J Hosp Infect 83: S11-S16.

28. Picheansathian W (2004) A systematic review on the effectiveness of alcohol-based solutions for hand hygiene. Int J NursPract 10: 3-9.

29. Haas JP, Larson EL (2007) Measurement of compliance with hand hygiene. J Hosp Infect 66: 6-14.

30. Scheithauer S, Lemmen SW (2013) How can compliance with hand hygiene be improved in specialized areas of a university hospital? J Hosp Infect 83 Suppl 1: S17-22.

# 27

# The Effects of Horticultural Therapy on the Well-Being and Hope of Women in Rural Korea

**Soon Min, Yun-Ju Ha, Jung-Hwa Kang and Hee-Young Kang**

*Chosun University, Gwangju, Korea, Republic of Korea.*

*Corresponding author: Hee-Young Kang, Chosun University, Gwangju, Korea, Republic of korea, E-mail: moohykang@naver.com

## Abstract

**Purposes:** Horticultural therapy (HT) is an enjoyable and accessible method of recreation that readily lends itself to a variety of healthful lifestyle activities. HT is valued for its physical, cognitive, social, emotional, and recreational benefits. This study was designed to examine the effects of HT on the psychological well-being and hope of rural women.

**Methods:** HT consists of three stages: establishing credibility (sessions 1-3), well-being and interpersonal relationships improvement (session 4-22), and maintenance (sessions 23-24). Participants consisted of 45 women from rural Korea, of which 21 were assigned to the experimental group and 24 to the control group. The experimental participants attended 24 sessions of HT.

**Results:** Two groups undergone the program had a significant difference in the psychological well-being and hope.

**Conclusions:** The findings of this study show that HT has positive effects on psychological and emotional health, and can be utilized as an intervention to help rural women.

**Keywords:** Horticultural therapy; Rural women; Well-being; Hope

## Introduction

The rural population of Korea is 3.43 million, accounting for 7.3 % of the total population. In 2010, the estimated rural population was 2.96 million, of which 1.51 million (51 %) are female [1].

In spite of the current situation of mechanized agriculture, fewer people working make the farmworks very dependent on rural women. In addition, they increase the hardship of rearing children, supporting parents-in-law due to aging of rural area, doing housework, and fulfilling the role of a wife [2].

Due to these multiple roles, rural women have experienced increasingly more frequent health problems compared to those who live in metropolitan areas [3]. Specifically, rural women have higher incidences of depression, anxiety, low self-esteem, and stress, as well as physical illnesses, such as arthritis and heart disease [3,4]. Furthermore, rural women often do not have sufficient time to nurture their children, and they lack confidence in their ability to parent. They have less income and cultural exposure in comparison to their metropolitan counterparts, resulting in a lower quality of life [5].

The quality of life encompasses the concept of well-being and hope. Well-being is defined as how satisfied an individual is with his or her own life [6]. Hope is the belief that one's situation may improve [7,8]. People who have a strong sense of well-being and hope are able to cope with stress and engage in relationships, and they typically have the motivation necessary to reach their goals [9]; however, the excessive burdens placed on rural women can negatively affect their psychological health by lowering their quality of life [4,10]. In order for rural women to improve their physical, psychological, and social health, it is necessary to implement activities that will positively affect these women's lives.

Recently, from a study investigating several activities for their effects on quality of life and cultural benefits on rural women, horticultural therapy (HT) is emerging due to its use of natural flowers and plants, and engages all of the sensory systems, and it has been used for the treatment of mental illnesses since 1879 [11]. HT is also a popular and accessible method of recreation that readily lends itself to a variety of healthful lifestyle activities [12].

In many Korean studies, the results of HT for teenagers showed that it decreases stress, depression, and anxiety [13], and improves achievement of goals and confidence [14], relieves depression, and improves self-esteem [15]. An overseas study [16] also stressed that viewing plants through windows can be very effective in promoting emotional stability and recovery from illness. In another study, 59 patients with coronary heart disease were treated with HT, which improved mood in these participants [12]. The results of these studies indicated that HT provides psychological benefits to its participants by stimulating interest in plants, improving social confidence, and promoting positive thinking [17-19].

Currently, it is used by the general public, as well as in residential facilities for people with mental illness, elderly patients with dementia, delinquent adolescents, and prisoners [20,21]. The field of use of HT, however, has not been studies of the use of HT for rural Korean women. The aim of this study of HT was to develop a practical system that positively affects the quality of life, such as increasing the well-being and hope, of rural Korean women.

## Methods

### Study design

A quasi-experimental design with a nonequivalent control group was used in a pre-post test. The independent variable is 24 sessions of HT, with sessions lasting 90 minutes at a frequency of twice a week. The dependent variable consists of psychological well-being and hope, as shown in Figure 1.

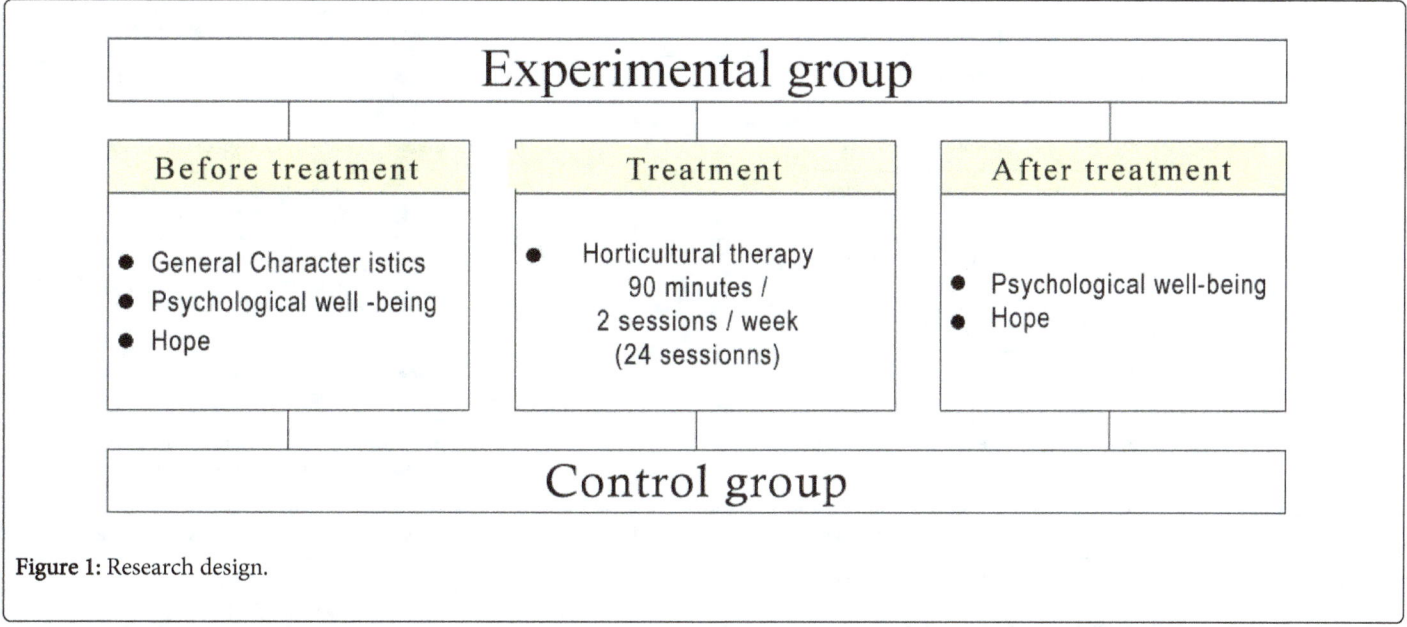

**Figure 1:** Research design.

### Participants

The participants were subjected to simple randomization using a random number of individuals recruited from the women's development center located in B district, J province, South Korea. The inclusion criteria for this study comprised the following: (a) women in a rural area, (b) 35-55 years old, (c) who was married, bereaved, or divorced, (d) were capable of understanding the information in the questionnaires and the objectives of the study, (d) gave consent to participate. The exclusion criteria were the following: (a) sensory deficits, (b) mental or physical disorders, and (c) participation in a similar intervention in the past.

G-power analysis program was used to calculate the power of the study. With 21 women in each group, the power of this study was .70 based on a medium effect size of .50 and a type 1 error of 0.05. A total of 50 women were initially recruited and randomly assigned to either an experimental or control group (25 women in each). In the experimental group, two women dropped out due to domestic problems, and two due to physical problems. In the control group, one woman dropped out because of domestic problem. The final number of participants was 21 in the experimental group and 24 in the control group, creating participation rates of 84% and 96% for the experimental and control group. Finally those in the control group were able to participate in the horticultural therapy after the study was completed.

### Treatment: Horticultural Therapy

The experiment was conducted over the course of 12 weeks, with two 90-minute HT sessions per week, for a total of 24 sessions. The contents of the program are shown in Table 1. HT was designed to help participants experience fulfillment from horticultural activities and be proud of their accomplishments.

| Stage | Session | Contents | Form | Purpose |
|---|---|---|---|---|
| Establishing credibility | 1 | Introduction to horticulture and self-introduction with name card | individual | Motivation for horticultural study and improvement in understanding team members |
| | 2 | Viewing flowers | | Motivation and self representation about horticultural |
| | 3 | Drinking herbal tea | group | Decreasing stress and increasing comfort |
| Improving well-being and relationships | 4 | Bulbous plant plantation | group | Mind tranquility, stimulating senses, decreasing stress, and increasing social skills through interpersonal relationships |
| | 5 | Grass doll topiary and seeding | | Importance of lives, increasing self-sufficiency, and decreasing psychological stress |

| | 6 | Making a rose basket | | Building relationships, stimulating senses, and increasing self-presentation |
|---|---|---|---|---|
| | 7 | Making a flower bag | | Stimulating senses and well-being, increasing self-sufficiency |
| | 8 | Water culture (tomato) | | Mind tranquility, stimulating senses, comforting stresses, mind tranquility, and increasing social ability through interpersonal relationships |
| | 9 | Barbola | | Increasing achieving sentiment through expectancy and interest |
| | 10 | Rosemary cottage | | Causing curiosity and psychological well-being |
| | 11 | Plant transportation | | Positive consideration improvement and strengthening active action |
| | 12 | Making a dish garden | | Increasing positive thinking through expectancy and interest, increasing self-esteem through self-sufficiency, increasing self-representation, and expectancy for life value |
| | 13 | Man doll topiary | | Planning for future, increasing self-sufficiency and satisfaction, and increasing positive thinking |
| | 14 | Making a fleshy plant garden | | Stimulating senses, recognizing life value, improving self-esteem, hope, and psychological well-being through repetition |
| | 15 | Making a cactus garden | | Finding hope through volition and expectancy for life |
| | 16 | Making a circular artificial flower lease | | Value of life, increasing positive thinking, increasing self-sufficiency, and decreasing stress |
| | 17 | Growing chrysanthemums | | Forming interpersonal relationships, stimulating senses, increasing positive emotions, and psychological well-being |
| | 18 | Making a corsage | individual | Forming interpersonal relationships, psychological well-being, and self-representation |
| | 19 | Group making a frame with dried flowers | group | Self-representation, increasing social skills through interpersonal relationships |
| | 20 | Cultivating sprouts | | Forming interpersonal relationships, improving motivation, and psychological well-being |
| | 21 | Making a collection flower arrangement | | Forming interpersonal relationships, improving self-representation, and increasing positive emotions |
| | 22 | Orchid-planting in volcanic stone | | Forming interpersonal relationships, psychological well-being, and hope |
| Maintenance | 23 | Making an invitation letter with a barbola card(card with decoration of colored flowers) | group | Increasing positive thinking, self-satisfaction, psychological well-being, and forming interpersonal relationships |
| | 24 | Drawing a flower picture and displaying it | | Increasing positive thinking and self-awareness through establishment and maintenance of interpersonal relationships |

**Table 1:** Horticultural Therapy Schedule.

HT consists of the following three stages: (a) establishing credibility (sessions 1-3), (b) well-being and interpersonal relationships improvement (session 4-22), and (c) maintenance (sessions 23-24).

### (a) Establishing Credibility through HT (sessions 1-3)

In the credibility-establishment stage, overall orientation for HT was conducted. To stimulate interest in HT, flower appreciation and an herbal tea was served to participants. The purpose of the HT was to motivate participants about life.

Sensory stimulation, improving social skills via relationships, and promoting emotional stability were the main goals. The purpose of HT is to help participants become attuned to their senses, improve their level of comfort, and relieve stress.

## (b) Improving well-being and relationships through HT (sessions 4-22)

To improve the participants' sense of well-being, the participants were asked to recall activities from historic rural life. HT provides opportunities to interact with nature, which revitalizes expressive skills and benefits physical and emotional well-being. The purpose of this stage was to help participants feel hopeful for a new life.

## (c) Maintenance stage of HT (sessions 23-24)

In the maintenance stage of HT, participants sent invitation letter with barbola card their friends and family in order to maximize the effect of the program by encouraging themselves with a sense of accomplishment and social relationship.

## Procedure

Before the intervention began, we collected baseline data from the study participants that included general characteristics, a sense of well-being, and hope. The intervention group was provided with HT for 12 weeks. Post-test data, which included senses of well-being and hope, were collected after completion of the intervention.

## Measures

Psychological well-being was measured using a self-reported questionnaire, the Psychological Well-being Scale (PWBS), developed by Ryff [22] and modified for use in Korea by Kim, Kim, and Cha [23]. The questionnaire included 46 items scored in a 5- point Likert- type scale. The items included self-acceptance, positive relationships with others, autonomy, environmental mastery, purpose in life, and personal growth dimensions. Higher scores indicated higher levels of well-being. Using Chronbach's α reliability measure, Kim et al. [23] achieved a Cronbach's α of 0.71. The Cronbach's α achieved in this study was 0.83.

Hope was measured using a self-reported questionnaire, the Dispositional Hope Scale (DHS), developed by Snyder et al. [24] and translated into Korean (K-DHS) by Kang [25]. Based on personal traits, the K-DHS consists of the following three content areas: 4 items for pathway thinking, 4 items for agency thinking, and 4 items for filter thinking. There were 12 items scored on a 4-point Likert-type scale. Higher scores indicated higher levels of hope. Using Chronbach's α reliability measure, Kang [25] achieved a Cronbach's α of 0.82. The Cronbach's α achieved in this study was 0.83.

## Data Analysis

SPSS PC (14.0) for Windows was used for data analysis. Demographic data were analyzed using descriptive statistics. The Chi-square test and Fisher's exact test were used to determine homogeneity of general characteristics of the experimental group in comparison to the control group. An independent t-test was used to compare differences between the groups' pre-test and post-test outcomes.

## Ethical Considerations

Ethical approval was obtained from the institutional review board of the affiliated institution (IRB-1-015). The participants were assigned to either the experimental group or the control group based on their preferences. All study participants were given both verbal information of the study, where a voluntary participation, guarantee of anonymity, free will of withdrawal from the participation, and no disadvantage upon withdrawal were explained. Upon both verbal and written consents from the women, data was collected.

## Results

### General characteristics of the participants

The characteristics of the experimental and control groups are shown in Tables 2 and 3. Two groups at pre-test had no significant differences in general characteristics, well-being and hope.

| Categories | | Exp.(n=21) | Cont. (n=24) | $\chi^2$ | p |
|---|---|---|---|---|---|
| | | n(%) | n(%) | | |
| Age (yr) | 39-45 | 3 (14.3) | 2 (8.3) | 0.402 | .652 |
| | 46-55 | 18 (85.7) | 22 (91.7) | | |
| Religion | Yes | 15 (71.4) | 10 (41.7) | 4.018 | .071 |
| | None | 6 (28.6) | 14 (58.3) | | |
| Education level | Middle school | 9 (42.9) | 8 (33.3) | 0.432 | .552 |
| | High school | 12 (57.1) | 16 (66.7) | | |
| Monthly income (US $) | < 1000 | 7 (33.3) | 6 (25.0) | 0.925 | .675 |
| | 1000-2000 | 11 (52.4) | 12 (50.0) | | |
| | 2000 | 3 (14.3) | 6 (25.0) | | |
| Marital state | Married | 20 (95.2) | 21 (87.5) | 0.828 | .611 |
| | Others | 1 ( 4.8) | 3 (12.5) | | |
| Occupation | Yes | 8 (38.1) | 8 (33.3) | 0.111 | .765 |
| | None | 13 (61.9) | 16 (66.7) | | |

**Table 2:** Homogeneity Test for General Characteristics of Participants (N=45).

| Variables | Exp.(n=21) | Cont. (n=24) | t | p |
|---|---|---|---|---|
| | Mean ± SD | Mean ± SD | | |
| Psychological well-being | 3.07 ± 0.71 | 2.98±0.20 | 0.56 | .576 |
| Hope | 3.45 ± 0.34 | 3.40±0.32 | 0.46 | .645 |

**Table 3:** Homogeneity Test for Outcome Variables at Baseline(N=45).

Exp.=Experimental group; Cont.=Control group

### Psychological Well-being

The psychological well-being score in the experimental group increased from 3.07 to 3.56 after treatment. The score for the control group was equal from 2.98 to 2.98. After implementation of HT, the experimental group's psychological well-being was significantly higher than the control group's (t=-2.01, p=.049), as shown in Table 4.

| Variables | Pre-test | Post-test | Difference | t | p |
|---|---|---|---|---|---|
| | M±SD | M±SD | M±SD | | |
| **Psychological well-being** | | | | | |

| | | | | | |
|---|---|---|---|---|---|
| Exp.(n=21) | 3.07 ± 0.71 | 3.56 ± 0.61 | -0.52 ± 1.27 | -2.01 | .049 |
| Cont..(n=24) | 2.98 ± 0.20 | 2.98 ± 0.20 | 0.00 ± 0.10 | | |
| **Hope** | | | | | |
| Exp.(n=21) | 3.45 ± 0.34 | 3.61 ± 0.33 | -0.16 ± 0.33 | -2.18 | .042 |
| Cont..(n=24) | 3.40 ± 0.32 | 3.39 ± 0.34 | 0.01 ± 0.18 | | |

**Table 4:** Changes of Outcome Variables between the Experimental and Control Group (N=45).

## Hope

The hope score in the experimental group increased from 3.45 to 3.61 after treatment. The score for the control group decreased from 3.40 to 3.39. After implementation of HT, the experimental group's hope was significantly higher than the control group's (t=-2.18, p=.042), as shown in Table 4.

## Discussion

Compared to women who live in metropolitan areas, rural women have an isolated lifestyle and comparatively more stress. This study investigated the effect of HT on well-being and hope in rural women, wherein it found that HT was very effective in improving well-being and hope in rural women.

HT is defined by the American Horticultural Therapy Association [26] as "a process utilizing plants and horticultural activities to improve the social, educational, psychological, and physical adjustment of persons, thus improving their body, mind, and spirits. HT uses gardening, plants, floral materials, and vegetation to stimulate clients' interest in their surroundings and to promote the development of leisure or vocational skills" [27]. In a meta-analysis of HT [28] in Korea, HT was determined to be a meaningful program since it is within the range of an effective size of 0.93, based on the standard established by Cohen [29]. In addition, the effective size of the independent variable was significant in regard to the outcomes of improved self-esteem, anxiety, and depression. Moreover, our study investigated psychological variables, such as well-being and hope, which had not been previously investigated. It has been reported that HT has a greater impact on adults, wherein groups of 4-6 or 11-20 for 21-25 sessions optimally maximize benefits to well-being and hope [28,30]. Our study was performed with a 21-subject group, and the experiments were conducted over 24 sessions.

The results of this study found that well-being, the first endpoint of the study, was significantly increased in the HT group. This result was consistent with a previous study conducted by Ha [11] , which reported that HT improves well-being by reducing physical and psychological stresses on elderly women. Söderback et al. [19] reported that, as a result of providing HT to 46 patients with brain damage, emotional, cognitive, and/or sensory motor functions were improved and socialization, health, well-being, and life satisfaction were increased.

Psychological well-being encompasses self-acceptance, positive relationships, autonomy, and control over one's environment, life purpose, and personal development. Results of the present study agree with the results of Lee, Hwang, Song, and Son's study [31], which reported that HT was effective to improve life purpose, self-identity and self-esteem for in middle-aged women.

In this study, the hope of the experimental group increased significantly. Most studies have focused on the use of HT in cancer patients [8,32] (Shin and Park, 2007; Sock and Jung, 2006). Since our study focused on rural women with hope as an endpoint and a comparable study does not exist, it is impossible to compare results; however, hope, social support, and quality of life have meaningful relations [8,33] . HT provides a great opportunity to improve hope and self-esteem by presenting achievements to family members at the end of the program.

In the view of nursing research, this research is meaningful in that it provides basic data derived from systemically executed positive intervention via the setting up study templates in psychological intervention. In the view of nursing practice, HT was proven to improve rural women's well-being and hope, such that it can be applied as a nursing intervention. In the view of nursing education, in practice, students can be directed to settle health problems with HT as a nursing process, and such a program can be contained within the curriculum.

## Limitation of the study

Participants were recruited from an agricultural development institute located in B district, J province, Korea. It is unlikely that this population represents all women in the rural areas of Korea which limits the generalization of the results. This study should be repeated on a larger scale with a randomly-selected sample of women from different populations in order to develop a protocol appropriate for nursing intervention. For rural women who have limited cultural exposure, HT is an enjoyable and accessible method of recreation; therefore, more systematic, longitudinal research into this promising therapeutic intervention is justified and necessary.

## Conclusions

The extraordinary workload of rural women often has a negative effect on their psychological health, causing a lack of sense of well-being and hope. HT has beneficial psychological effects, like stimulating interest in nature, improving social confidence, and promoting positive thinking. This study found that HT enhances well-being and hope in rural women. Through relationships developed during HT among participants and between participants and the researchers, interpersonal relationships, positive sentiments, and self-expression improved. These findings suggest that HT can be very beneficial to improving the quality of life of women in a rural community setting.

## References

1. Statistics Research Institute (2008) Analysis report on agriculture, forestry and fishery using the 2005 census data.

2. Lee EH, Choi JH (2004) A study on the mental health of middle aged woman living in rural community. J Welf for the Aged 23:231-251.

3. Park JH, Eun Y, Back KS, Lee SS, Shin SC (2007) Determinants of factors influencing health-promotion behaviors of middle-aged rural women. Korean Public Health Research, 33:175-187.

4. Shin KR, Yang JH (2003) Influencing factors on quality of life of middle-aged women living in rural area. J Korean AcadNurs 33:999-1007

5. Choi C H, Kim J H (2008) The relationship between leisure satisfaction and mental health of middle aged women living in rural communities. J Sport and Leisure Studies 34:607-16.

6. Kim HY, Kim MS (2000) Analyses on the structure of psychological well-being (PWB) and relationship between PWB and subjective well-being (SWB) among Korean married women. Korean J Psychol: Woman 5:27-41.

7. Herth KA (2001) Development and implementation of a hope intervention program. OncolNurs Forum 28:1510.

8. Shin AM, Park JS (2007) The effects of hope intervention on hope and depression of cancer patients staying at home. J Korean AcadNurs 37:994-1002.

9. Snyde CR, Sheavens J, Sympson SC (1997) Hope: An individual motive for social commerce, Group Dynamics: Theory, Res Pract 1:107-118.

10. Hemard JB, Monroe PA, Atkinson ES, Blalock LB (1998) Rural women's satisfaction and stress as family health care gatekeepers. Women Health 28:55-77.

11. Ha SY (2008) The effects of horticulture welfare program on well-being in the female elderly. Chosun University, Master thesis, Gwangju.

12. Mattew W, Jonathan W, Francois H, Ana M, Mariano JR (2005) Effect of horticultural therapy on mood and heart rate in patients participating in an inpatient cardiopulmonary rehabilitation program. J CardiopulmRehabil 25:270-274.

13. Kim RB, Kim HY (2009) Effect of horticultural therapy on stress and stress coping strategy of juvenile delinquents. J Korean Soc People Plants Envir 12:17-23.

14. Kweon YH (2006) Effect of horticultural therapy on the changes of mentality, sociality of mental disorder persons. Seoul National University, Master thesis, Seoul.

15. Jung HJ (2002) Effect of horticultural therapy on the changes of self-esteem and anxiety of the mentally retarded students in high school. KonKuk University, Master thesis, Seoul.

16. Ulrich R S (1984) View though their window may influence recovery from surgery. Science 224:420-421.

17. Mackenzie ER, Agard B, Portella C, Mahangar DJ, Barol J, et al. (2000) Horticultural therapy in long-term care settings. J Am Med DirAssoc 1:69-73.

18. Page M (2008) Gardening as a therapeutic intervention in mental health. Nurs Times104:28-30.

19. Söderback I S, Söderström M, Schälander E (2004) Horticultural therapy: the 'healing garden' and gardening in rehabilitation measures at Danderyd Hospital Rehabilitation Clinic, Sweden. PediatrRehabi 7:245-60.

20. Kim JH, Jo MK, Park HS, Joo SH, Son GC (2008) Effects of horticultural therapy based on social skill on the improvement of interpersonal relationship and sociality of women with mental retardation. Korean J HortSciTechnol 25:81-89.

21. Sim YE, Seo JK, Lee SH (2008) Effect of horticultural therapy program for improvement of work adjustment skill in people with mental retardation. J VocatRehabil 18:89-115.

22. Ryff CD (1989) Happiness is everything, or is it? Explorations on the meaning of psychological well-being. J PersSocPsychol 57:1069-1081.

23. Kim MS, Kim HW, Cha KH (2001) Analyses on the construct of psychological well-being (PWB) of Korean male and female adults. Kor J SocPersPsychol 15:19-39.

24. Snyder CR, Harris C, Anderson JR, Holleran SA, Irving LM, et al. (1991) The will and the ways: development and validation of an individual differences measure of hope. J PersSocPsychol 60:570-585.

25. Kang LY (2002) Development and application of counseling process hope scales. Sunkyunkwan University, Master thesis, Seoul.

26. American Horticultural Therapy Association (2010) The history and practice of horticultural therapy.

27. Morgan B (1989) Growing together. (5thedn). Pittsburgh: Pittsburgh Civic Garden Center.

28. Hong SH (2006) A meta-analysis of the effects of horticultural therapy. Hanyang University, Master thesis, Seoul.

29. Cohen, J. 1988. Statistical power analysis for the behavioral sciences. (2ndedn). New Jersey : Lawrence Erlbaum Associates.

30. Heliker D, Chadwick A, O'Connell T (2001) The meaning of gardening and the effects on perceived well being of a gardening project on diverse populations of elders. Activities, Adaptation & Aging 24:35-56.

31. Lee YA, Hwang HJ, Song JE, Son KC (2007) Effect of horticultural therapy using pressed flower based upon logotherapy on the improvement of the purpose in life and ego identity of middle-aged women. Hort Environ Biotechnol 25:277-290.

32. Sock TY, Jung Y S (2006) Effects of a forgiveness nursing intervention program on hope and quality of life in woman cancer patients. Korean OncolNursSoc 6:111-120.

33. Perrins-Margalis NM, Rugletic J, Schepis NM, Stepannski HR, Walsh MA (2000) The immediate effects of a group-based horticulture experience on the quality of life person with chronic mental illness. OccupTherMent Health 16:15-32.

# 28

# "The Thing with Non-Physical Fatigue is that you can't Get Rid of it with Rest": Psychosocial Nursing Students Reflect on their Clinical Placement, South Africa

**Anna E Van den Heever***

*University of the Witwatersrand, South Africa*

*Corresponding author:** Anna E Van den Heever, P.O Box 1654, Pinegowrie, 2123, Johannesburg, South Africa, E-mail: annalie.vandenheever@wits.ac.za

## Abstract

The emotions of childhood are intense and difficult to control, but over the years, they are mixed and moulded into more subtle and expressed feelings full of meaning and under cognitive control. During this process, people use certain defense mechanisms to deal with the pressure of their emotions, or deceive themselves about the actual conditions so that they can view reality as non-threatening. While the community's attitude towards people who live with a mental, physical or emotional disability or those who have been abused has been ranging from disregard, rejection and stigmatization to apathy; for health professionals and families of traumatized children, there seemed to be little opportunity to escape from the emotional and physical effects of being face to face with reality. Suggestions are that compassion fatigue could be due to psychological and physiological responses when working with and caring for traumatized people. A problem was identified during visits to the clinical facilities, when despite four years of exposure to general nursing, midwifery and community health; psychosocial nursing students expressed their fears of being traumatized by their experiences. Despite theoretical knowledge and practical training, they seemed to be in a state of emotional exhaustion. The question was asked: are nursing students emotionally prepared to work with severely emotionally, intellectually or physically traumatized children in the community?

The qualitative, descriptive study and psychodynamic approach was to explore and describe final year psychosocial nursing students' reflections and experiences during clinical placement with children who are traumatized by accidental or non-accidental injury or abuse. A purposive sample comprised of written and marked narratives from psychosocial reflective journals of 16 final (4th) year students until saturation of information was reached. Thematic analysis of the written narratives highlighted an emotional rollercoaster of feelings, ethical and professional conflict between the abused and being the abuser.

**Keywords:** Mental health; Student nurse; Abuse; Trauma; Defense mechanisms

## Introduction and Background

People who suffered severe injuries or abuse need help and protection as a consequence of their cognitive, emotional and behavioral difficulties but what is often seen, is that those who care for them may suffer emotional and physical exhaustion. There is a tendency in society on the other hand, to stigmatise or deny the effects of traumatic events, which could be seen as an attempt to view reality as a non-threatening event [1].

There are many factors which may contribute to the prevalence of intellectual disabilities or neurodevelopmental disorders. Birth injuries are currently the most frequent cause of intellectual disabilities in South Africa. This means that adequate antenatal and maternity care is the first line of prevention and could decrease the incidence of intellectual disabilities [1].

In a study done in South Africa factors that predispose adults and children to violent injuries include poverty, unemployment, income inequality, patriarchal notions of masculinity, risk taking, defense of honor, weak parenting, firearms, alcohol, drug abuse, weakness in law reinforcement. Exposure to rape, child neglect, abuse, and partner violence are only some of the risk factors to the country's prevalence of health problems, which subsequently result in substance abuse, common mental disorders, post-traumatic stress disorders, depression and suicidality [2].

According to Manglio [3], the result of sexual abuse, particularly among girls is the risks associated with unprotected sex with multiple partners and sex trading. In addition, child sexual abuse is significantly related to depression, low self-esteem, psychological problems such as personality disorders, dissociative disorders, self-injurious behavioural problems in adolescence.

Traumatized family members require professional support, parenting skills and on-going therapy, while physical and financial strain can cause high levels of stress in families and children with disabilities. The caring process relies on the nurses' knowledge, understanding and insights but also on the ordinariness of being a human being [4]. On the other hand, in 1991, Wakley found that it was not uncommon for doctors when faced with a sexual abuse case to feel a sense of panic, or not being fully equipped to deal with the emotive problems which are evoked by hearing about abusive episodes [5].

A study done in the United Kingdom by Harrison and Zohhadi [6] revealed that the impact of failing to fully understand the role of mental health needs and the provision of emotional care was apparent, while in Australia, the mixed attitudes of nurses to caring for people with mental illness such as their lack of knowledge and fear of saying the wrong thing resulted in people receiving limited mental health care from nurses [7].

Increasingly nursing students come into contact with severely traumatized people and it is not always possible to effectively discuss the physical and emotional impact that these experiences have on them. A consequence of this is that student nurses could be left with unresolved issues and a sense of failure, while the conflicting attitudes towards people with disabilities often ranges from disregard to rejection but then also shift towards wanting to make a positive contribution or sympathy [1]. Reflecting on experiences is therefore an important aspect for nurses and could help to overcome this problem.

Reflective journal writing can be viewed through many different lenses: as a form of self-expression, a record of events or a form of therapy [8]. Although much can be learned from reflections, it is also a way to make sense of and exploring often messy and confused events while focusing on the thoughts and emotions that accompany them. A psychodynamic approach therefore includes all the theories in psychology that see human functioning based upon the interaction of drives and forces within the person particularly unconscious and between the different structures of a person [9]. Mentally revisiting and portraying the experience in writing can be an important first step in focusing on the feelings and emotions which accompanied those experiences and an opportunity to get rid of negative feelings while learning from the positive ones [10].

Mental illness is not only a major psychosocial problem in South African society but the consequences of child abuse affect children and adults in various ways. Nurses are not only responsible for recognizing and identifying, but are bound by law to report child abuse of any nature [11]. Psychosocial nursing forms an integral part of training at the University, towards a bachelor's degree and registration as a Professional Nurse. Students complete 4,000 clinical hours during four years of study in general hospitals, midwifery, community clinics and psychiatric units. Because of the sensitivity around children, only final year students are placed in a children's psychiatric ward of a psychiatric facility, an outpatient unit for emotionally, sexually and physically traumatized children as well as in a residential care facility for intellectually disabilities.

A problem was identified when, despite theoretical knowledge of diagnosis and predisposing factors regarding child abuse and practical experience in general, psychiatric, community nursing and midwifery, students expressed their fear, anxiety and reluctance to work in those institutions. The facilitator was challenged about the need to work there and what they could possibly learn from those people whom they cannot even imagine having a conversation with. The question then was whether student nurses were emotionally prepared for the reality of coming face to face with severe emotionally, intellectually or physically traumatized children in the community?

## Purpose and Objective of the Study

The purpose of this study was to explore and describe final year psychosocial nursing students' reflections, feelings and experiences during clinical placement with intellectually, emotionally and physically traumatized children.

## Research Design and Method

The purpose of the qualitative, descriptive study was to explore and describe final year psychosocial nursing students' reflections, personal feelings and experiences during clinical placement with children who are traumatized by accidental, environmental and non-accidental injury or abuse. A purposive sample comprised of written and marked narratives applicable to the experiences while in particular institutions and extracted from psychosocial reflective journals of final (4th) year students until saturation of information was reached. Qualitative methods focus on the qualitative aspects of meaning, experience and understanding, and they study human experience from the viewpoint of the research participants in the context in which the action takes place [12]. The researcher used bracketing by becoming the writer of the students' reflections and a psychodynamic approach to make sense of the interactions within and between people's unconscious structures [9].

## Data Collection

Permission was granted and ethical clearance obtained from the Human Research Ethics Committee of the University (M150636). The ethical principle of non-maleficence [13] was applied to ensure that no harm occurred to the respondents during the research process. An information leaflet was handed to the students and informed consent was obtained from 16 students to use the narratives from their reflective journals. The data was collected from their reflective journals after the final marks were published; therefore their responses could not be detrimental to their progress. Because of the small number of students and only a few male students in the course, confidentiality and anonymity was ensured by not using names or student numbers. Biographical data which may identify students was therefore not collected.

## Rigor

Only one group's experiences were explored, which limits the transferability of the findings, but students' reflections and feelings were truthfully represented [14].

Credibility refers to the confidence in the truth of the data and interpretations of them, but truth of the data in this study may be subjective due to emotional involvement of the students.

Confirmability is concerned with establishing that data represents information participants provided and findings reflect the participants' voice and not that of the inquirer/researcher. However when bracketing was used, the researcher's voice was identified in the narrative. Reflection on negative feelings and difficulties in practice confirmed the data collected and did not seem to influence how the students recorded such feelings.

## Analysis of Information

Embedded in Reissman's [15] approaches to narrative analysis, is thematic analysis which relies on categorizing accounts or aspects of accounts that are being told. In this study, written narratives were explored; however there is a possibility that the product of the narrative analysis also becomes a narrative by the researcher [16]. Data collection and thematic analysis occurred concurrently as the journals were read and re-read to extract the following themes and sub-themes (Table 1) that stood out from the narratives:

| Themes | Subthemes | Narratives |
|---|---|---|
| The students were disillusioned | Disillusions<br><br>Making sense of the world, of themselves, life and people; us and them?<br><br>Annoyed by their own inability to respond | "People just turn a blind Eye" |
| An emotional rollercoaster ride | Physically demanding; tired; emotionally exhausting;<br><br>Can't get rid of it with rest To feel or not to feel?<br><br>Mixed emotions and conflicting feelings pity, crying, angry, happy, smiling, "disgusting", empathy, fear | "Negative feelings weighed me down" |
| They struggled with unresolved ethical issues | Ethical and moral dilemmas; Ashamed to be a nurse; Being a man<br><br>Unresolved feelings; Abused or Abuser? Regress to own childhood<br><br>Think about their own childhood | "Talk about it or not?" |
| Conflicting professional and moral dilemmas | On being a Carer:<br><br>Good enough nurse and midwife?<br><br>Bad mother or parent, abused or the abuser? Who is to blame?<br><br>Negligence? nurse, midwife, parents, carers, child, society or legal system | "I was angry at the mother" |
| Moving from disgust to gratitude | Eye opener, admiration for those who do good; they helped me; appreciation, understanding of lessons learned; Some justice restored; Restored faith in humanity | "I am grateful for the experience" |

**Table 1**: Themes and subthemes derived from the narritives of students' reflective journals.

## The students were disillusioned

Most of the students were disillusioned because things were not as good as they believed it could be. They felt shocked and disappointed and they no longer believed in people while the world felt unreal to them:

*"It had never occurred to me that anybody can do that to another"*

*"As sad and harsh as it might sound, not everyone is meant to be a parent"*

*"It is unfair to feel this way about all people. I felt as if I lost hope in humanity"*

Some students lost faith in their own judgement and abilities, while most of the students identified with the patients' inabilities, disabilities or being "retarded". How could they help someone to pick up the pieces if they themselves are also falling apart?

*"It was a shocking experience and made me ask questions about me as a man"*

*"Little did I know that I would not only be frustrated but I would also feel extremely incompetent?"*

## An emotional rollercoaster ride

The sudden and extreme changes in their emotions, angry and scared the one moment just to feel happy the next moment, were physically and emotionally exhausting.

*"It was a scary, frustrating and sad place to be in the beginning."*

*"Through something as small and simple as remembering my name, he gave me so much"; "It made me happy to see her smile"*

Emotional exhaustion is a chronic state of physical and emotional depletion which could result from excessive job and personal demands or continuous stress; a person may lose interest and motivation in what let them to become a nurse in the first place [17].

A number of students felt trapped and wanted to escape from intolerable feelings and a rollercoaster of emotions; others did not know how to feel or how not to feel at all. However, by suppressing those feelings, they dissociated into a state of not feeling and not knowing.

*"I curled tighter into myself and blocked all my thoughts out. I refused to continue feeling and thinking, my emotions ceased to develop, they were retarded"*

Some students seemed scared and in an attempt to tolerate their fear and bottled up aggression they seemed to project the rage into their colleagues.

"I could have STRANGLED this doctor"

In Freud's theory [18], the ego uses defense mechanisms to handle conflict between the id and the superego to reduce tension, for example being scared of a dog, is seen as anxiety of something in reality. But on the other hand an unconscious fear could be seen as students being unaware of the nature of the threat, and uncertainty whether a threat exists at all:

"I was worried that I would not cope emotionally"; "It raised terrifying feelings in me"

## They struggled with unresolved ethical issues

One student wanted to get out of there. *"Free me!"; "Let me out of here!"; "End a life or save a life?"* Most of the students were worrying, questioning and thinking a lot but found it hard to make sense of the patients and themselves. They felt responsible for what happened to the patients, while others felt guilty to feel those feelings.

*".......and we continue to infringe on these children's rights"*

*"Sterilisation: do good no harm - I am still uneasy about this law"*

*"I remember thinking to myself that if I gave birth to such a child, I would end its life"*

*"These children are a full-time job, they require chronic therapy and they stress finances"*

*"I ask myself questions but could not get the answers"*

*"It can be questioned if it is ethically correct to resuscitate a child who might end up with some sort of disability?"*

Some students felt disgusted by the damaged bodies and minds in some of the patients and seemed to be ashamed about their reaction or guilty about questioning whether someone with a severe disability should be resuscitated. This is confirmed by the shame and toxic shame that patients can identify with about their own deformed bodies and that they can feel as a result of physical and sexual abuse [19]. A similar process of projective identification described by Klein [20] could also get into the nursing students and therefore genuine awareness of the way we feel about a situation can help us to understand ourselves and the patients in that moment [21].

### Conflicting professional and moral dilemmas

*"Who am I? The abused or the abuser?"*

Being in their fourth year, the general expectation was that students had been exposed to most illnesses and conditions. Some of them were mothers themselves, and delivered at least 15 babies at that point of their training. Above all, they wondered whether they are being abused by the system or are they seen as the abusers.

The students wanted to blame someone, but who was to blame? They projected their own feelings of incompetence and disabilities into the system, but they themselves were part of the health system. Most students or doctors further denied the existence of those feelings by not saying anything or avoid talking about it.

*"The child wants to speak, but her jaw is tight"*

*"The doctor ignored her"*

*"Not only one of us asked how the mother was feeling"*

*"The mother knew about the abuse and wouldn't do anything"*

With the unconscious use of projection, the students could defend against their own anxiety and unpleasant feelings by attributing the badness into the abused, but also identified with the abusive and neglectful feelings that were projected onto them by the patients. Defense mechanisms can falsify reality [20], therefore in their minds; the students became the neglectful abuser, bad mother or midwife.

*"My anger was directed towards midwives" "I felt pushing the blame onto the midwife"*

*"She was in labour for 24 h, then forceps - he is now profoundly mentally handicapped"*

*"You need to ensure as a midwife to give proper care - because most of them are due to some negligence during pregnancy or birth"*

*"It was stark reality and this was close to home - I was generally disappointed at the care during antenatal visits"*

### From disgust to gratitude

Their eyes opened slowly and most of the students expressed surprise at how these unfortunate people and their circumstances could teach them facts about life that they were unaware of. The sense of denigration that they felt in the beginning, changed to admiration of the carers and those parents who were committed to care for their unfortunate children. Eventually their own roles were idealised by wanting to be good mothers, and good nurses.

*"An eye opener as I journeyed in the shoes of the innocent"*

*"This inspired me – I too want to be so caring"*

*"You walk out of here every day with great appreciation for life"*

*"It restored some of my faith in humanity"*

*"I gave her a doll and she stopped crying; it was quite a nice feeling"*

Some students thought about their own childhood and regressed to a helpless state of infancy by feeling insignificant or unskilled and incompetent but had renewed appreciation for their own parents and a happy childhood [10].

*"I am grateful for my parents and the way I was raised"*

*"It once again made me reflect on my childhood and to see the emotions I experienced when I was young"*

Others somatised their emotions by feeling physically paralyzed, disabled or retarded on the one hand and realizing that they are human after all on the other hand realised that this was a journey of discomfort, exhaustion, growth and revelation and what became clear, is that they learned a lot about themselves and remembered the reasons for choosing to be a nurse.

*"I learned a lot about psychiatry and myself"; "I will be a better midwife because of psychiatry"; "I need to be more aware of myself and my personality"*

*"I am too hard on myself"; "I realised that I am a sensitive being"*

### Results and Discussion

The researcher became the reflective writer of the students' story while having to question her own role in the transference. The apparent psychodynamic pattern of defense mechanisms [1] used by the students and my own anxiety may have influenced the ability to think or to answer the many questions. Have I also become part of the abusive system in the students' minds?, therefore also angry with me? Or, like society in general, also became desensitized? What were the students' expectations of psychosocial nursing? I wondered whether the students felt that their voices were not heard? Did we even listen to each other?

*"I think the mother felt like she had not been 'heard' ..."*

*"I silently shed a tear" "The child wants to speak, but her jaw is tight – how much dignity and grace does she have!"*

Have they also been failed or were their own rights and need for care disrespected in any way?

*"We deny many kids their right and freedom to be loved and cared for"*

*"I was almost in tears because all along I thought he was unable to speak or comprehend what was happening around him"*

The challenge to become a reflective practitioner was not without its hurdles. It was no longer possible for the nurses to accept everything at face value, and the effort required to do this should not be underestimated. At times there seemed not much of a difference between the students and the patients with hidden bits of themselves showing from time to time. A build-up of emotions made them feel physically and emotionally sick and incapable of helping one another. Although younger, inexperienced nurses are less genuine with patients or themselves [21], by reflecting on their experiences, the students in this study had an opportunity to express their feelings in an honest attempt to make sense of their experiences.

It is not uncommon for an abused person to feel helpless, fearful and insignificant [19] . Emotional abuse, deliberate humiliation, the instillation of fear and shame similar to what students in this study experienced, can damage emotional health [19]. Commonly survivors of trauma and sexual abuse blame themselves very harshly and feel responsible for what happened to them. Further suggestions are that compassion fatigue could be due to psychological and physiological responses when working with and caring for traumatized people and can lead to secondary trauma, or vicarious traumatization and burnout [17]. The only way the students seemed to protect them against the unbearable anxiety, and to cope with feelings of guilt, shame and anger, was to unconsciously made use of defense mechanisms [1].

However, as one student said: *"You can defend against it but you can't get rid of it with rest".*

The students' use of defense mechanisms were as a result of what they have experienced in their environment, which did not leave them feeling good; [1] instead they were left with a vague, low-level anxiety which was difficult to explain, but never the less seemed to be associated with feelings of confusion and helplessness. This might have had an effect on the way they viewed themselves and the world as well as on their belief systems and emotional well-being [17].

Having to endure and experience the effects of trauma could have resulted in symptoms of vicarious traumatization which are parallel to the post-traumatic stress suffered by survivors: [17]. However, a person's reaction when exposed to an emotionally loaded event could be amplified, which is grounded in a traumatic past or present experience [17] and can drain emotional energy.

It was hard for the researcher to make sense of the blur between what was the patients' or the students' words, and how that tied in with their experiences. She was left wondering how student nurses could be emotionally empathetic and mindful, while they themselves felt like falling apart? But on the other hand, how could their confusion and frustration be known, unless they had a space to talk?

## Limitation

The reflections of only one group of students were explored.

## Recommendations

The use of reflective journal writing should be encouraged during clinical placement. Langley and Brown [22] write that the practice of reflective journaling contributes to important learning outcomes for online graduate nursing students. They identify four learning outcomes that are evident in nursing and education literature; professional development, personal growth, empowerment, and facilitation of the learning process. Reflective journaling strengthened their self-

confidence, thereby helping the students become change agents in their work environments [22].

By analysing the narratives of these journals, the importance of supervision, self-reflection and support became clear:

*"What I liked was how all our allocations ended with a de-briefing session from the sister in charge – that helped with reflection and clarification" and that is why "I need to have someone I can talk to and confide in when I feel overwhelmed by work"*

- Support in the form of group discussions before placement as well as empathetic listening and understanding while in placement to process their fears is recommended
- The staff of the clinical facilities should be supported to create an understanding of the students' emotions and vulnerabilities while in practice
- A follow up study should explore the effects on students' views after supportive measures were implemented

## Conclusion

Although for some students, *"Writing this journal was more enriching than just telling a story",* others expressed emotional fatigue and internal conflict between life and just being alive. The students struggled with the role they might play as a midwife in the lives of babies that they deliver, and being a good-enough mothers to protect their own children from abuse. But they had renewed admiration for carers, parents and institutions that become their homes. Their relief was recognised when they eventually understood the reasons for placement and when the factors influencing these events became clearer.

*"The exciting part for me was to be able to make the connection between theory and practice and the ability to reflect on it in a meaningful way"*

Although the placement was not what the students have anticipated it to be, they seemed free from mistaken beliefs or foolish hopes about people and life as a whole, in other words, free from illusion towards the end of their clinical placement.

## References

1. Uys LR, Middleton L (2014) Mental health nursing: A South African perspective 6thedition, Cape Town, Juta, 226-228.

2. Stein DJ, Seedat S, Herman A (2008) Lifetime prevalence of psychiatric disorders in South Africa. Br J Psych 192: 112-117.

3. Manglio R (2009) The impact of child sexual abuse on health: A systematic review of reviews. Clin Psychol Rev 29: 647-657.

4. Berg A, Hallberg IR, Norberg A (1998) Nurses' reflections about dementia care, the patients, the care and themselves in their daily caregiving. Int J Nurs Stud 35: 271-282.

5. Wackely G (1991) Sexual abuse and the primary care doctor; the problem in primary health care: Springer Science and Business media, Psychosexual Medicine Series, pp: 1-10.

6. Harrison A, Zohhadi S (2005) Professional influences on the provision of mental health care for older people within a general hospital ward. J Psychiatr Ment Health Nurs 12: 472-480.

7. Reed F, Fitzgerald L (2005) The mixed attitudes of nurses to caring for people with mental illness in a rural general hospital. Int J Ment Health Nurs 2005: 249-257.

8. Chase S (2005) Narrative inquiry: Multiple lenses, approaches, voices. In: Denzin, NK, LincolnYS (eds.,) The SAGE handbook of qualitative

research. 3rdedition. Thousand Oaks, London, Sage Publications, New Delhi, pp: 651-679.

9. McLeod SA (2007) Psychodynamic approach.

10. Boud D (2001) Using journal writing to enhance reflective practice: New directions for adult and continuing education, Summer 2001, John Wiley and Sons, Inc.

11. South Africa Government Gazette (2007) Children's Act No. 38 of 2005, Juta Ltd.

12. Polit DF, Beck CT (2012) Nursing research generating and assessing evidence for nursing practice. Lippincott Williams and Williams, USA

13. Dhai A, McQuoid-Mason D (2011) Bioethics, human rights and health law: Principles and practice, Juta, Cape Town, pp: 14-15

14. Begley AM (2008) Truth-telling, honesty and compassion: A virtue-based exploration of a dilemma in practice. Int J Nurs Pract 14: 336-341.

15. Reissman CK (2008) Narrative methods for the human sciences. Thousand Oaks, Sage Publications, London.

16. Clandinin DJ, Connelly FM (2000) Narrative enquiry: Experience and story in qualitative research, Jossey-Bass publishers, San Francisco.

17. Phillips SB (2004) Group interventions for treatment of psychological trauma. Module 7: Countertransference, Effects on the group therapist working with trauma, New York, pp: 196-222

18. Freud S (1856-1939) Psychodynamic perspective.

19. Mollon P (2002) Shame and Jealousy: The Hidden Turmoils, Karnac Books (Ltd.,), USA

20. Klein M (1946) 'Notes on some schizoid mechanisms.' In: The Writings of Melanie Klein, Volume III, Hogarth, 1-24.

21. Van den Heever AE, Poggenpoel M, Myburgh CPH (2015) Nurses' perceptions of facilitating genuineness in a nurse-patient relationship. Health SA Gesondheid 20: 109-117.

22. Langley ME, Brown ST (2010) Perceptions of the use of reflective journals in online graduate nursing education. Nurs Educ Perspect 3 1: 12.

# 29

# The use of 4G Android Tablets for Enhanced Patient Activation of Chronic Disease Self-Management in People with Heart Failure

Judith Kutzleb*,Nancy Elmann, Andrew Fruhschien, Stephen Angeli, Angel Mulkay , Jarrett Bauer, Rohan Udeshi and Dan Priece

*Advanced Practice Professionals at Holy Name Medical Center, 718 Teaneck Road, Teaneck, New Jersey, USA*

*Corresponding author: Judith Kutzleb, et al. Advanced Practice Professionals at Holy Name Medical Center, 718 Teaneck Road, Teaneck, New Jersey, 07666, USA, E-mail: kutzleb@mail.holyname.org

## Abstract

### Problem

The purpose of this research was to evaluate the impact of an advanced practice nurse-directed patient education approach to heart failure treatment integrating the use of an interactive 4G android tablet, will enable patients to experience enhanced patient activation and engagement in chronic disease self-management and fewer 30-day rereadmissions.

### Data source

This was a prospective patient randomization, multi-center quasi-experimental design study of 50 patients comparing an advanced practice nurse-directed education of disease self-management and use of a 4G android tablet (TC) group (n = 25) and routine medical management (MC) group. The study length was 12 months.

### Conclusions

Descriptive statistics were computed, and the intervention and control groups were compared for differences. Descriptive statistics using ANOVA was conducted to calculate for statistical significance of readmissions between the two groups at 30 days. T-tests showed that the 30-day readmissions rate was significantly lower for the tablet groups compared to the medical group at 30 days (8% and 28% respectively; P=0.010).

### Implications for Practice

The results support that integrating 4G android tablet technology does have a significant impact on enhancing patient activation and engagement in chronic disease self-management and correlated to reduced 30-day readmissions in people with heart failure.

**Keywords** Heart failure; Patient education; Mobile technology in chronic disease; Patient activation; Patient engagement; Disease self-management

## Introduction

Heart Failure (HF) is a major public health problem in the United States and is the most common discharge diagnosis in the population of people over 65 years. The prevalence of heart failure continues to rise involving approximately 6.6 million Americans, with 550,000 newly diagnosed cases each year [1,2]. Because of the aging population and despite the successful treatment of underlying conditions that cause heart failure, such as coronary artery disease and hypertension, the number of people with heart failure continues to increase. The annual number of hospitalizations for the primary diagnosis of heart failure has increased from 800,000 to over 1 million over the last 20 years [3]. Economically, heart failure is the most costly healthcare problem, with direct cost for diagnosis and treatment being approximately $39.2 billion in 2012 [1]. Of particular concern to healthcare organizations, are the frequent readmissions despite the advancements in HF-related medical care [2]. Approximately one fifth of Medicare beneficiaries discharged from a hospital are readmitted within 30 days; and 50% of patients with HF are readmitted within 6 months of discharge, with 70% of the rehospitalizations being related to worsening HF symptomatology [4].

Many healthcare organizations are focusing on improving performance and patient outcomes in HF paying particular attention to better chronic disease management so as to prevent readmissions, decrease costs, and improve quality of life [5-7]. As of October 2013, the Centers for Medicare and Medicaid Services (CMS) have implemented decreased reimbursement with additional penalties for patients who require readmission for any cause within 30 days of their initial admission [8]. A decrease in healthcare reimbursement can be a threat to most hospitals' mission of patient care. Financial pressures may stem from reduced insurance reimbursement, capitation, and changes in public funding. Pressures for innovation result from increasing numbers of patients, higher acuity, and the aging population with complex chronic disease processes [9-11].

Primary care providers, not cardiologists, treat most patients and play a key role in improving clinical outcomes in patients with and at risk for heart failure. Educating patients about their disease; motivating adherence to a course of therapy through patient activation of disease self-management are critical aspects in promoting positive outcomes. The purpose of this project was two-fold: first, to evaluate the impact of nurse-directed patient education on chronic disease self-management; second, to evaluate the extent to which 30 day hospital readmissions decreased by patient activation in disease self-management through the use of a 4G android tablet. Patient activation is defined as, an individual being able to self-manage symptoms and problems; engage in activities that maintain physical function; and maintain involvement in clinical decision-making as their overall reduced health declines [11,12].

## Literature Review

Mobile technology has expanded dramatically around the world. The integration of 3G, 4G, and bluetooth technology has had a huge impact on chronic disease management [13,14]. Technology has been used to support lifestyle modification for diabetes and COPD disease management [15,16]. Researchers have developed mobile phone software applications that can help COPD patients self-manage their disease [17-19]. The aim is to provide software applications that are available any time and any place to help individuals improve their health status and obtain social support while at the same time providing ready access to a health professional if an emergency arises [20,21]. One of the biggest problems for elderly patients is forgetting to take their prescription medications. It is estimated that only 50 percent of patients take their medication as prescribed [22,23]. They either forgot to take their medication or did not take them at the time or dosage set by their primary care provider. This means that half of the benefit of prescription medications is lost through human error. Research has found that individuals who have access and used technology that allows for self-management of disease, have been able to obtain some level of success in terms of improving their health outcomes [24,25].

Liu et al., conducted a study on mobile phones plus COPD-specific software. The results of this study did show improvement with incremental shuttle walk test distances, walking endurance, compliance with home-based exercise programs, inspiratory capacity, quality of life scores, exercise time, physical functioning and self-efficacy in managing dyspnea. The results also showed decreased hospital length of stays for disease exacerbations as well as the number of unscheduled visits to physician offices.

Cotter et al. 2013, did a systematic review of evidence on internet interventions to support lifestyle modification for diabetes management. The results of the systematic review demonstrated improvements in diet and or physical activity, and improvements in glycemic control when comparing web-based intervention with control cohorts. Therefore, in conclusion, web-based strategies provided a valuable option for facilitating diabetes self-management.

Johnston et al., examined whether the use of a Blackberry-based daily symptom diary would detect 95% or more COPD exacerbations and enable characterization of seasonal differences among daily diary entries. An alert system was triggered when symptoms changed, missed diary transmissions occurred, or there was need for medical intervention. The results showed that of the 28,514 possible daily symptoms diary entries, the participants transmitted 99.9% of the possible entries. In conclusion, smart-phone based collection of COPD symptom diaries enabled near-complete identification of exacerbations at inception.

## Treatment Approaches

Pharmacotherapeutic treatments for heart failure have improved outcomes in the past 10 years, and evidence-based guidelines provide a structured approach to the treatment of heart failure. Clinical trials have shown that maximizing pharmacotherapy in conjunction with patient education and activation reduces hospital admissions, decreases morbidity and mortality, and improves the quality of life for patients with heart failure. An advanced practice nurse-directed multidisciplinary approach to heart failure management incorporates both patient monitoring and patient self-management of symptoms as a central strategy. Active patient activation is paramount in the effective management of chronic conditions. Various self-management initiatives have been developed to assist patients to optimize the management of their health. The objective of these programs is to provide patients with information and skills that will enhance their ability to participate in their health care. Targeting risk factors for unplanned readmissions in concert with protocol driven medical management are the tenets for achieving successful outcomes.

## Hypothesis

Patients who participate in an advanced practice nurse-directed patient education approach to heart failure treatment in concert with the use of an interactive 4G android tablet will experience enhanced patient activation and engagement in disease self-management and fewer 30 day hospital readmissions.

## Research Methods

This study is a prospective multi-center quasi-experimental design with patient randomization to an advanced practice nurse-directed disease self-management with the use of a 4G Android Tablet (TC) group and a routine medical management (MC) group.

## Sample

All adult patients 20 to 89 years of age admitted to the hospital with the principal diagnosis of heart failure were considered for inclusion in the study. The design flow chart (Figure 1) was developed to identify the process of patients through the study. Patient referrals were from either cardiologists or primary care physicians. Both sites were comparable in the medical management and patient population mix of heart failure admissions.

All patients enrolled had a diagnosis of heart failure confirmed by a cardiologist based on echocardiography with evidence of left ventricular systolic dysfunction or diastolic dysfunction. Patients who were not literate in English were excluded. Patients presenting with heart failure in the setting of myocardial infarction or unstable angina or in whom failure was not thought to be the primary problem, or for whom heart failure was a secondary diagnosis in conjunction with multiple chronic comorbidities, were excluded. Also, patients with illnesses that could compromise survival over the duration of the study (e.g. cancer) or with cognitive impairment, or who were taking mood-altering medications (antipsychotics, antianxiety, and antidepressant agents) were excluded. The baseline characteristics gathered on the total population, TC group and MC group included gender, age, average ejection fraction percentage, New York Heart Association (NYHA) classification, etiology, risk factors, and medications (Table 1).

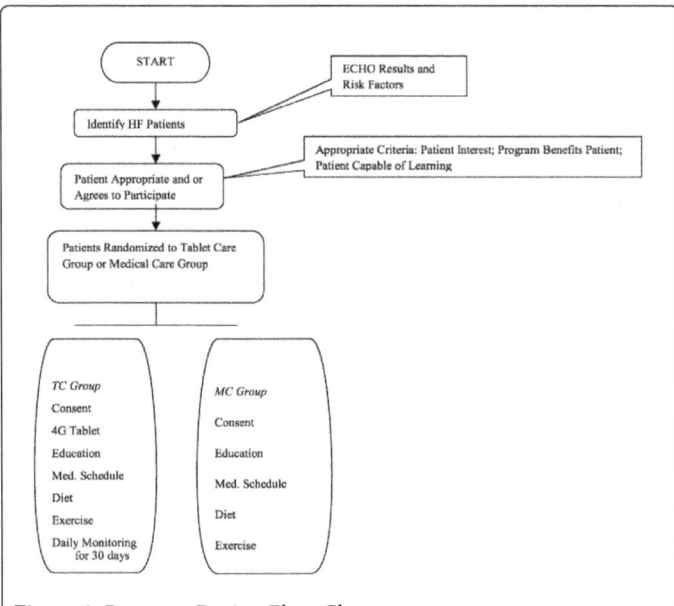

Figure 1: Program Design Flow Chart.

| Demographics | TC group | % | MC group | % |
|---|---|---|---|---|
| Gender | | | | |
| Male | 14 | 28% | 13 | 26% |
| Female | 11 | 22% | 12 | 24% |
| Average Age | 71 | | 72 | |
| Average EF (%) | 37% | | 41% | |
| NYHA class | | | | |
| Class I | 0 | | 0 | |
| Class II | 12 | 24% | 15 | 30% |
| Class III | 9 | 18% | 7 | 14% |
| Class IV | 4 | 8% | 3 | 6% |
| Etiology of HF | | | | |
| Ischemic CM | 4 | 8% | 1 | 2% |
| Hypertension | 10 | 20% | 15 | 30% |
| Alcoholic CM | 3 | 6% | 0 | 0% |
| Idiopathic | 5 | 10% | 3 | 6% |
| Valvular | 2 | 4% | 4 | 8% |
| Risk Factors | | | | |
| Hypertension | 21 | 42% | 14 | 28% |
| DM | 11 | 22% | 11 | 22% |
| Smoking | 8 | 16% | 11 | 22% |
| Alcohol abuse | 1 | 2% | 3 | 6% |
| CAD | 16 | 32% | 12 | 24% |
| COPD | 7 | 14% | 5 | 10% |
| Renal Insufficiency | 4 | 8% | 3 | 6% |
| Medications | | | | |
| ACE inhibitor | 23 | 46% | 24 | 48% |
| Diuretic | 25 | 50% | 23 | 46% |
| Beta-blocker | 25 | 50% | 25 | 50% |
| Digoxin | 5 | 10% | 7 | 14% |
| Other | 10 | 20% | 8 | 16% |

Table 1: Baseline demographic characteristics of total population, TC group, and MC group

Note: N=50; CM: Cardiomyopathy; NYHA: New York Heart Association; EF: Ejection Fraction; ACE: Angiotensin-Converting Enzyme; DM: Diabetes Mellitus; CAD: Coronary Artery Disease; COPD: Chronic Obstructive Pulmonary Disease

After blind randomization, all patients who participated were told the purpose of the study and signed an informed voluntary written consent form (approved by the institutional review boards) indicating their willingness to participate. Patients were informed that their responses would be kept confidential and that under no circumstances would their participation or lack of participation influence treatment decisions or jeopardize their care. Patients were interviewed to determine their hospitalization history and the length and nature of symptoms associated with heart failure. Severity of symptoms was assessed by categorizing the patients according to the NYHA functional classifications: class I, unlimited activity without cardiac symptoms; class II, ordinary physical activity causes fatigue, dyspnea, or palpitations; class III, marked limitation of activity and symptoms with less than usual activity but no symptoms at rest; and class IV, any physical activity is accompanied by symptoms and symptoms may occur at rest.

## Setting and Plan of Action

The patients were evaluated by the advanced practice nurse after admission in each study site. At the time of evaluation, patients randomized to the TC group were informed of the following for study inclusion: education on the use of the 4G android tablet for recording of daily weights; daily exercise; and daily medication administration for the duration of 30 days. The TC group also received comprehensive disease education with a patient education pamphlet describing heart failure, listing recommendations to maintain a heart healthy lifestyle and signs and symptoms of changes in condition status that warrants medical notification. Medication compliance counseling consisted of a personalized medication schedule. Each individual schedule was programmed into the tablet where the patient was required to record his/her administration of medications within the established parameters. The tablet also contained pre-recorded videos and power points for educational support for both the patient and family members reinforcing the importance of medication adherence; daily weight monitoring; meal planning and managing a low-sodium diet. Predischarge counseling also concentrated on smoking cessation and elimination of alcohol intake. Interventions were monitored by the advanced practice nurse on a daily basis by review of the computer generated program of the data obtained from the android tablets.

The MC group was informed of the following criteria: review of the patient education booklet that included daily weight charting; diet and nutrition counseling incorporating food exchange list, food preparation tips, and a four-step approach to managing a low-salt diet. A medication administration schedule was designed for each patient, listing medications, dosage strengths, and mechanism of action. Individualized counseling concentrated on exercise, smoking cessation, and elimination of alcohol intake. Interventions were monitored by telephone follow-up on a weekly basis by the call center from each site. A standard questionnaire was utilized to maintain consistency in patient response.

## Functional Capacity

The objective measure of functional capacity was obtained using a 6-minute walk test. Patients were told to walk at a brisk pace as far as they could within the allotted time, resting as needed. The limitation of the 6-minute walk test is the inability to standardize it with regard to step length and pace. However, differences were minimized in the method at each site by using the same physical area each time, and by standardizing the directions given to the patients.

## Results

### Characteristics of Sample

Out of 83 eligible patients, 50 patients (25 from site #1 and 25 from site #2) consented for study participation. The mean age of the study participants was 71 years old; 46% were women and 54% were men. Average ejection fraction for participants in the TC group was 37% versus 41% in the MC group, which represents a significantly higher risk population in the TC group. There was no significant difference found by group membership regarding gender or race. The average number of medications taken was six and is consistent with the complex treatment that is characteristic of this illness. In terms of illness management, 80% of the MC either reported never being placed on or did not follow a strict low-sodium diet, and compliance to medication adherence was low. Seventy-seven percent of the TC groups and 20% of the MC group engaged in daily exercise activity. Eighty percent of the MC group managed their illness by restricting their activities and taking frequent rests. There were no deaths, nor any patients lost to follow-up in either group during this study. Age, race, and economic status did not differ significantly between patients who participated in the study.

The data was analyzed using the Statistical Package for Social Sciences 21 (IBM Corp.) for analysis. Descriptive statistics were computed, and the intervention and control groups were compared for differences. Descriptive statistics using ANOVA was conducted to calculate for statistical significance of readmissions between the two groups at 30 days. T-tests showed that the 30-day readmissions rate was significantly lower for the tablet group compared to the medical group at 30 days (8% and 28% respectively; P = 0.010) (see Table 2).

| Variable (Tablet Care%/ Medical Care %) | F | df | 95% CI | Standard Deviation | P |
|---|---|---|---|---|---|
| 30 days (8%/ 28%) | 1.40 | 1 | 1.4209-1.6286 | .40118 | .010 |

**Table 2:** One-Way ANOVA Statistical Analysis of HF Readmissions between Tablet Care group and Medical Care group at 30 days

Note: F=ratio; df=degrees of freedom. *P<.05 (two-tailed test)

The results support that integrating 4G android tablet technology does have a significant impact on enhancing patient activation and engagement in chronic disease self-management and correlated to reduced 30-day readmissions in people with heart failure.

## Discussion

The research interventions in this study were directed toward increasing patient activation and engagement with the use of technology as an adjuvant modality to patient education of chronic disease self-management. This study focused specifically on patients with heart failure who were identified to be at high-risk for early readmissions, and the intervention with technology addressed targeted causes of re-hospitalization (life-style, medication and diet noncompliance, exercise noncompliance, and lack of engagement for self-care disease management). The study sites were initiated in hospitalized heart failure patients who were discharged home, whereas prior studies focused on interventions on hospitalized heart failure patients not including post-acute discharge management or monitoring. The literature has theorized that outpatient management should be successfully provided by primary care providers, not cardiologists. This study did prove that successful management of heart failure patients was provided by advanced practice nurses in concert with primary care providers. The outcome of this study also demonstrated that patient engagement did correlate with reduced 30-day readmissions.

The TC group patients described their most positive changes in their overall well-being as relating to their ability to self-manage their medications and diet which stemmed from the daily engagement with the 4G interactive android tablet. The physiological changes experienced as a result of pharmacological and non-pharmacological regimens improved their overall exercise tolerance and ability to maintain independence. The improved adherence to treatment modalities as observed in this population has proven to be a predictor of adjustment to illness and disease self-management. The mean exercise time in the TC group increased from 6 minutes to 23 minutes daily. The 6-minute walk test proved to be an inexpensive and uncomplicated but limited clinical measure of exercise capacity.

## Future Research

Further evaluation of functional capacity and NYHA classification to test for sensitivity for differences in clinical status of heart failure patients would require further study. Studies directed at integrating 4G android technologies for monitoring multiple disease processes in concert with HF management are required to identify if timely treatment of multiple disease exacerbations are associated with decreased risk for mortality and heart failure related hospitalizations. A number of patients could not be included in this study because of either language barrier or lack of health literacy. This represents a significant limitation of the present study given the high rate of functional illiteracy in the United States, along with the complexity of the illness management regimen needed for most heart failure patients. It is imperative that the needs of these patients be described and interventions for technology integration for chronic disease be developed for future studies. Last, further development of reliable and sensitive self-report and observer-related specific measures for study population would also be useful in the future.

## Conclusion

In our opinion, the improved patient activation in our patients was a direct result of the study intervention with the use of 4G interactive android tablet. Patients were never without questions, and several patients were averted from either emergency room visits or rehospitalizations by timely interactions with the study team. The focused nature of the intervention, the close monitoring of patient activation through a web portal, and follow-up, support our hypothesis and explanations for our findings. A significant portion of patient crises are avoided through interventions that improve patient activation and compliance with prescribed management protocols and improve recognition of early warning signs of clinical problems.

Thus, as management of symptoms and the work associated with the regimen needed to achieve symptom control are necessary elements in successful management of any chronic illness, heart failure patients participating in an advanced practice nurse symptom management program in concert with interactive technology can be expected to achieve better outcomes than patients who do not learn to actively engage in disease self-management. The participants in this study were able to demonstrate disease self-management through daily entry of prescribed activities of daily weights, medication regimens (dosages and administration), low sodium diet adherence, and lifestyle modification via the use of 4G android tablets. The study demonstrated the use of interactive technology significantly improved patient engagement, and prevented 30-day rehospitalizations in patients with heart failure.

## References

1. Roger VL, Go AS, Loyd-Jones DM, Benjamin EJ, Berry JD (2012) Heart disease and stroke statistics: 2012 update: a report from the American Heart Association. Circulation 125: e2-e220.

2. Butler J, Kalogeropoulos A (2008) Worsening heart failure hospitalization epidemic we do not know how to prevent and we do not know how to treat! J Am Coll Cardiol 52: 435-437.

3. Ross JS, Chen J, Lin Z, Bueno H, Curtis JP, et al. (2010) Recent national trends in readmission rates after heart failure hospitalization. Circ Heart Fail 3: 97-103.

4. Jencks SF, Williams MV, Coleman EA (2009) Rehospitalizations among patients in the Medicare fee-for-service program. N Engl J Med 360: 1418-1428.

5. Kutzleb J, Reiner D (2006) The impact of nurse-directed patient education on quality of life and functional capacity in people with heart failure. J Am Acad Nurse Pract 18: 116-123.

6. Fang J, Mensah GA, Croft JB, Keenan NL (2008) Heart failure-related hospitalization in the U.S., 1979 to 2004. J Am Coll Cardiol 52: 428-434.

7. Dickson VV, Riegel B (2009) Are we teaching what patients need to know? Building skills in heart failure self-care. Heart Lung 38: 253-261.

8. Medicare Payment Advisory Commission (2008) Report to Congress: Reforming the delivery system.

9. Kim, S, Han H (2013). Evidence-based strategies to reduce readmissions in patients with heart failure. The Journal for Nurse Practitioners, 9: 224-232.

10. Jessup M, Abraham W, Casey D, Arthur M. Feldman, Theodore G Ganiats, (2009) Focused Update: ACCF/AHA guidelines for the diagnosis and management of heart failure in adults: A report of the American College of Cardiology Foundation/American Heart Association Task Force on Practice Guidelines: Developed in collaboration with the international society of Heart and lung transplantation. Circulation 119: 1977-2016.

11. Hibbard JH, Stockard J, Mahoney ER, Tusler M (2004) Development of the patient activation measure (PAM): Conceptualizing and measuring activation in patients and consumers. Health Services Research 39: 1005-1026.

12. Gerber LM, Barrón Y, Mongoven J, McDonald M, Henriquez E, et al. (2011) Activation among chronically ill older adults with complex medical needs: challenges to supporting effective self-management. J Ambul Care Manage 34: 292-303.

13. Noh JH, Cho YJ, Nam HW, Kim JH, Kim DJ, et al. (2010) Web-based comprehensive information system for self-management of diabetes mellitus. Diabetes Technol Ther 12: 333-337.

14. Yu CH, Bahniwal R, Laupacis A, Leung E, Orr MS (2012) Systematic review and evaluation of web-accesible tools for management of diabetes and related cardiovascular risk factors by patients and healthcare providers. J Am Med Inform Assoc 19: 514-522.

15. Polisena J, Tran K, Cimon K, Hutton B, McGill S (2010) Home telehealth for chronic obstructive pulmonary disease: a systematic review and meta-analysis. J Telemed and Telecare, 16: 120-127

16. Trappenburg J, Niesink A, de Weert-van Oene G, vander Zeijden H, van Snippenburg R, (2008) Effects of telemonitoring in patients with chronic obstructive pulmonary disease. Telemedicine Journal e-Health 14: 138-146.

17. Nguyen HQ, Wolpin S, Chiang KC, Cuenco D, Carrieri-Kohlman V (2006) Exercise and symptom monitoring with a mobile device. AMIA Annu Symp Proc .

18. Wang H, Liu J (2009) Mobile phone based health care technology. Recent patents on Biomedical Engineering 2: 15-21.

19. Feil EG, Glasgow RE, Boles S, McKay HG (2000) Who participates in Internet-based self-management programs? A study among novice computer users in a primary care setting. Diabetes Educ 26: 806-811.

20. Sala E, Alegre L, Carrera M, Ibars M, Orriols FJ, et al. (2001) Supported discharge shortens hospital stay in patients hospitalized because of an exacerbation of COPD. Eur Respir J 17: 1138-1142.

21. Bischoff EW, Boer LM, Molema J, Akkermans R, van Weel C, et al. (2012) Validity of an automated telephonic system to assess COPD exacerbation rates. Eur Respir J 39: 1090-1096.

22. World Health Organization (2003) Adherence to long-term therapies: evidence for action 7-10

23. Kaufman N (2010) Internet and information technology use in treatment of diabetes. Int J Clin Pract Suppl : 41-46.

24. Glasgow RE, Kurz D, King D, Dickman JM, Faber AJ, et al. (2010) Outcomes of minimal and moderate support versions of an internet-based diabetes self-management support program. J Gen Intern Med 25: 1315-1322.

25. Welch G, Shayne R (2006) Interactive behavioral technologies and diabetes self-management support: recent research findings from clinical trials. Curr Diab Rep 6: 130-136.

26. Liu WT, Wang CH, Lin HC, Lin SM, Lee KY, et al. (2008) Efficacy of a cell phone-based exercise programme for COPD. Eur Respir J 32: 651-659.

# 30

# Treatment Outcomes of Tuberculosis Patients at Bale Robe Hospital Oromia Regional State, Ethiopia: A Five Year Retrospective Study

**Erdaw Tachbele**[1*], **Biruhalem Taye**[2], **Begna Tulu**[3] and **Gobena Ameni**[3*]

[1]*Department of Nursing and Midwifery, College of Health Sciences, Addis Ababa University, Ethiopia*

[2]*Aklilu Lemma Institute of Pathobiology, Addis Ababa University, Addis Ababa, Ethiopia*

[3]*Microbiology, Immunology and Parasitology Department, Bahir Dar University, Ethiopia*

*Corresponding author:** Erdaw Tachbele, P.O. Box 11240, Addis Ababa, Ethiopia, E-mail: Erdaw.tachbele@aau.edu.et

## Abstract

**Objective:** Monitoring of tuberculosis treatment outcome is scarcely done in Ethiopia. This study investigated the outcomes of tuberculosis treatment at Bale Robe Hospital in Oromia, Ethiopia.

**Methods:** A retrospective analysis of the profile and treatment outcome of all tuberculosis patients registered from September, 2007 to August, 2012 at tuberculosis Clinic was conducted. Patients' socio-demographic, clinical, laboratory and treatment outcomes were were extracted from registration document. Bivariate and multivariate logistic regression was used to determine treatment outcomes predictor variables.

**Results:** We analyzed treatment outcomes of 916 tuberculosis patients, of which 544 (59.6 %) were males. Of these 180 (19.7%) were cured, 536 (58.5%) were found completed their treatment, while 82 (9%) were died, in addition, 55 (6.0%) and 54 (5.9%) were defaulters and transferred out respectively. Overall, 716 (78.2%) had a successful and 200 (21.8%) a poor treatment outcome. Being female (AOR 1.23, P=0.05), HIV positive (0.48, P<0.001) and new TB patients (AOR 2.17, P=0.002) were significantly associated with treatment outcome. Patients aged ≤ 14 had significantly high treatment success rate (AOR 4.99, P=0.003) followed by 35-44 years (AOR 3.5, P=0.009) and 25-34 years (AOR 2.52, P=0.029). Tuberculosis patients with HIV co-infection (AOR 4.32, P=<0.001), smear negative pulmonary tuberculosis (AOR 2.00, P=0.05) and age ≥ 65 years (AOR 5.50, P=0.03) were more likely to experience death than their counter parts.

**Conclusion:** The treatment success rate of 78.2% tuberculosis patients was fairly good. However, a high proportion of patients (9%) death and 22.2% of HIV prevalence among TB patients is a serious public health concern that needs to be addressed urgently in the area.

**Keywords:** Treatment outcomes; Tuberculosis; DOTS; Bale robe; Ethiopia

**Abbreviations:** AFB: Acid Fast Bacilli, AOR: Adjusted Odds Ratio, CDR: Case Detection Rate, DOTS: Directly Observed Treatment, Short Course, GTB: Global Tuberculosis Programme, HBCs: High-Burden Countries, HIV: Human Immunodeficiency Virus, MDR: Multiple Drug Resistance, NTLCP: National Tuberculosis and Leprosy Control Program, TSR: Treatment Success Rate

## Introduction and Background

Despite great effort is exerted globally to combat tuberculosis (TB), still it remains the major cause of mortality worldwide and accounts for 25% of all avoidable deaths in developing countries and 2.5% of the world diseases Burdon [1].

The WHO 2013 report indicated that Ethiopia stands eighth among the world's 22 high tuberculosis Burdon countries [2]. Tuberculosis is the leading cause of morbidity, the third cause of hospital admission and the second cause of death in Ethiopia [3].

Without treatment, TB mortality rates are high. Natural history of disease studies showed that around 70% of sputum smear positive HIV-negative pulmonary TB cases died within 10 years , and 20% of culture positive (but smear negative) cases died within 10 years [4].

Since 1990 the WHO Global Tuberculosis Programme (GTB) has promoted the revision of national tuberculosis programmes to strengthen the focus on directly observed treatment, short-course (DOTS) and close monitoring of treatment outcomes. Patients treated by DOTS at the start of therapy had a significantly higher cure rate and decreased tuberculosis- related mortality compared with patients treated by self-administered therapy [5]. The implementation of DOTS and its subsequent surveillance system of treatment outcomes revealed 82% global treatment success rate in DOTs areas in comparison to only 67% in non-DOTs areas [6].

Routine recording and reporting of the numbers of TB cases diagnosed and treated by National Tuberculosis Programmes (NTPs) and monitoring of treatment outcomes was one of the five components of the global TB strategy (DOTS) launched by WHO in the mid-1990s and it remains a core element of its successor, the Stop TB Strategy [2], with set targets of 84% case detection rate (CDR) and 87% treatment success rate (TSR) by 2015. Between 1995 and 2012, 56 million people were successfully treated for TB in countries that had adopted the DOTS/Stop TB Strategy which saved approximately 22 million lives [2]. In 2011, the global treatment success rate was 87% among all new TB cases, except the European Region where the treatment success rate ranges from 65% for new smear positive cases to 72% for new smear negative cases [2].

In Ethiopia, Directly Observed Treatment, Short Course (DOTS), was started in 1992. Since then, the DOTS programme has been successively scaled up in the country with a 100% geographical coverage, and 95% health facility coverage [3]. The implementation of DOTS in Ethiopia has been associated with high rate of successful treatment outcome and reduced development of drug resistance [7]. According to WHO report, in 2011 Ethiopia reported treatment success rate of 90% for new smear positive, 87% for smear negative/ extra pulmonary, and 78 % for retreatment cases with case detection rate of 64% [2]. In reference to the updated global TB plan (2011-2015) with a set targets of 87% treatment success rate and 84 case detection rate, Ethiopia achieved the treatment success rate but needs to work hard to reach the global plan of case detection rate.

Monitoring the outcome of treatment by cohort analysis of tuberculosis patients is essential in order to evaluate the effectiveness of DOTS program and serves as a proxy of quality of TB treatment in a health care system [7,8]. In addition to this, understanding the determinant factors of unsuccessful treatment outcomes is crucial to improve the TB control system.

To this end, very few studies have reported treatment outcomes of DOTS in different parts of Ethiopia from 2005 to 2013 [7-18]. The studies conducted so far in different parts of the country (Southern region, Addis Ababa, Gambella and Northern region) documented different rate of treatment success rates ranging from 29.5% in Gondar, North west Ethiopia [15], to 89.2% in Tigray, Northern Ethiopia [17]. According to these studies, being male, older age, place of treatment, smear negative pulmonary TB, HIV positive, smear positive pulmonary TB at 2nd month follow up and retreatment cases were found to be the determinant factors of unsuccessful treatment outcomes [7,8,11,13,15-20].

Although Ethiopia has fully implemented DOTS program across the whole nation, information on epidemiological cohort analysis of TB treatment outcomes, especially in Oromia National Regional State is severely lacking. Therefore, this study was designed to investigate the treatment outcomes of TB patients and assess the association of demographic and clinical factors with treatment success of patients enrolled in Directly Observed Treatment Short Course (DOTS) program in Bale Robe Hospital Oromia, Ethiopia over the course of five consecutive years (From Sep 2007 to Aug 2012).

## Methods

### Study setting

Bale Robe is a regional hospital serving the population of Robe town and that of South West Ethiopia. Thetotal population served by the hospital is about 569,707.In the hospital a Directly Observed Therapy; Short-Course (DOTS) clinic is operating under the National Tuberculosis and Leprosy Control Program (NTLCP) of Ethiopia, under which the diagnosis of pulmonary TB is followed by examination of three sputum smears by Zihel-Nielsen staining method for acid fast bacilli (AFB). Chest radiographs and pathological investigations are also used to support the diagnosis. Patients

diagnosed with tuberculosis are referred to the DOTS clinic where they are registered and treated according to the NTLCP guideline [3,21].

### Study design and data collection

Institution based retrospective analysis of the profile and treatment outcome of all tuberculosis patients (cohort) registered from September, 2007 to August, 2012 at DOTS Clinic was conducted. The registration documents reviewed contain patient's age, sex, residence, weight, Acid Fast Bacilli smear result at base line, HIV status, 2nd 5th and 7th months follow up AFB smear result and weight, treatment regimen, treatment started and completed dates and treatment outcomes. The required information was extracted from TB treatment log books (registration document) using structured data reviewing formats by the investigators.

### Dependent and independent variables

**Dependent variables:** Treatment success (cured or completed treatment) and Unsuccessful treatment (either treatment failure, defaulter, died, or transferred out).

**Independent variables** for treatment outcomes were: TB Patients' age, sex, weight, residence HIV status, type of TB, patient category at the start of treatment and AFB smear-positive at baseline, 2 month, 5 month and 7 months.

### Data management and statistical analysis

Data were entered, cleared and analyzed using the statistical package SPSS for windows, version 20. For categorical data, we used proportions with 95% confidence intervals, Odds ratio and Chi-square test to compare different groups. Multivariate analysis using logistic regression model was used to analyze the association between treatment outcome and potential predictor variables. P values of less than 0.05 were considered statistically significant.

### Ethical consideration

Institutional ethical clearance was obtained from the Institutional Review Board (IRB) of Addis Ababa University and permission was received from Bale Robe Hospital to use the data. Informed consent from study participants was not required as the survey was based on retrospective data with no patient interaction and the report is part of standard public health practice. In order to ensure confidentiality of the information, names or identification numbers of TB patients were not included in the data sheet.

## Results

### Demographic and clinical characteristics of study participants

A total of 916 tuberculosis patients were registered for DOTs program at Bale Robe Hospital, Oromia, between September 2007 and August 2012.Of these, 544 (59.6 %) were males and 372 (40.4%) were females with the mean, standard deviation and median age of 28.84, 14.65 and 25 years, respectively. More than half (59.9 %) of the study participants were concentrated between the age group of 15-34 years, which is believed to be the productive segment of the society. With regard to their residence majority 623 (68%) live in urban area where as 293 (32%) reside in rural setting. Of the total study participants, 373

(40.7%), 305 (33.3%), and 238 (26%) were smear negative pulmonary tuberculosis, extra pulmonary tuberculosis, and smear positive pulmonary tuberculosis cases respectively. With regard to treatment categories, 808 (88.2%) of the patients were new cases, 86 (9.4%) were transferred in patients while 16 (1.6%) were relapse cases. HIV serostatus of 711 (77.6%) study participants was known, out of which 158 (22.2%) were found to be positive (Table 1).

| Characteristics | Frequency(N) | Percentage (%) |
|---|---|---|
| **Sex** | | |
| Male | 544 | 59.6 |
| Female | 372 | 40.4 |
| **Residence** | | |
| Urban | 623 | 68 |
| Rural | 293 | 32 |
| **Age Group** | | |
| ≤14 | 101 | 11 |
| 15-24 | 296 | 32.3 |
| 25-34 | 253 | 27.6 |
| 35-44 | 124 | 13.5 |
| 45-54 | 64 | 7 |
| 55-64 | 39 | 4.3 |
| ≥65 | 39 | 4.3 |
| **Category of Patients** | | |
| New Cases | 808 | 88.2 |
| Transfer in | 86 | 9.4 |
| Relapse | 15 | 1.6 |
| Failure | 5 | 0.5 |
| Defaulter | 1 | 0.1 |
| Transferred out | 1 | 0.1 |
| **Tuberculosis Type** | | |
| SPPTB | 238 | 26 |
| SNPTB | 373 | 40.7 |
| EPTB | 305 | 33.3 |
| **HIV Status (N=711)** | | |
| HIV Positive | 158 | 22.2 |
| HIV Negative | 553 | 77.8 |
| **Treatment Outcomes** | | |
| Cured | 180 | 19.7 |
| Treatment completed | 536 | 58.5 |
| Died | 82 | 9 |
| Failure | 9 | 1 |
| Defaulter | 55 | 6 |
| Transferred out | 54 | 5.9 |
| **Total** | 916 | 100 |

**Table 1:** General characteristics of study participants (n=916), Bale Robe Hospital, 2007-2012, N=916, SPPTB= Smear positive pulmonary TB, SNPTB=Smear Negative Pulmonary TB, EPTB=Extra Pulmonary TB.

## Acid fast staining follow up result of registered TB patients during treatment

From the total of 238 (26%) smear positive pulmonary tuberculosis patients, 199 (83.60%) had AFB staining laboratory result at the end of the 2nd month of treatment, out of which only 3 (1.5%) were AFB positive. At the end of 5th month of treatment 193 (81%) smear positive pulmonary tuberculosis patients had AFB result, out of which 4 (2.1%) were remained positive. At the end of the 7th month a total of 173 (72.70%) had AFB laboratory result, of which all of them were AFB negative.

## Treatment outcomes

We examined treatment outcomes of 916 tuberculosis patients who were registered on DOTs program at the Bale Robe hospital during the study period. Out of which 180 (19.7%) were cured, 536 (58.5%) were found completed their treatment, while 82 (9%) were died, in addition, 55 (6.0%) and 54 (5.9%) were defaulters and transferred out respectively. Overall, 716 (78.2%) had a successful and 200 (21.8%) a poor treatment outcome. Of those with a poor treatment outcome, 82 (41%) patients died, 55 (27.5%) defaulted and 54 (27%) transferred out (Table 1).

The result in Table 2 indicates that as age of tuberculosis patients increased death rate of patients was increased from 4 (4%) to 19 (6.4%), 21 (8.3%) to 14 (11.3%), 10 (15.5%) to 7 (17.9) and 7 (17.9) in the age group of 0-14 years, 15-24 years, 25-34 years, 35-44 years, 45–54 years, 55-64 years and 65 years, respectively. Whereas the age of tuberculosis patients increased, treatment success rate of patients decreased from 91 (90.1%) to 229 (77.4%) to 99 (79.8%), 50 (78.1%), to 25 (64.1%), and 26 (66.7%), respectively.

| Characteristics | Treatment Outcomes | | | | | |
|---|---|---|---|---|---|---|
| | Treatment Success N (%) | Transferred out N (%) | Default N (%) | Death N (%) | Failure N (%) | Total |
| **Sex** | | | | | | |

| | | | | | | |
|---|---|---|---|---|---|---|
| Male | 413 (75.9) | 38 (7) | 39 (7.2) | 45 (8.3) | 9 (1.7) | 544 (100) |
| Female | 303 (81.5) | 16 (4.3) | 16 (4.3) | 37 (9.9) | 0 (0) | 372 (100) |
| **Residence** | | | | | | |
| Urban | 495 (79.5) | 35 (5.6) | 35 (5.6) | 52 (8.3) | 6 (1.0) | 623 (100) |
| Rural | 221 (75.4) | 19 (6.5) | 20 (6.8) | 30 (10.2) | 3 (1.0) | 293 (100) |
| **Age Groups(years)** | | | | | | |
| ≤14 | 91 (90.1) | 2 (2.0) | 4 (4.0) | 4 (4.0) | 0 (0) | 101 (100) |
| 15-24 | 229 (77.4) | 22 (7.4) | 22 (7.4) | 19 (6.4) | 4 (1.4) | 296 (100) |
| 25-34 | 196 (77.5) | 17 (6.7) | 16 (6.3) | 21 (8.3) | 3 (1.2) | 253 (100) |
| 35-44 | 99 (79.8) | 6 ((4.8) | 5 (4.0) | 14 (11.3) | 0 (0) | 124 (100) |
| 45-54 | 50 (78.1) | 3 (4.7) | 1 (1.6) | 10 (15.5) | 0 (0) | 64 (100) |
| 55-64 | 25 (64.1) | 2 (5.1) | 4 (1.6) | 7 (17.9) | 1 (2.6) | 39 (100) |
| ≥65 | 26 (66.7) | 2 (5.1) | 4 (10.3) | 7 (17.9) | 1 (2.6) | 39 (100) |
| **Patient Category** | | | | | | |
| New | 645 (79.8) | 44 (5.4) | 39 (4.8) | 73 (9) | 7 (0.9) | 808 (100) |
| Relapse | 10 ( 67.7) | 3 (20) | 0 (0) | 2 (13.3) | 0 (0) | 15 (100) |
| Failure | 3 (60) | 1 (20) | 0 (0) | 1 (20) | 0 (0) | 5 (100) |
| Defaulter | 1 (100) | 0 (0) | 0 (0) | 0 (0) | 0 (0) | 1 (100) |
| Transferred in | 56 (65.1) | 6 (7) | 16 (18.6) | 6 (7) | 2 (2.3) | 86 (100) |
| Transferred out | 1 (100) | 0 (0) | 0 (0) | 0 (0) | 0 (0) | 1 (100) |
| **Tuberculosis Type** | | | | | | |
| SPPTB | 190 (79.8) | 16 (6.7) | 11 (4.6) | 16 (6.7) | 5 (2.1) | 238 (100) |
| SNPTB | 284 (76.1) | 19 (5.1) | 19 (5.1) | 49 (13.1) | 2 (0.5) | 373 (100) |
| EPTB | 242 (79.3) | 19 (6.2) | 25 (8.2) | 17 (5.6) | 2 (0.7) | 305 (100) |
| **HIV Status( N=711)** | | | | | | |
| HIV positive | 106 (67.1) | 10 (6.3) | 10 (6.3) | 31 (19.6) | 1 (0.6) | 158 (100) |
| HIV Negative | 447 (80.8) | 30 (5.4) | 38 (6.9) | 33 (6.0) | 5 (0.9) | 553 (100) |
| **Year of Treatment** | | | | | | |
| 2008 | 152 (78.4) | 15 (7.7) | 6 (3.1) | 18 (9.3) | 3 (15) | 194 (100) |
| 2009 | 156 (81.7) | 5 (2.6) | 18 (9.4) | 12 (6.3) | 0 (0.0) | 191 (100) |
| 2010 | 158 (79.4) | 7 (3.5) | 14 (7.0) | 17 (8.5) | 3 (1.5) | 199 (100) |
| 2011 | 144 (75.8) | 12 (6.3) | 16 (8.4) | 15 (7.9) | 3 (1.6) | 190 (100) |
| 2012 | 106 (78.2) | 15 (10.6) | 1 (0.7) | 20 (14.1) | 0 (0.0) | 142 (100) |

**Table 2:** Treatment outcomes by sex, residence, age group, patient category, TB type, HIV status, and year of treatment Bale Hospital, Oromia regional State, 2007-2012, N=916, SPPTB=Smear Positive Pulmonary TB, SNPTB=Smear Negative Pulmonary TB, EPTB=Extra Pulmonary TB, N=Number.

Table 3 indicated that as age of tuberculosis patients increased, prevalence of smear negative pulmonary tuberculosis cases showed increasing pattern from 35.6% in the age group of 0-14 years to 71.8% in the age group of 66-99 years, whereas prevalence of Extrapulmonary tuberculosis (EPTB) showed decreasing pattern from 57.4% in the age group of 0-14 years to 17.9 % in the age group of 65 -99 years ($x^2$=71.36, p. value=0.00). In multi variate analysis, younger ages ($\leq$ 14 years) were more likely to develop EPTB than their older counter parts (AOR=8.81, CI=3.03-25.65) result not shown.

| Variables | Type of Tuberculosis | | | | Total number of TB patient's n (%) | $X^2$ (P. value) |
|---|---|---|---|---|---|---|
| | SPPTB n (%) | | SNPTB n (%) | EPTB n (%) | | |
| **Sex** | | | | | | |
| Male | 141 (25.9) | | 233 (41.1) | 180 (33.1) | 544 (100) | 0.044 (0.98) |
| Female | 97 (26.1) | | 150 (40.3) | 125 (33.6) | 372 (100) | |
| **Age Categories** | | | | | | |
| 0-14 | 7 (6.9) | | 36 (35.6) | 58 (57.4) | 101 (100) | |
| 15-24 | 102 (34.5) | | 102 (34.5) | 92 (31.1) | 296 (100) | 71.36 (00) |
| 25-34 | 76 (30.0) | | 95 (37.5) | 82 (32.4) | 253 (100) | |
| 35-44 | 29 (23.4) | | 56 (45.2) | 39 (31.5) | 124 (100) | |
| 45- 54 | 11 (17.2) | | 36 (56.2) | 17 (26.6) | 64 (100) | |
| 55-64 | 9 (23.1) | | 20 (51.3) | 10 (25.6) | 39 (100) | |
| 65-99 | 4 (10.3) | | 28 (71.8) | 7 (17.9) | 39 (100) | |
| **TB patient categories** | | | | | | 46.47 (00) |
| New | 192 (23.8) | | 343 (42.5) | 273 (33.8) | 808 (100) | |
| Relapse | 13 (86.7) | | 1 (6.7) | 1 (6.7) | 15 (100) | |
| Failure | 4 (80) | | 1 (20.0) | 0 (0.0) | 5 (100) | |
| Default | 1 (100) | | 0 (0.0) | 0 (0.0) | 1 (100) | |
| Transferred in | 28 (32.6) | | 28 (32.6) | 30 (34.9) | 86 (100) | |
| Transferred out | 0 (0.0) | | 0 (0.0) | 1 (100) | 1 (100) | |
| **Total** | 238 (26.0) | | 373 (40.7) | 305 (33.3) | 916 (100) | |

Table 3: Association of TB type with sex, Age category and TB patient categories, Bale Robe Hospital, Oromia, September, 2007-August, 2012, N=916SPPTB=Smear Positive Pulmonary TB, SNPTB=Smear Negative Pulmonary TB, EPTB=Extra Pulmonary TB, N=Number.

As shown in Table 4, female tuberculosis patients had significantly higher treatment success rate (81.5% versus 75.9%) than male (AOR=1.23, CI=1.10-1.75). In addition, patients in the age group of 0-14 years (AOR=4.99, CI=1.75-14.27), 25-34 years (AOR=2.52, CI=1.10-8.91) and 35-44 years (AOR=3.50, CI=1.37-8.91) had significantly higher treatment success rate compared to the other age groups. With regard to patient category at the start of treatment, new TB patients had significantly higher treatment success rate (AOR=2.17, CI=1.32-3.57) than retreated cases including relapse, failures, defaulters, transferred in cases. Whereas, HIV positive tuberculosis patients had significantly lower treatment success rate (AOR= 0.43, CI=0.28-0.65) than HIV negative ones (Table 4).

| Characteristics | Frequency | Treatment success | | COR | 95% CI | P-Value | A OR * | 95% CI | P-value |
|---|---|---|---|---|---|---|---|---|---|
| | | Yes N (%) | No N (%) | | | | | | |
| **Sex** | | | | | | | | | |
| Male | 544 (59.6) | 413 (75.9) | 131 (24.1) | ----- | ---- | -- | 1 | ------ | |
| Female | 372 (40.4) | 303 (81.5) | 69 (21.8) | 1.4 | 1.04-1.93 | 0.05 | 1.23 | 1.10-1.75 | 0.05 |

| HIV Sero Status(711) | | | | | | | | | |
|---|---|---|---|---|---|---|---|---|---|
| HIV Positive | 158 (22.2) | 106 (67.1) | 52 (32.9) | 0.48 | 0.33-0.72 | 0.05 | 0.43 | 0.28-0.65 | <0.001 |
| HIV Negative | 553 (77.8) | 447 (80.8) | 106 (19.2) | 1 | ------ | ----- | 1 | ------ | --- |
| **Patient Category** | | | | | | | | | |
| New | 808 | 645 (79.8) | 163 (20.2) | 2.06 | 1.34-3.18 | 0.001 | 2.17 | 1.32-3.57 | 0.002 |
| Retreated | 108 | 71 (65.7) | 37 (34.3) | 1 | ------ | ------ | 1 | ----- | ---- |
| **Age Group (years)** | | | | | | | | | |
| 0-14 | 101 (11.0) | 91 (90.1) | 10 (9.9) | 4.55 | 1.79-11.56 | 0.02 | 4.99 | 1.75-14.27 | 0.003 |
| 15-24 | 296 (32.3) | 229 (77.4) | 67 (22.6) | 1.71 | 0.83- 3.51 | 0.14 | 1.95 | 0.87-4.36 | 0.1 |
| 25-34 | 253 (27.6) | 196 (77.5) | 57 (22.5) | 1.72 | 0.83-3.56 | 0.14 | 2.52 | 1.10-8.91 | 0.029 |
| 35-44 | 124 (13.5) | 99 (79.8) | 25 (20.2) | 1.98 | 0.89-4.40 | 0.09 | 3.5 | 1.37-8.91 | 0.009 |
| 45-54 | 64 (7.0) | 50 (78.1) | 14 (21.9) | 1.79 | 0.73-4.35 | 0.2 | 2.22 | 0.81-6.06 | 0.121 |
| 55-64 | 39 (4.3) | 25 (64.1) | 14 (35.9) | 0.89 | 0.35-2.27 | 0.81 | 0.92 | 0.31-2.73 | 0.881 |
| ≥ 65 | 39 (4.3) | 26 (66.7) | 13 (33.3) | 1 | ---- | ---- | 1 | ---- | ---- |

**Table 4:** Crude and Adjusted odds ratios for various factors that might affect treatment outcomes among tuberculosis patients, Bale Robe Hospital, September 2007-August 2012, N=916, TB=Tuberculosis, OR=Odds Ratio, CI=Confidence Interval, N=Number, *=All the variables in the table are included in the model.

Of the total 916 registered patients in the cohort, 834 (91%) survived, while 82(9%) were died in the entire follow-up period. In this study, the proportion of death from pulmonary negatives, pulmonary positives and extra pulmonary TB patients were 13.1 %, 6.7 and 5.6%, respectively.

Participants' HIV sero-status, tuberculosis type, and age, were significantly associated with patients' death (p<0.05). In multivariate logistic regression older ones (age ≥ 65) were more likely to die than the younger groups (AOR=5.50, CI=1.21-25.01). HIV positive tuberculosis patients were four times more likely to die than HIV negative TB patients (AOR=4.32, CI=2.45-7.64). In addition, smear negative pulmonary tuberculosis patients were two times more likely to die than smear positive and extra pulmonary tuberculosis patients (AOR=2.56, CI=1.44-4.55, AOR=2.00, CI=1.05-3.84) Table 5.

| Characteristics | Death Status | | Crude OR | 95% CI | P-Value | Adjusted OR * | 95% CI | P-Value |
|---|---|---|---|---|---|---|---|---|
| | Alive N (%) | Died N (%) | | | | | | |
| **HIV Status** | | | | | | | | |
| HIV Positive | 127 (80.4) | 31 (19.6) | 3.85 | 2.27-6.52 | 0 | 4.32 | 2.45-7.64 | <0.001 |
| HIV Negative | 520 (94.4) | 33 (6.0) | 1 | ---- | --- | 1 | | |
| **TB Types** | | | | | | | | |
| SPPTB | 222 (93.3) | 16 (6.7) | 1.22 | 0.60-2.47 | 0.58 | 1.17 | 0.52-2.57 | 0.72 |
| SNPTB | 324 (86.9) | 49 (13.1) | 2.56 | 1.44-4.55 | 0 | 2 | 1.05-3.84 | 0.05 |
| EPTB | 288 (94.4) | 17 (5.6) | 1 | ------- | --- | 1 | --- | ---- |
| **Age Group (years)** | | | | | | | | |
| ≤ 14 | 97 (96) | 4 (4.0) | 1 | ---- | ----- | 1 | --- | -- |
| 15-24 | 277 (93.6) | 19 (6.4) | 1.66 | 0.55-5.01 | 0.36 | 2.04 | 0.56-7.39 | 0.28 |
| 25-34 | 232 (91.7) | 21 (8.3) | 2.2 | 0.73-6.56 | 0.59 | 1.5 | 0.41-5.54 | 0.55 |
| 35-44 | 110 (88.2) | 14 (11.3) | 3.09 | 0.98-9.70 | 0.05 | 1.31 | 0.32-5.35 | 0.71 |

| 45-54 | 54 (84.4) | 10 (15.5) | 4.5 | 1.34-15.00 | 0.01 | 3.53 | 0.86-14.50 | 0.08 |
| 55-64 | 32 (82.1) | 7 (17.9) | 1.46 | 1,46-19.31 | 0.01 | 4.5 | 0.95-21.28 | 0.06 |
| ≥65 | 32 (82.1) | 7 (17.9) | 1.46 | 1,46-19.31 | 0.01 | 5.5 | 1.21-25.01 | 0.03 |

**Table 5:** Crude and Adjusted odds ratios for various factors that might affect, Death rate among tuberculosis patients, Bale Robe Hospital, 2007-2012, N=916, TB=Tuberculosis, OR=Odds Ratio, CI=Confidence Interval, N=Number, AOR= adjusted OR. * =All variables showed significant association in the bivariate analysis are included in the model.

## Discussion

According to the WHO 2013 report on global tuberculosis control [2], the treatment success rates under the DOTS programs among 22 high-burden countries (HBCs) varied from 65% in Russian Federation to 95% in China, with an average of 88%. In the same year, the global treatment success rate was 87% among all new TB cases. Of the 22 HBCs, 15 reached or exceeded a treatment success rate of 85% among all new cases in 2011, including Ethiopia, following a major improvement from 77% in 2010 to 89% in 2011 [2].

In agreement with previous study conducted in Gonder, Ethiopia [15] and in Italy [22], in this study, larger proportion of male patients (59.6%) than female patients (40.4%) and lower proportion of patients older than 55 years of age (8.6%), registered for TB treatment, but this finding is in contrary to a study done by Beza in the same region [16].

More than half (59.9%) of the study participants were concentrated between the age group of 15-34 years, which is believed to be the productive segment of the society. This is in agreement with a study done in South Ethiopia [9] and Addis Ababa [13].This indicates the negative impact of TB on the socio-economic condition of the society.

Studies conducted in different parts of Ethiopia documented different rate of treatment success rates ranging from 29.5% in Gondar, North west Ethiopia [15], to 89.2% in Tigray, Northern Ethiopia [17]. In our study, the overall treatment success rate was 78.2% among a cohort of tuberculosis patients registered for DOTs in Bale Robe Hospital between 2007 to 2012, which is lower than the NTLCP and WHO target of 85%.In our study treatment success rate among all new TB patients was found to be 78.9%. Treatment success rate of 78.2% of the study is in agreement with the previous study conducted in South Ethiopia [9] and much better than that of a study conducted in Gondar which is 29% [15], in Gambella 63.4% [23], and in South Ethiopia 73% [8], low income areas of Italy 56.5% [22] and Europe 74.4% [24]. However, TSR of 78.2% is slightly lower than most studies done in different parts of Ethiopia which is ranging from 80.5% in Gonder [7] to 89.2% in Tigray Region [17].

In agreement with several local studies, being female, younger in age and HIV-negative TB patients more likely result in good treatment outcome than their counter part [7-9,11,15,17,25,26]

In the present study, HIV sero-status of 711 (77.6%) of study participants was determined, out of which 158 (22.2%) of were found to be HIV sero-positive. Treatment outcomes are worse among HIV-positive TB patients compared with HIV-negative TB patients. In2011, the TSR for all new HIV-positive TB patients was 73% compared with 87% among HIV negative TB patients (2). In this study, treatment success rate among HIV negative TB patients was 80.8 % compared with 67.1% among HIV positive ones.

In the current study, from the total of 200 (21.8%) TB patients with a poor treatment outcome, the largest proportion (41%) was caused by death followed by defaulters (27.5%) and transferred out (27%). The overall death rates of TB patients in this study was found to be 82 (9%), which is greater than 3.3 % in Northwest Ethiopia [25], 3.7% in a study done in Addis Ababa [12], 3.6% in Gambella [20] and 2.6% in Southern Ethiopia [8] but slightly lower than a study conducted in Gondar University Hospital [15] with death rate of 10.1%.

It is evident that, as the age of the study subjects advanced, the death rate of patients was steadily increased from 4% in the age group of ≤ 14 years to 17.9% in the age group of ≥ 55 years (Table 2). This is in agreement with the finding of a study done in Gonder and Addis Ababa [13,15]. Older age ≥ 65 years has been found to be an independent factor to determine death, due to increasing co morbidities as well as the general immunological deterioration with age [15],

In agreement with previous studies done in different part of the world, in the present study, older ages, smear negative [12,15] and HIV positive [7,10] pulmonary TB patients were more likely to die than their counter parts.

## Conclusion

Being female, younger age and HIV negative were predictor variables for treatment success of TB patients. Although the treatment success rate is fairly good, a high proportion of patients death (9%) and 22.2% of HIV prevalence among TB patients is a serious public health concern that needs to be addressed urgently in the area.

## Authors Contribution

BT: Conceived, designed the project and collected the data, and reviewed the manuscript.

ET: Developed the proposal, analyzed, interpreted the data and prepared the manuscript for publication.

Begna T: Designed the project, collected the data and reviewed the manuscript. All of these authors provided critical comments for revision and approved the final version of the manuscript.

GA: Developed the proposal, analyzed, interpreted the data and prepared the manuscript for publication.

## Acknowledgement

We are very grateful for the TB clinic staff of the study site, and Addis Ababa University for financial support.

# References

1.  Woldeyohannes D, Kebede N, Erku W, Tadesse Z (2011) Ten years' experience of directly observed treatment short-course (dots) therapy for tuberculosis in Addis Ababa, Ethiopia. Ethiop Med J 49: 221-229.

2.  WHO: Global tuberculosis report 2013. WHO Report 2013 Geneva 2013.

3.  FMOH: Guidelines for Clinical and Programmatic Management of TB, TB/HIV and Leprosy In Ethiopia, Addis Ababa, Ethiopia 2013.

4.  Tiemersma EW (2011) Natural history of tuberculosis: Duration and fatality of pulmonary tuberculosis in HIV negative patients: A systematic review. PLoS ONE 6.

5.  Robert M, Jasmer CBS, Leah C Gonzalez, L Masae Kawamura, Dennis H Osmond, et al. (2004) Tuberculosis treatment outcomes directly observed therapy compared with self-administered therapy. Am J Respir Crit Care Med 170: 6.

6.  Faustini A, Hall AJ, Perucci CA (2005) Tuberculosis treatment outcomes in Europe: A systematic review. Eur Respir J 26: 503-510.

7.  Zelalem Addis WB, Alemu A, Mulu A, Ayal G, Negash H (2013) Treatment outcome of tuberculosis patients in Azezo Health Center, North West Ethiopia. Int J Biomed Adv Res 4: 7.

8.  Shargie EB, Lindtjorn B (2005) DOTS improves treatment outcomes and service coverage for tuberculosis in South Ethiopia: A retrospective trend analysis. BMC Public Health 5: 62.

9.  Munoz-Sellart M, Cuevas LE, Tumato M, Merid Y, Yassin MA (2010) Factors associated with poor tuberculosis treatment outcome in the Southern Region of Ethiopia. Int J Tuberc Lung Dis 14: 973-979.

10. Sileshi Balewgizie ND, Belaineh Girma, Muluken Melese, Pedro Suarez (2013) Predictors of mortality among TB-HIV Co-infected patients being treated for tuberculosis in Northwest Ethiopia: A retrospective cohort study. BMC Infect Dis 13: 10.

11. Nigatu T, Abraha M (2010) Epidemiological analysis of tuberculosis trends in Ethiopia: 2000-2009. Tuberk Toraks 58: 375-384.

12. Getahun B, Ameni G, Biadgilign S, Medhin G (2011) Mortality and associated risk factors in a cohort of tuberculosis patients treated under DOTS programme in Addis Ababa, Ethiopia. BMC Infect Dis 11: 127.

13. Getahun B, Ameni G, Medhin G, Biadgilign S (2013) Treatment outcome of tuberculosis patients under directly observed treatment in Addis Ababa, Ethiopia. Braz J Infect Dis 17: 521-528.

14. Datiko DG, Lindtjorn B (2009) Tuberculosis recurrence in smear-positive patients cured under DOTS in southern Ethiopia: Retrospective cohort study. BMC PUBLIC health 9: 348.

15. Tessema B, Muche A, Bekele A, Reissig D, Emmrich F, et al. (2009) Treatment outcome of tuberculosis patients at Gondar University Teaching Hospital, Northwest Ethiopia. A five year retrospective study. BMC Public Health 9: 371.

16. Beza MGMTW, Teferi MD, Getahun YS, Bogale SM, Tefera ASB (2013) Five years tuberculosis treatment outcome at Kolla Diba Health Center, Dembia District, Northwest Ethiopia: A retrospective cross-sectional analysis. J Infect Dis Ther 1: 6.

17. Berhe G, Enquselassie F, Aseffa A (2012) Treatment outcome of smear-positive pulmonary tuberculosis patients in Tigray region, Northern Ethiopia. BMC Public Health 12: 537.

18. Munoz-Sellart M, Yassin MA, Tumato M, Merid Y, Cuevas LE (2009) Treatment outcome in children with tuberculosis in southern Ethiopia. Scand J Infect Dis 41: 450-455.

19. Nigatu T, Abraha M (2010) Epidemiological analysis of tuberculosis trends in Ethiopia: 2000-2009. Tuberk Toraks 58: 375-384.

20. Demeke D, Legesse M, Bati J (2013) Trend of tuberculosis and treatment outcomes in Gambella region with special emphasize on Gambella Regional Hospital, Western Ethiopia. J Mycobac Dis 3: 8.

21. FMOH: Tuberculosis, Leprosy and TB/HIV prevention and Control program manual. Manual 2008, 4th ed.

22. Baussano I, Pivetta E, Vizzini L, Abbona F, Bugiani M (2008) Predicting tuberculosis treatment outcome in a low-incidence area. Int J Tuberc Lung Dis 12: 1441-1448.

23. Demeke D, Legesse M, Bati J (2013) Trend of tuberculosis and treatment outcomes in Gambella region with special emphasize on Gambella Regional Hospital, Western Ethiopia. J Mycobac Dis 3: 1-8.

24. Faustini A, Hall AJ, Perucci CA (2005) Tuberculosis treatment outcomes in Europe: A systematic review. Eur Respir J 26: 503-510.

25. Beza MG WM, Teferi MD, Getahun YS, Bogale SM, et al. (2013) A five years tuberculosis treatment outcome at Kolla Diba Health Center, Dembia District, Northwest Ethiopia: A retrospective cross-sectional analysis. Infect Dis Ther 1: 6.

26. Demeke D LM, Bati J (2013) Trend of tuberculosis and treatment outcomes in Gambella region with special emphasize on Gambella Regional Hospital, Western Ethiopia. J Mycobac Dis 3.

# 31

# Usefulness of Nursing Documentations in Multi-Professional Collaboration and Information Exchange in Finland

**Anne Kuusisto[1], Pirkko Nykänen[2] and Johanna Kaipio[3]**

[1]*Satakunta Hospital District, 28500 Pori, Finland*

[2]*University of Tampere, School of Information Sciences, 33014 Tampere, Finland*

[3]*Aalto University, School of Science, 00076 Aalto, Finland*

\*Corresponding author: Anne Kuusisto, Satakunta Hospital District, 28500 Pori, Finland, E-mail: anne.kuusisto@satshp.fi

## Abstract

**Background:** Efficient collaboration and information exchange among care givers is essential during patient's hospital period for the high quality and safety of patient care. Nursing documentation plays important role in effective collaboration and information exchange. One prerequisite for efficient and productive multidisciplinary collaboration is the nursing documentation when it is in appropriate format and easily accessible. In Finland, nursing documents are produced, stored and represented with a nursing documentation system (NDS), which is part of an electronic health record (EHR). The nursing model applied in this study is based on a nursing process, a nationally defined nursing core data set and the Finnish Care Classification (FinCC).

**Research design and method:** This study is a part of the research where we evaluated the feasibility and usability of the structured nursing documentation model and four widely used NDSs. One perspective in evaluation was the study of the usefulness of the nursing model and NDSs in multi-professional collaboration and information exchange. The materials were collected with thematic interviews with seven physicians and 20 nurses in spring 2010 in the clinical contexts of primary, specialized and private health care.

**Results:** Nursing documentation model and NDSs supported poorly electronic multi-professional care and information exchange. Physicians found nursing documentations difficult to access and to understand. Information was documented as small, separate items and thus a comprehensive picture of the patient's situation was not present. Collaborative care aspects were either not supported. The nursing model used could not be utilized by the physicians and NDSs did not take into account the needs of the physicians who require information on patient care provided by nurses.

**Conclusion:** Experiences from our study can be used by other hospitals, care givers and countries for better design of nursing documentation. In the future, better utilization of information requires that the nursing documentation model and NDSs are designed to support not just documentation but also information exchange and multi-professional collaboration.

**Keywords:** Nursing documentation; Nursing documentation system; Multi-professional communication; Multi-professional collaboration

## Introduction

Health information exchange and collaboration between nurses and physicians is essential to improve patient care and an important priority among usability requirements. Efficient information exchange and collaboration among care givers during patient's hospital period is an important goal for the high quality and safety of patient care [1]. One effort to increase interdisciplinary communication and information exchange among care providers is to standardize the data content of the electronic health record (EHR) for achieving semantic interoperability between different health information systems [2,3]. Terminologies are used to structure data content in the records, i.e. classifications, vocabularies, nomenclatures or codes [4].

Also nursing documentation and production of patient care plan in EHR are moving towards standardization. The most common model to structure the nursing notes in EHRs in European countries is the nursing process model [5]. There are several products such as NANDA-I [2], Nursing Intervention Classification (NIC) [2], Nursing Outcome Classification (NOC) [2], VIPS model [4,6] and Clinical Care Classification (CCC) [7] for standardizing nursing language in the care plan activity [4]. When using standardized nomenclatures, the nurses are no longer able to document care problems, goals (expected outcomes) and interventions only by entering free text data. However, the records do include a free text description field where a user can individualize the patient care plan based on his or her particular needs [2].

Different health care professional groups have their own roles, needs and professional responsibilities. For example the role of nurses is to care and that of a physicians is to cure [8]. Professionals need to communicate effectively with each other in the workplace. Multi-professional collaboration in the health care between nurses and physicians requires that nursing documentations support communication and fluent information exchange. Physicians' and nurses' perspectives in health care terminologies differ [6] and currently, no multi-professional terminology for practical health care use exists [4,6] despite of the global efforts to develop unifying multi-professional terminologies [6].

Usability of a nursing classification system and a NDS is paramount for the continuous documentation of task effectively, efficiently and fluently [9]. Multi-professional collaboration in health care between nurses, physicians and other health professionals requires that the tools and systems, including EHRs and NDSs, support work flows, communication and information exchange. The systems should enable collaborative care and division of work between health professionals. For example Green and Thomas [10] found that physicians saw detailed assessments and well-described interventions of nurses' as essential to their ability to effectively practice medicine. Also Klehr et al. [2] perceived after implementation of the standardized nomenclature in EHR that at worst both nurses and physicians have rejected reading nursing care plans when the nomenclature did not completely meet the hospitalized patient's care plan needs.

In Finland, nursing documents are produced, stored and represented using a NDS which is part of an EHR system. The often applied nursing model is the national Finnish model of standardized documentation. It is based on a nursing process, a nationally defined nursing core data set and the Finnish Care Classification (FinCC) [11]. FinCC is based on Clinical Care Classification (CCC) [7].

The FinCC consists of the Finnish classification of nursing diagnoses (FiCND), the Finnish classification of nursing interventions (FiCNI) and the Finnish classification of nursing outcomes (FiCNO). FiCND and FiCNI have similar hierarchical structures (component, main category and sub-category levels). The component level is the most abstract. The most concrete main categories and sub-categories of the FiCND and FiCNI have been aggregated under the components, and they are actually used in nursing documentation. In version 3.0 of the FinCC, both FiCND and FiCNI have 17 components. The number of main categories and sub-categories under each component varies. FiCND has 88 main categories and 150 subcategories, while FiCNI has 127 main categories and 180 sub-categories. In all, there are 215 main categories and 330 sub-categories, totalling 545. [12]

The nursing model covers four phases of the nursing process: (1) data collection and needs assessment, (2) nursing diagnosis and setting nursing care aims, (3) planning and delivering the nursing interventions and (4) evaluation of the outcomes. Nursing diagnoses are documented using the FiCND, the planned and delivered nursing interventions are documented with the FiCNI. The outcomes are documented using the care components of the FiCNO [11]. The NDS offers the user an interface for the nursing care process phases and the nursing classification. The flexibility and usability of the NDSs are dependent on the nursing process model, the nursing classification and the EHR and its implemented functionalities.

The national Finnish model of standardized documentation is widely used in Finland, although it is not normative like the Austrian model where legal requirement to document nursing diagnoses may have stimulated the use of standardized terminologies for nursing diagnoses and the implementation of NDSs [13]. An important objective for implementation of the national nursing model in NDSs has been to enable multi-professional collaborative work and information exchange between health professionals. One motivation for this evaluation study was that its usefulness for interdisciplinary collaboration had been questioned. Internationally interdisciplinary collaboration via electronic medical record has been studied [10]. But

study findings about usefulness of nursing documentations in multi-professional collaboration do not exist.

## Materials and Methods

This study is part of the research where we evaluated the feasibility and usability of the structured nursing documentation model and four widely used NDSs in Finland. Research and its findings have been published [14-18], but earlier publications do not cover this particular point of view which is the focus of this paper. In this paper we report the results of evaluating the usefulness of the nursing model and NDSs in multi-professional collaboration and information exchange. The study was carried out in spring 2010 in the clinical contexts of primary, specialized and private health care. The materials were collected with thematic interviews with seven physicians in five health care organization (2 in public specialized care, 2 in public primary care and one from a private hospital) and 20 nurses (10 nurses from public specialized care, seven from public primary care and, three from a private hospital). Thematic interviews covered the following issues: Participation in education and training to use the national nursing model and nursing documentation systems, utilization of the documents from the nursing documentation system, the nursing documentation model, problems in nursing documentation and differences between nurses' and physicians' documentation practices.

## Results

The results show that nursing documentation model and NDSs supported poorly the multi-professional care and information exchange. The physicians' opinions on the nursing documentations were very suspicious and negative. In three health care organizations the five physicians did not read the nursing documentations and did not consider them useful. Physicians found nursing documentations difficult to access and to understand. Information was documented as small, separate items, following the FinCC classification and thus a comprehensive picture of the patient's situation was not present. The physicians would prefer to have a more holistic view of the patient's nursing care. This was not possible because the information had been documented using a very detailed and multi-layered nursing classification.

Collaborative care aspects were either not supported. The nursing model and NDSs did not take into account the needs of the physicians requiring information on patient care provided by nurses. Physicians primarily require a broad, overall view of the patient's condition and status, in particular they want to see that changes in the patient's status are clearly presented. When information is presented in many layers and divided into small pieces, it is not easy for the physician to utilize the documentation. Additionally, the physicians considered that the layering of the documentation was not logical from the care perspective. The physicians had also difficulties in accessing nursing documentations from NDSs and they had troubles in understanding the information because it was documented and presented in a very complex and detailed manner, following the FinCC classification. However, there were two situations where the information exchange was found successful: Home care services and in a community health centres. There physicians even made treatment decisions based on the nurses' documentation and utilized the information while preparing the discharge summaries. In a health centre one physician regularly red the nursing documentations and assessed them useful and important for her own work. In the case of home care services, the patients are at home and the nurses go there to see them and report the status and condition of the patient to the physician through the NDS after returning back to their offices. The nurses interviewed agreed with the physicians about information exchange and support for collaborative care.

## Conclusion

We evaluated the usefulness of the nursing documentation model and NDSs in multi-professional collaboration and information exchange. Efficient collaboration and information exchange among care givers is essential during patient´s hospital period. Nursing documentation has an important role in this process. We concluded that the FinCC nursing documentation model used could not be utilized by the physicians and the studied, widely used NDSs did not support collaboration and information exchange between the nurses and the physicians effectively. To our knowledge this kind of research has not been carried out elsewhere. Hence these experiences are valuable and could be used by other hospitals, care givers and countries for better design of nursing documentation.

In the future, better utilization of information requires that both the nursing documentation model and NDSs are designed and implemented to support not just documentation but also information exchange and utilization. The needs of nurses and other relevant health professionals should be taken into account in the system design. The applied models and terminologies should enable nursing information representation in such a way that information is useful for the nurses and also for the physicians and even for the patients. This requires that the classifications should be generic and reflect the work flows and processes of the patient care. Our results underline like [6] the need for sufficient coverage and level of nursing content to support different professional perspectives in health care terminologies. The principle guideline for the development work should be to guarantee secure continuity of patient care, which necessitates efficient information exchange both intradisciplinary among nurses and also interdisciplinary between various professional groups. So each of the professional group of internal, but also interprofessional communication needs should be taken into account in development work [4].

## Acknowledgement

We acknowledge the funding of this research by the Finnish Work Environment Fund and by Ministry for Social Affairs and Health.

## References

1. Joint Commission 2013. Available at: http://www.jointcommission.org/assets/1/18/NPSG_Chapter_Jan2013_HAP.pdf. Accessed 29.7.2013

2. Klehr J, Hafner J, Spelz LM, Steen S, Weaver K (2009) Implementation of standardized nomenclature in the electronic medical record. Int J Nurs Terminol Classif 20: 169-180.

3. Collins SA, Stein DM, Vawdrey DK, Stetson PD, Bakken S (2011) Content overlap in nurse and physician handoff artifacts and the potential role of electronic health records: a systematic review. J Biomed Inform 44: 704-712.

4. Häyrinen K, Saranto K, Nykänen P (2008) Definition, structure, content, use and impacts of electronic health records: a review of the research literature. Int J Med Inform 77: 291-304.

5. Thoroddsen A, Saranto K, Ehrenberg A, Sermeus W (2009) Models, standards and structures of nursing documentation in European countries. Stud Health Technol Inform 146: 327-331.

6. Florin J, Ehrenberg A, Ehnfors M, Björvell C (2013) A comparison between the VIPS model and the ICF for expressing nursing content in the health care record. Int J Med Inform 82: 108-117.

7. Saba VK (2013) Clinical Care Classification System. Available at: http://www.sabacare.com Accessed 1.8.2013

8. McKay KA, Narasimham S (2012) Bridging the gap between doctors and nurses. Journal of Nursing Education and Practice 2: 52-55.

9. Ala-Hiiro T, Lemmetty K, Pitkänen S, Häyrinen E (2010) Adopting the national structure of nursing documentation is consequential in the development of care. Stud Health Technol Inform 160: 421-423.

10. Green SD, Thomas JD (2008) Interdisciplinary collaboration and the electronic medical record. Pediatr Nurs 34: 225-227, 240.

11. Häyrinen K, Lammintakanen J, Saranto K (2010) Evaluation of electronic nursing documentation--nursing process model and standardized terminologies as keys to visible and transparent nursing. Int J Med Inform 79: 554-564.

12. Liljamo P, Kinnunen UM, Ensio A (2012) FinCC classification system, user's guide. FiCND 3.0, FiCNI 3.0, FiCNO 1.0. National Institute for Health and welfare (THL). Classifications, terminologies and statistic guidelines 2/2012. 85 pages. Helsinki.

13. Hübner U, Ammenwerth E, Flemming D, Schaubmayr C, Sellemann B (2010) IT adoption of clinical information systems in Austrian and German hospitals: results of a comparative survey with a focus on nursing. BMC Med Inform Decis Mak 10: 8.

14. Viitanen J, Nykänen P, Kuusisto A (2011) Usability in the nursing context - Considerations on the methodological approach. Proc. of 5th Human Factors Engineering in Health Informatics Symposium, pp. 183-188. August 26-27, 2011. Trondheim, Norway.

15. Viitanen J, Nykänen P, Kuusisto A (2011) Evaluation of the usability of electronic nursing documentation systems (ENDs). International Hospital, vol. 37, May/June 2011, pp. 8-9.

16. Viitanen J, Kuusisto A, Nykänen P (2011) Usability of electronic nursing record systems: definition and results from an evaluation study in Finland. Stud Health Technol Inform 164: 333-338

17. Kuusisto A, Kaipio J, Nykänen P (2012) The national nursing documentation model from the nursing practice perspective – Results from a Finnish evaluation study. NI2012: 11th International Congress on Nursing Informatics, AMIA Proceedings 2012, pp. 233-237.

18. Nykänen P, Kaipio J, Kuusisto A (2012) Evaluation of the national nursing model and four nursing documentation systems in Finland -- Lessons learned and directions for the future. Int J Med Inform 81: 507-520.

# 32

# Using Clinical Microsystems to Implement Care Coordination in Primary Care

Daren Anderson*, Khushbu Khatri and Mary Blankson

*Weitzman Institute, Community Health Center, Inc. Middletown, CT, USA*

*Corresponding author: Daren Anderson, VP/Chief Quality Officer, Community Health Center, Inc., Director, Weitzman Institute, Associate Professor of Medicine, Quinnipiac University, 631 Main St, Middletown, CT 06457, E-mail: daren@chc1.com

## Abstract

**Objective:** Care coordination is a core competency for primary care nurses and an essential element of the Patient Centered Medical Home (PCMH) model. Implementing care coordination in primary care is challenging and requires changes in roles, staffing, and culture. Clinical Microsystems are frontline teams of healthcare staff that, when engaged in quality improvement, can make important contributions towards practice redesign. We used a Microsystem team to develop an effective model to integrate nurse care coordinators into a busy primary care center.

**Methods:** A Clinical Microsystem team, supported by an improvement coach, met weekly for one year to develop and test a new nurse staffing model in a large Federally Qualified Health Center. Intervention uptake and impact on workflow was tracked by direct observation of nurses and by measuring volume of nursing visits and virtual contacts. Nurses in a non-participating site with similar characteristics served as a comparison group.

**Results:** The Microsystem team developed and implemented a new nurse care coordination model for their site. The intervention emphasized patient self-management, independent nursing visits, and hospital and emergency room transition support. The nurse care coordinator in this new role managed 335 patients over a nine-month study period. The nurse in this new role spent 276 minutes over two days of observation engaged in direct care coordination work while two nurses at the comparison site spent only 94 minutes and 149 minutes, respectively, over the same time period.

**Conclusion:** Engaging front line staff is an effective way for organizations to make changes in delivery systems, improve quality and spread innovations. In this study, a Microsystem team developed a model to provide key components of care coordination to support PCMH practice redesign at a large community health center.

**Keywords** Clinical microsystems; Primary care; Quality improvement; Medical home; Care coordination

## Background

Primary care is at the forefront of efforts to reform the healthcare system in America, and the Patient-Centered Medical Home (PCMH) model of primary care is a promising example of such reform [1]. One of the objectives of the PCMH is to reduce the potentially negative effects of the fragmentation of the health system on patients and their families, especially for those with chronic or complex health conditions who are at high risk for adverse outcomes associated with complications of their conditions [2-5]. To that end, care coordination is one of the core functions of the PCMH [2]. Care coordination is defined broadly as "the deliberate organization of patient care activities between two or more participants involved in a patient's care to facilitate the appropriate delivery of health care services" [4]. Care coordination can improve patient health outcomes, reduce hospitalizations and readmissions, and can lower overall costs [5-14].

Providing effective care coordination poses significant challenges. The current healthcare system is disjointed, with multiple sources of care and inadequate exchange of patient information between primary care providers (PCPs) and specialists [15]. A typical PCP may share patient care with over 200 other medical providers with whom care must be coordinated [16]. Few primary care practices have developed standardized approaches to coordinating care. Recent surveys suggest that fewer than 3% of small to medium sized primary care practices use care managers [17], and only 46% of larger practices coordinate care for patients with chronic illnesses [18]. Part of the challenge has been financial, as most care coordination activities are not reimbursable in traditional fee-for-service models.

Primary care nurses are ideally suited to provide care coordination. The American Nurses Association states that "patient-centered care coordination is a core professional standard and competency for all nursing practice" [19]. Furthermore, the Institute of Medicine, in its report on the future of nursing, noted the need for an effective, well-trained nursing staff that practices to the full extent of their education and training [20]. Unfortunately, the role of the primary care nurse has not been well defined.

Efforts to implement a nurse-driven care coordination model face several challenges. First, care coordination remains a poorly defined concept with few models to guide the integration of these services into the primary care staffing model of most health centers. In addition, adopting elements of the PCMH model such as care coordination requires substantial system redesign work and represents a significant change in workplace culture [21].

Clinical Microsystems is a quality improvement methodology emphasizing the engagement of frontline staff to design, test and implement changes in their work environment [22]. A microsystem is a team of healthcare staff who regularly work together to provide care to patients. Such frontline teams, when supported by a trained improvement coach, can play an important role improving the quality of care [23-26]. The Clinical Microsystem approach has resulted in improvements in a wide range of areas including hypertension control [27], cystic fibrosis [28], and perinatal care. With its emphasis on frontline staff engagement and coaching for effective process improvement, this model may be a useful approach to help practices implement the PCMH [29].

As part of an effort to improve the coordination of care and overall health outcomes for complex patients in a large, multi-site Federally Qualified Health Center (FQHC) we conducted a collaborative quality improvement initiative using Clinical Microsystems to design and implement a nurse-led care coordination model. In a previous study, we demonstrated that despite a well-functioning team of PCPs, nurses, and medical assistants, primary care nurses were only able to devote a small amount of each day (15%) to engage in care coordination work. Most of their time was spent on other nursing tasks such as vaccination and medication administration, triage, and paperwork [30]. The goal of this project was to develop a new model that would allow nurses to devote more time and effort to coordination care and improving outcomes for the most complex patients in the practice. In this paper, we describe the quality improvement approach and the care coordination model that was developed.

## Methods

### Setting

Community Health Center, Inc. (CHCI) is a multi-site FQHC located in Connecticut. CHCI provides comprehensive primary care services in 12 primary care health centers across the state and over 200 additional sites of care including school-based clinics, homeless shelters, and mobile outreach sites. CHCI cares for over 140,000 medically underserved patients. Over 68% are racial/ethnic minorities; over 90% are below 200% of the federal poverty level; 70% have state Medicaid insurance, and 22% are uninsured. Primary care at CHCI is provided by a team of healthcare professionals that includes PCPs, medical assistants (MAs), registered nurses (RNs) and behavioral health providers. PCPs include family practice, pediatric or internal medicine physicians, adult, pediatric or family nurse practitioners, and physician assistants. This study was reviewed and approved by the Institution Review Board of the Community Health Center, Inc.

### Clinical microsystems

In 2011 CHCI began using the Clinical Microsystems quality improvement methodology [22,24-26,31-34] as part of an agency-wide effort to improve the quality of patient care and empower frontline staff to play an active role in systems redesign. A Clinical Microsystem is a team whose members work together on a regular basis providing clinical care or other services and have been provided with appropriate training, support, and guidance to work together to improve performance. Microsystems generate new ideas and serve as early adopters of new processes and approaches to patient care. Microsystems provide front line staff opportunities to take ownership of process changes and improvement work at their individual practice location. As part of this initiative, Microsystem teams were recruited

and trained across the agency and provided with an improvement coach and a regular time to meet. Each team was expected to identify areas for improvement in their local site, conduct tests of change, and report regularly on their progress to members of the senior leadership team.

Microsystem teams follow the Clinical Microsystems Improvement Ramp for all improvement projects (Figure 1). The Improvement Ramp provides a structured approach that emphasizes careful review and evaluation of data, global and specific goal setting, measurement of outcomes, and the use of rapid cycle tests of change, Plan Do Study Act (PDSA) cycles, to test and refine new ideas for improvement. All teams start at the bottom of the ramp with a comprehensive analysis of their site's performance and characteristics, which is referred to as the 5P's. The 5P's stand for Purpose, Providers, Patients, Patterns and Processes. The 5P analysis provides teams a structure to use to help identify themes and establish global and specific aims to address areas in need of improvement. Teams can establish a wide range of aims focused on improving care for a specific condition, addressing areas of dissatisfaction for patients and staff, improving a specific performance measure, or improving the efficiency of a specific process. Once the aims and measures have been established, teams conduct flow mapping and brainstorming activities to fully evaluate a process and develop a specific intervention to test. PDSA cycles are rapid tests of change that allow teams to implement new, testable ideas on a small scale and learn from the test before implementing a new process on a larger scale. Teams conduct successive PDSA cycles, refining and making modifications until a new process is developed with demonstrable improved results. Use of this schematic helps teams focus and separate larger issues into well-scoped projects that can be effectively measured and managed.

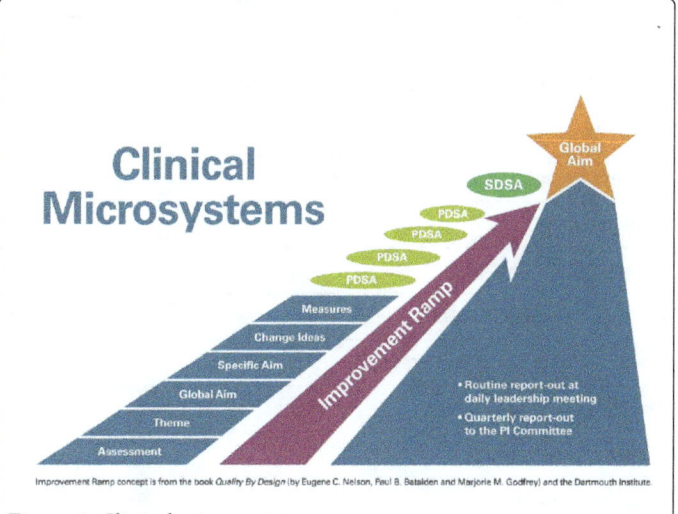

**Figure 1:** Clinical microsystems.

For this project, a Microsystem team based in one of CHCI's largest sites, serving approximately 21,000 patients, analyzed its 5Ps and identified hospital transitions and poorly controlled chronic illnesses as areas in need of improvement. They chose to design a more effective model to allow nurses to devote time to care coordination and improving outcomes for patients with complex medical needs, particularly those transitioning from hospital to home and those with poorly controlled hypertension. The team was granted dedicated time each week during the workday to meet and conduct improvement work under supervision and guidance of a trained improvement coach. The project lasted approximately 12 months.

## Outcome measures

To assess the workload of care coordination and understand the potential patient impact, we tracked the number of patients who had face-to-face visits with the designated nurse care coordinator (RNCC) and the number of patient and patient-related phone calls made by the RNCC. The RNCC documented telephone and non-face-to-face encounters using a "virtual visit" feature in the electronic health record (EHR). "Virtual visits" and face-to-face contact volume was determined through queries of the EHR. Lastly, we directly observed and recorded all activities carried out by nurses following the implementation, noting the total amount of time each nurse dedicated to care coordination tasks versus other types of work. Nurses working in another practice site with similar staff composition, size, and patient demographics that did not implement the new care coordination

model were used as a comparison group. Using a standardized data collection tool and a stopwatch, the evaluator identified each task completed by the nurse; the time spent completing the task, and the type or category of each task. Five broad categories were defined: 1) Team interaction (discussions with on-site care team members); 2) Patient interaction (direct nurse contact with patient in person or by phone); 3) Outside interaction (discussing patient with non-CHCI personnel such as specialists, visiting nurses, or hospitals); 4) Computer/paperwork (documenting patient encounters, form completion, etc.) and 5) Other. Each category contained multiple subcategories to give as much specificity to the task as possible (Table 1). Tasks that could not be classified by the observer were recorded as "other" and reviewed and classified by the research team using a consensus process during the analysis. In total, the research observer shadowed five nurses for two full eight-hour workdays each. All nurses involved in the study signed informed consent to participate.

| Team Interaction | |
|---|---|
| Pre-Huddle prep work[*] | |
| Morning Huddle[*] | |
| Discuss patient with primary care physician[*] | |
| Discuss patient with another nurse[*] | |
| Discuss patient with medical assistant | |
| Discuss patient with pharmacist[*] | |
| Discuss schedule with front desk | |
| Meeting/committee work | |
| Discuss patient with behavioral health clinician/licensed clinical social worker[*] | |
| Other interpersonal interaction (non-patient related) | |
| **Patient Contact** | |
| Vaccines | Spirometry |
| Patient triage at CHC | Suboxone follow up |
| Medical emergency ("Code Blue") | Tobacco cessation counseling[*] |
| Associated or Independent nurse visit | Tuberculin skin test plant or read |
| Blood pressure check[*] | Urine toxicology screen |
| Depo-Provera injection | Urinary tract infection |
| Diabetic foot exam | Unstable patient |
| Ear lavage | Women, Infants and Children (WIC) support |
| Electrocardiogram | Wound care |
| Home blood pressure monitoring[*] | Other |
| International normalized ratio (INR) check | Patient phone call |
| Insulin titration[*] | Complaint |
| Lab results review[*] | Initial visit prep |

| | |
|---|---|
| Lead check | Review Lab results* |
| Medication administration | Medication question |
| Medication reconciliation* | Medication refill needed |
| New-born screening visit | Symptoms |
| Patient education and self-management* | Needs paperwork |
| Peg-Interferon Hepatitis C treatment | Needs appointment |
| Phlebotomy | Pain-related complaint |
| Pregnancy test | Referral question |
| Prescription pick up | Other |
| Retinopathy screening | |
| **Outside Interaction** | |
| Make visiting nurse referral | |
| Discuss patient with visiting nurse* | |
| Make specialty referral | |
| Discuss patient with specialist* | |
| Discuss patient with hospital* | |
| Discuss patient with emergency department* | |
| Discuss patient with school nurse* | |
| Discuss patient with Department of Children and Families* | |
| Pharmacy call | |
| Prior authorization for insurance | |
| Other (patient related) | |
| Other (non-patient related) | |
| **Computer/Paperwork** | |
| Web INR online tracking system | |
| Pediatric lead screening log | |
| Addressing EHR internal messages from other staff | |
| Charting patients' encounters | |
| Pharmacy patient assistance forms | |
| Reportable communicable disease forms | |
| Other patient form completion | |
| Joint Commission work | |
| Department of Children and Families work | |
| Adolescent chart audit | |
| Email/faxing/scanning/letter writing (patient related) | |
| Personal organization (i.e., Human Resource forms, time cards, etc.) | |

| Restock/ organize dispensary |
| --- |

**Table 1:** Nursing activities.

Using a well-established framework for care coordination [35] we classified the following tasks as representing care coordination work: communication amongst care team members or with outside specialists, nurses, and hospitals that related to coordinating a specific patient's care, and direct patient contact via phone or in-person that focused on disease management, self-management, or follow up after a hospitalization or visit to another care provider. Examples of tasks that did not represent a care coordination activity included completing forms and other paperwork, administering vaccinations and medications, and conducting triage.

## Analysis

We used simple statistics to tally and average the time spent completing various tasks by the RNCC, other nurses at the same site, and nurses at the comparison site. Given the small sample size, statistical tests for significance were not performed.

## Results

### Clinical microsystems

The Microsystem team met weekly for the duration of the study. Based on their analysis of baseline data they chose to develop a team based approach focused on coordinating care more efficiently. With the assistance of a coach they developed and refined a new nursing care coordination model by conducting approximately 10 PDSA cycles focused on areas such as workflow, developing a new vaccine administration process, devising a new clerical assistant role, testing a new patient intake process, developing a nursing visit focused on patient self-management, and designing a new process to improve follow-up of patients with recent hospital discharges. The final model divided the nursing staff into two discreet roles RNCC, and a primary care nurse (PCRN).

### Care coordinator role

The job of care coordination was assigned to one designated nurse, the RNCC, who supported eight primary care clinicians. This nurse was given dedicated time each day to coordinate care for specific patients assigned to her. All other routine daily tasks requiring a nursing license, such as administering immunizations and other injections, medications and nebulizer treatments, as well as point of care testing, triage, basic patient education, medical care under standing orders, and telephone follow up, were provided by the PCRNs.

**Specific functions of the RNCC included:** Using data from the EHR to identify complex patients (those with uncontrolled diabetes, hypertension, recent hospital discharge, and frequent emergency rooms visits) who needed additional support, conducting weekly "panel management" team meetings with providers to review and discuss care plans, contacting patients within 48 hours from a hospital discharge to provide transition care support, contacting patients recently discharged from an emergency room, coordinating office follow-up care for complex patients, managing abnormal cancer screening follow up, coordinating care with home health care agencies/ social services, hospital discharge planners, hospitalists and emergency room staff, conducting nursing visits with patients for chronic disease support, medication adherence, medication reconciliation, self-management training and education, supporting group medical visits, and assisting patients to attend scheduled medical visits.

### Care coordinator workload

The RNCC at the intervention site accepted referrals from the patient panels of eight PCPs and over nine months provided care coordination for 335 patients. During this period the RNCC created or responded to 675 virtual visit encounters. Of these patients, 74 had one documented virtual encounter each, 100 patients had 2 to 5 each, 30 patients with 6 to 10 each, 6 patients had greater than 11 encounters and 125 patients did not have virtual visit encounters recorded in the EHR. These virtual visits included patient-related contact with CHCI providers, outside providers, pharmacies, and other supportive services and represent a broad measure of workload for the RNCC. In addition, the RNCC conducted 198 independent nurse visits for 99 unique patients, ranging from one to eleven visits per patient.

### Workflow observation

To gain a better understanding of how much time nurses in different roles devoted to different tasks we observed five nurses, including the RNCC from the intervention site, PCRNs from the intervention site, and two nurses from a matched comparison for site two full workdays each to determine the amount of time they each devoted to care coordination activities. The RNCC at the intervention site spent 276 minutes over two days of observation engaged in direct care coordination work (Table 2), while two nurses at the comparison site spent only 94 minutes and 149 minutes, respectively, over the same time period , engaged in care coordination work. Two PCRNs at the intervention site assigned to routine primary care (non-care coordination) work spent only 87 and 85 minutes over two days engaged in activity classified as care coordination. The increase in care coordination work by the RNCC was largely accounted for by more time spent more time on hospital transition care coordination, medication reconciliation, blood pressure follow up, communication with visiting nurses (VNA), and self-management support. Little or no time was devoted to these activities in the comparison site, despite there being a similar population of patients with high hospitalization rates and high rates of poorly controlled chronic illness.

| | | Comparison RN 1 (min) | Comparison RN 2 (min) | PCRN 1 (min) | PCRN 2 (min) | RNCC (min) |
|---|---|---|---|---|---|---|
| **Team Communication** | Morning huddle | - | 17 | 7 | 9 | 22 |
| | Discuss patient with Primary Care Provider | 6 | 14 | 1 | 9 | 10 |
| | Discuss patient nurse | - | 13 | 1 | 1 | 2 |
| **Direct Patient Care** | Patient education/self-management | 17 | - | - | 4 | - |
| | Blood pressure check | 32 | 34 | - | 20 | 78 |
| | Home blood pressure monitoring | - | - | 4 | - | - |
| | Insulin Titration | 16 | 48 | - | - | - |
| | Lab results review | - | - | 23 | 19 | - |
| | Medication Reconciliation | - | - | 29 | - | 14 |
| **Patient Communication (Telephone)** | Self-Management goal follow up (diabetes) | - | - | - | - | 11 |
| | Hospital discharge follow up | 4 | - | - | - | 44 |
| | Lab results | 6 | 11 | 23 | 19 | 10 |
| | Medication Reconciliation | - | - | - | - | 12 |
| **External Communication** | Discuss patient with Visiting Nurses Association | 11 | 13 | - | - | 50 |
| | Discuss patient with specialist | 2 | - | - | - | 5 |
| | Discuss patient with hospital | - | - | - | 3 | 4 |
| | Discuss patient with emergency department | - | - | - | - | - |
| | Discuss patient with school nurse | - | - | - | - | - |
| | Discuss patient with Dept. of Children and Families | - | - | - | - | 15 |
| Total minutes on CC over two days | | 94 | 149 | 87 | 85 | 276 |

**Table 2:** Time engaged by nurses in care coordination work.

## Discussion

In this study, we used a formal quality improvement process, Clinical Microsystems, to engage front line healthcare staff to redesign their staff roles to improve the coordination of care for complex patients. By following a structured improvement method the team was able to address critical issues and determine how best to integrate care coordination activities into its clinic workflow. The team developed a new allocation of work and task assignments for the nursing team, with a designated nurse to focus on care coordination tasks, and routine nursing tasks assigned to other nurses. The resulting model did not require any additional staff time, funding, or external support.

This new model was based on the conceptual framework of the Chronic Care Model (CCM) [36]. The CCM proposes that improved patient outcomes can be achieved with a prepared, proactive healthcare team working together with an informed, activated patient. The new nursing intervention heavily emphasized proactive planning and coordination of care to ensure that the care team was optimally prepared to meet the needs of the patients. In addition, self-management support was a key part of the RNCC's new role. This team based intervention focused on coordinating care broadly for a wide range of patients rather than a more specific case management-type intervention. The team felt that care coordination was a core function that should be embedded in primary care, while case management was often accomplished by specially trained staff working outside the front line team.

The new model had substantial impact on nursing workflow. Prior to implementation of the model, nurses engaged in care coordination work but those tasks accounted for only about 15% of their total workload [30]. Care coordination tasks were often overshadowed by the need to address more immediate tasks such as triage and vaccine administration. After implementation, PCRNs continued to spend about the same amount of time involved with care coordination activity (14%) while RNCC spent nearly half of her time engaged directly in coordinating care and supporting 335 complex patients over the nine month study period. These results suggest that with dedicated time and focus, a primary care team can carry out all needed nursing tasks while still incorporating essential elements of care coordination into its daily work to provide additional support for complex patients. This support includes critical activities such as reconciling medication, teaching self-management skills, and supporting patients transitioning from a recent hospitalization. Based on the work of this microsystem team, CHCI is now implementing a nursing-based care coordination model across all 12 of its primary care practices.

Improving the ability of primary care practices to meet the needs of complex patients is critical to the success of the PCMH model. The current healthcare system is characterized by disjointed care between primary care, multiple specialists, hospitals, emergency rooms, pharmacies and other sources of care [37]. There are large gaps in the exchange of appropriate patient information between specialists and PCPs [15] and poorly coordinated care amongst multiple care sources leads to inefficiency, reduced quality of care, and errors [38,39].

Healthcare reform efforts are shifting the emphasis to accountable care and value-driven payment models. This shift, combined with incentives to implement the PCMH model, is leading to a growing interest in improving care coordination across the healthcare continuum. However, integrating care coordination into the primary care delivery system is challenging for primary care practices [37] and requires substantial workflow and practice redesign [21]. Many practices struggle to make such significant changes [40]. In this study, we demonstrate how a frontline Microsystem improvement team supported by an improvement coach can tackle these challenges and make fundamental changes in their daily workflow.

Our study has several limitations. The study was observational and not designed to draw statistical comparisons between different nurses with different roles. As a quality improvement project the goal was principally to evaluate the uptake of the intervention and understand how it was impacting nursing work flow. Future studies are underway to capture a wider range of data and longer term patient outcomes to further evaluate the impact of care coordination in primary care.

An additional limitation is the potential inaccuracy in our method for designating specific tasks as representing care coordination. This inaccuracy is partly due to the lack of a formal, widely accepted definition of care coordination. We used a broad definition of the types of tasks that constituted care coordination, based on the framework presented by the Agency for Healthcare Research and Quality [35]. This may have overestimated the amount of time spent truly coordinating care. Additionally, we did not count time spent engaged in documentation and handling messages as part of care coordination. One could argue that such tasks, when related to the care of complex patients; constitute work that should be "counted" as care coordination. Our decision to exclude this work in the definition of care coordination may underestimate the true amount of work spent coordinating care.

Clinical Microsystems represents a powerful tool for practice transformation specifically because it engages frontline staff in the change process. Microsystem teams benefit from the model's formal structure and the support of a trained improvement coach and actively participate in the design, testing, and implementation of new processes. Front line staff provides key insights and take ownership over new processes, and in so doing becoming powerful change agents and ambassadors when spreading these new processes to other locations.

Quality improvement work is often not published in peer-reviewed journals [41]. The quality improvement process is iterative, empiric and often not amenable to controlled designs and structured evaluation. Work such as this however, represents the critical element of practice redesign on the front lines of healthcare reform. Healthcare staff working together to design better ways of caring for patients, following a process such as Clinical Microsystems, is the key to making meaningful, lasting change that is needed to move healthcare care towards a more effective, efficient, and patient-centered system.

## References

1.  Rich E, Lipson D, Libersky J, Parchman M (2012) Coordinating care for adults with complex care needs in the patient-centered medical home: Challenges and solutions. Rockville, MD: Agency for Healthcare Research and Quality.

2.  AHRQ. Patient-centered medical home resource center.

3.  American Nurses Association (2013) Framework for measuring nurses' contributions to care coordination.

4.  McDonald KM, Sundaram V, Bravata DM, Lewis R, Lin N, et al (2007) Closing the Quality Gap: A Critical Analysis of Quality Improvement Strategies. Technical Review 9.

5.  Meyers D, Peikes D, Genevro J, Peterson Greg TE, Tim Lake T, et al. (2010) The roles of patient-centered medical homes and accountable care organizations in coordinating patient care. Agency for Healthcare Research and Quality Rockville, MD.

6.  Au M, Simon S, Chen A, Lipson D, Gimm G, et al (2011) Comparative Effectiveness of Care Coordination for Adults with Disabilities. Mathematica Policy Research.

7.  Paulus RA, Davis K, Steele GD (2008) Continuous innovation in health care: implications of the Geisinger experience. Health Aff (Millwood) 27: 1235-1245.

8.  Friedberg MW, Lai DJ, Hussey PS, Schneider EC (2009) A guide to the medical home as a practice-level intervention. Am J Manag Care 15: S291-299.

9.  Reid RJ, Fishman PA, Yu O, Ross TR, Tufano JT, et al. (2009) Patient-centered medical home demonstration: A prospective, quasi-experimental, before and after evaluation. Am J Manag Care 15: e71-87.

10. Dorr DA, Wilcox AB, Brunker CP, Burdon RE, Donnelly SM (2008) The effect of technology-supported, multi-disease care management on the mortality and hospitalization of seniors. J Am Geriatr Soc 56: 2195-2202.

11. Leff B, Reider L, Frick KD, Scharfstein DO, Boyd CM, et al. (2009) Guided care and the cost of complex healthcare: A preliminary report. Am J Manag Care 15: 555-559.

12. Jack BW, Chetty VK, Anthony D, Greenwald JL, Sanchez GM, et al. (2009) A reengineered hospital discharge program to decrease rehospitalization: A randomized trial. Ann Intern Med 150: 178-187.

13. Peikes D, Chen A, Schore J, Brown R (2009) Effects of care coordination on hospitalization, quality of care, and health care expenditures among Medicare beneficiaries: 15 randomized trials. JAMA 301: 603-618.

14. Boult C, Groves C, Novak T (2011) Coordination of care by guided care interdisciplinary teams. Comprehensive Care Coordination for Chronically Ill Adults. John Wiley and Sons.

15. O'Malley AS, Reschovsky JD (2011) Referral and consultation communication between primary care and specialist physicians: Finding common ground. Archives of Internal Medicine 171: 56-65

16. Pham HH, O'Malley AS, Bach PB, Salontz-Martinez C, Schrag D (2009) Primary care physicians' links to other physicians through medicare patients: The scope of care coordination. Annals of Internal Medicine 150: 236-242.

17. Rittenhouse DR, Casalino LP, Shortell SM, McClellan SR, Gillies RR, et al. (2011) Small and medium-size physician practices use few patient-centered medical home processes. Health Aff (Millwood) 30: 1575-1584.

18. Rittenhouse DR, Shortell SM, Gillies RR, Casalino LP, Robinson JC, et al. (2010) Improving chronic illness care: findings from a national study of care management processes in large physician practices. Med Care Res Rev 67: 301-320.

19. Camicia M, Chamberlain B, Finnie RR, Nalle M, Lindeke LL, et al. (2013) The value of nursing care coordination: A white paper of the American Nurses Association. Nurs Outlook 61: 490-501.

20. Institute of Medicine (US). Committee on the Robert Wood Johnson Foundation Initiative on the Future of Nursing; 2011The future of nursing: Leading change, advancing health. National Academies Press.

21. Nutting PA, Miller WL, Crabtree BF, Jaen CR, Stewart EE, et al. (2009) Initial lessons from the first national demonstration project on practice transformation to a patient-centered medical home. Ann Fam Med 7: 254-260.

22. McKinley KE, Berry SA, Laam LA, Doll MC, Brin KP, et al. (2008) Clinical microsystems, Part 4. Building innovative population-specific mesosystems. Jt Comm J Qual Patient Saf 34: 655-663.

23. Batalden PB, Nelson EC, Edwards WH, Godfrey MM, Mohr JJ (2003) Microsystems in health care: Part 9. Developing small clinical units to attain peak performance. Jt Comm J Qual Saf 29: 575-585.

24. Nelson EC, Batalden PB, Homa K, Godfrey MM, Campbell C, et al. (2003) Microsystems in health care: Part 2. Creating a rich information environment. Jt Comm J Qual Saf 29: 5-15.

25. Wasson JH, Godfrey MM, Nelson E, Mohr JJ, Batalden PB (2003) Microsystems in health care: Part 4. Planning patient-centered care. Joint Commission Journal on Quality and Patient Safety 29: 227-237.

26. Nelson EC, Batalden PB, Huber TP, Mohr JJ, Godfrey MM, et al. (2002) Microsystems in health care: Part 1. Learning from high-performing front-line clinical units. Jt Comm J Qual Improv 28: 472-493.

27. Wasson JH, Bartels S (2009) CARE Vital Signs supports patient-centered, collaborative care. J Ambul Care Manage 32: 56-71.

28. Kraynack NC, McBride JT (2009) Improving care at cystic fibrosis centers through quality improvement. Semin Respir Crit Care Med 30: 547-558.

29. Anonymous Maine Quality Counts.

30. Anderson DR, St Hilaire D, Flinter M (2012) Primary care nursing role and care coordination: An observational study of nursing work in a community health center. Online J Issues Nurs 17: 3.

31. Nelson EC, Godfrey MM, Batalden PB, Berry SA, Bothe AE Jr, et al. (2008) Clinical microsystems, part 1. The building blocks of health systems. Jt Comm J Qual Patient Saf 34: 367-378.

32. Godfrey MM, Nelson EC, Wasson JH, Mohr JJ, Batalden PB (2003) Microsystems in health care: Part 3. Planning patient-centered services. Joint Commission Journal on Quality and Patient Safety 29: 159-170.

33. Batalden PB, Nelson EC, Mohr JJ, Godfrey MM, Huber TP, et al. (2003) Microsystems in health care: Part 5. How leaders are leading. Jt Comm J Qual Saf 29: 297-308.

34. Mohr JJ, Barach P, Cravero JP, Blike GT, Godfrey MM, et al. (2003) Microsystems in health care: Part 6. Designing patient safety into the microsystem. Jt Comm J Qual Saf 29: 401-408.

35. McDonald KM, Schultz E, Albin L, Pineda N, Lonhart J, et al (2010) Care Coordination Atlas Version 3.

36. Wagner EH, Austin BT, Davis C, Hindmarsh M, Schaefer J, et al. (2001) Improving chronic illness care: translating evidence into action. Health Aff (Millwood) 20: 64-78.

37. Anderson DR, Olayiwola JN (2012) Community health centers and the patient-centered medical home: challenges and opportunities to reduce health care disparities in America. J Health Care Poor Underserved 23: 949-957.

38. Mehrotra A, Forrest CB, Lin CY (2011) Dropping the baton: specialty referrals in the United States. Milbank Q 89: 39-68.

39. Bodenheimer T (2008) Coordinating care--a perilous journey through the health care system. N Engl J Med 358: 1064-1071.

40. Nutting PA, Crabtree BF, Stewart EE, Miller WL, Palmer RF, et al (2010) Effect of facilitation on practice outcomes in the National Demonstration Project model of the patient-centered medical home. Ann Fam Med 8 Suppl 1: S33-S44, S92.

41. Thomson RG (2005) Consensus publication guidelines: The next step in the science of quality improvement? Qual Saf Health Care 14: 317-318.

# 33

# Virtual Patients in Emergency Nursing Training

**Tudor Calinici***

*Iuliu Hatieganu" University of Medicine and Pharmacy Cluj-Napoca· Romania*

**\*Corresponding author:** Tudor Calinici, Department of Medical Education, Medical Informatics and Biostatistics Discipline, Louis Pasteur Street, No 6, 400012, Cluj-Napoca, Romania, E-mail: tcalinici@umfcluj.ro

## Abstract

Emergency nurses are specialized to provide rapid assessment and treatment to patients in the initial phase of illness or trauma and often in life-threatening situations. They are required to have a lot of knowledge –not only in medical area - and to possess multiple abilities which will enable them to face different situation that may occur. Due to different constrains – time, money, ethical considerations, etc., the institutions which provide training for emergency nurses are forced to find alternative methods to reach all the outcomes required in real life situations. One of the methods is the use of virtual patients. The scope of this paper is to present the concept of virtual patients, to describe their main characteristics which recommend them to be used for training the emergency nurses and to present the main types of virtual patients.

**Keywords:** Emergency nursing training; Virtual patients

## Introduction

Emergency nurses are specialized to provide rapid assessment and treatment to patients in the initial phase of illness or trauma and often in life-threatening situations. Practicing not only in emergency departments of the hospitals, but on cruise ships, crisis intervention centers or prisons, they must have a lot of knowledge about general as well as specific health issues in order to assess, intervene and stabilize a variety of trauma and illness with decisive action. [1]

One of the actions in which the emergency nurses are involved is the triage. [2] An emergency nurse must have the ability to make quick and accurate assessments about incoming patients, including both physical and mental health conditions and find and record relevant information about incoming patients like medical problem, any allergies that the patient may have, the current medication, if exists, body temperature, blood rate, etc. The emergency nurses are expected also to perform other different actions like to clean and bandage wounds, to administer medication, to move patients, to take blood samples, so on.

Emergency nurses are expected to comply with protocols, procedures and safety policies of a health care facility. Emotional stability, communication, leadership, sympathy and attention to detail are characteristics expected and appreciated for emergency nurses. [1]

Patient contact with medical and healthcare trainee is at the heart of gaining the clinical competency. However this vital contact is declining. [3] The training of emergency nurse using the patient contact is hampered by two important factors: the healthcare budget constraints that increasingly limit clinical teaching and the specific of the emergency which leave no room for practice and little time for explanations.

A method for increasing the level of knowledge and clinical abilities for emergency nurses is the use of e-learning applications: simulations, virtual worlds, virtual patients, games and many more, applications with proven impact in medical education. [4] The uses of those methods provide repeated practice opportunities in dispersed locations with uncommon, life-threatening trauma cases in a safe, reproducible, flexible setting. [5] The goal of those methods is not to replace the contact with the patient which is indispensable for medical education, but to provide to the trainees more opportunities to practice specific tasks in order to obtain specific outcomes. [6]

## Virtual patients

A virtual patient is defined as "an interactive computer simulation of real-life clinical scenarios for the purpose of medical training, education or assessment" [7]. Generally, the virtual patients have two components, the patient case, and the educational activities leading to a specific educational goal [8].

The virtual nature of the patient allows emergency nurses to practice in a virtual – safe – environment. Each virtual patient will be designed for learning specific learning outcomes or for assessing the knowledge. Because of their limitations – the impossibility of performing real maneuvers on them –this method could be located between first two steps on a scale which contain the main sources for gaining clinical abilities, as is shown in Figure 1

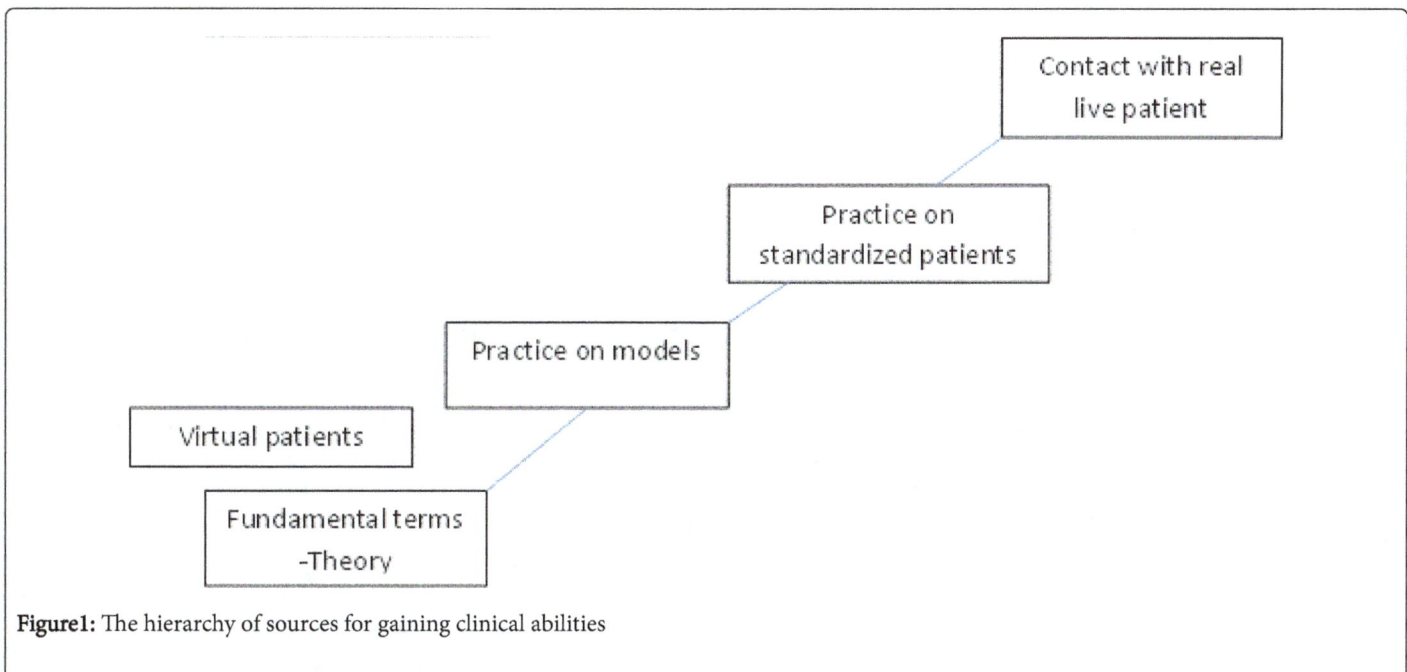

**Figure1:** The hierarchy of sources for gaining clinical abilities

Virtual patients are associated with large positive effects compared with no intervention. Effects in comparison with non- computer instruction are on average small. [9] The increase is evident in clinical reasoning – the critical analysis of patients' symptoms, signs, laboratory results and imaging, to support the determination of a diagnosis, and the planning of an appropriate attitude. [10]

The authors of the virtual patients can imagine many emergency scenarios in which the trainees are able to see the consequences of their actions. Those actions, which sometimes are wrong, will build experiences which can increase awareness and serve as powerful teaching strategies. [11]

The main advantages of the virtual patients in training of emergency nursing are:

### Availability and accessibility

In contrast to real emergency cases which could happen in any moment and must be resolved at the time, the virtual patients are available any time. The emergency nurse could choose the moment in which he/she wants to train by solving a specific virtual patient. Most of the virtual patients management systems are implemented to be accessible online, so, in those situations, the trainee only need equipment connected on internet. More, the trainee has the opportunity to select the type of the situation (pathology) which wants to practice, this thing being impossible in real-life emergency room.

### Diversity

Using virtual patients the authors have the chance to present a lot of situations that the emergency nurses may face. They can build scenarios based by rare but big impact incidents - as earthquakes or terrorist attacks; they can introduce patients with rare pathologies; they can combine different parts of real-life events in order to cover as many situations as it is possible. In case of a similar real-life event, it is a big possibility that the emergency nurse to react in an adequate manner.

### Reusability

Once it was created, a virtual patient could be a source for different clinical scenarios. By doing small changes - like changing the value of biological parameters - the user will face different situations, triggering changing in attitude and different decisions. More, a study conducted by Muntean et al [12] indicated that the virtual patients could be used in multicultural and multilingual environment, with small efforts for adaptation. The development of the standards for exchange between different applications [13] made virtual patients more popular, being easier to find a proper virtual patient for a specific outcome.

The main disadvantage of this method consists in the amount of time consumed for creating a virtual patient. Major collaborative studies in Europe have suggested that the mean time spent on creation of a virtual patient is about 20–80 hours. [14] Having this in mind, it is easy to realize that the cost in money could vary from cheap to very expensive [15].

## Types of virtual patients

There are three main categories of virtual patients: linear, demi-linear and branched virtual patients. The difference between those categories is given by the way in which the user interacts with the clinical scenario. The way of interacting is related with the purpose of use of different types of virtual patients – learning, training, assessing.

## Linear virtual patients

In this case, each sequence of the clinical scenario is presented as a slide. The user has only one option to advance, only when the actions related to the side were finished, as it is presented in Figure 2.

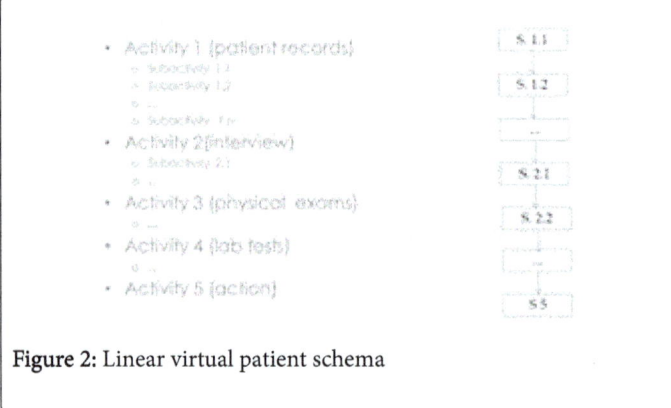

**Figure 2:** Linear virtual patient schema

The feedback could be available to the users any time when the author of the scenario considers that is necessary. The design of those virtual patients makes them suitable for learning – protocols, simple procedures, etc.

CAMPUS [16] and CASUS [17] are the most common applications for creating and using linear virtual patients.

### Demi-linear virtual patients

In this situation, like in precedent, each sequence of the clinical scenario is presented as a slide, but on each slide there are mandatory or optional things to do, or actions to perform. The user can move between the slides and choose the time when to perform the actions. The demi-linear virtual patient schema is presented in Figure 3.

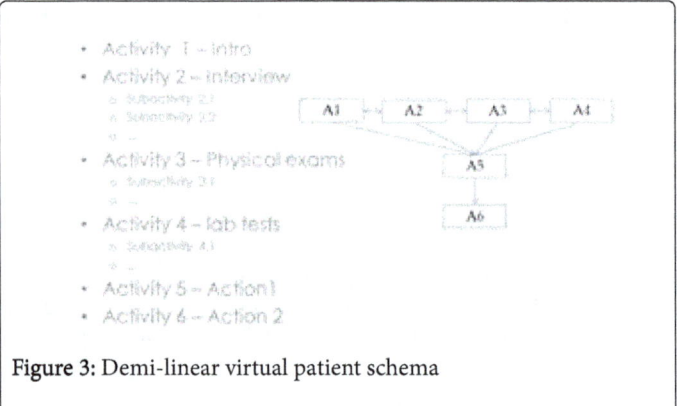

**Figure 3:** Demi-linear virtual patient schema

The feedback will be available to the user only when the case is finished. These virtual patients are usually used for learning – clinical thinking and resource planning and using.

WebSp [18] is most representative demi-linear virtual patient system, being in the same time probably the most geographically widespread virtual patient system. [6]

### Branched virtual patients

In this case, on each slide of the clinical scenario, the user could choose to perform between different actions or take different attitudes, and the scenario is changing according to the selected action. The user is able to see the consequences of his/her choice. The schema for branched virtual patients is presented in figure 4.

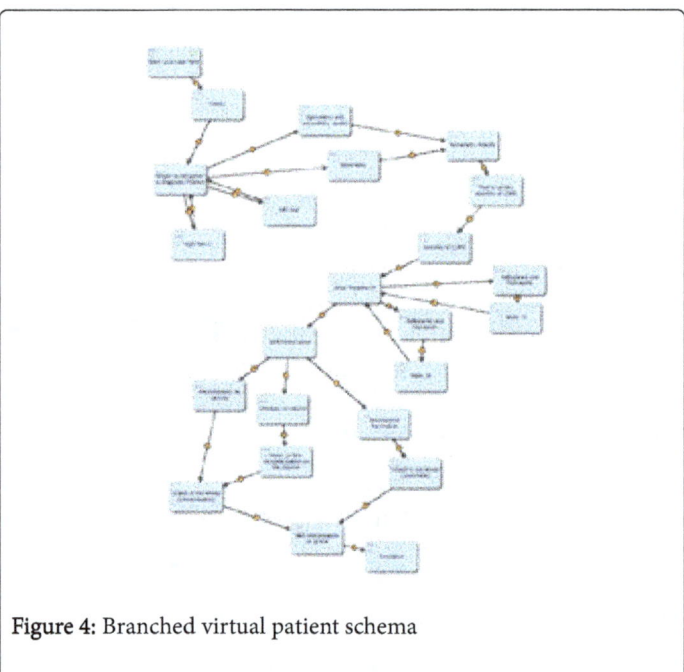

**Figure 4:** Branched virtual patient schema

The user has a lot of freedom of choice. Each action could modify the scenario. The feedback could be available any time. This structure makes this type of virtual patients to be used for self-training or assessment and it seems to be an alternative for the classical problem base learning paper-based cases. [19]

One of the most representative applications for creating and managing branched virtual patients is OpenLabyrinth. [20]

### Conclusion

Because of their characteristics, virtual patients could be a useful tool to be used in emergency nurses training. Without having the purpose to replace the rest of methods of training, the use of virtual patients together with all the available methods could increase the performance and the level of knowledge of the emergency nurses both on undergraduate or postgraduate level.

### References

1.  Emergency Nurse: Job Description, Duties and Requirements, Glossary of Career Education Programs / Medical and Health Professions

2.  Definition of triage

3.  Bombeke K, Symons L, Debaene L, De Winter B, Schol S, et al. (2010) Help, I'm losing patient-centredness! Experiences of medical students and their teachers. Med Educ 44: 662-673.

4.  Ruiz JG, Mintzer MJ, Leipzig RM (2006) The impact of E-learning in medical education. Acad Med 81: 207-212.

5.  LeRoy Heinrichs W, Youngblood P, Harter PM, Dev P (2008) Simulation for team training and assessment: case studies of online training with virtual worlds. World J Surg 32: 161-170.

6.  Poulton T, Balasubramaniam C (2011) Virtual patients: a year of change. Med Teach 33: 933-937.

7.  Cook DA, Triola MM (2009) Virtual patients: a critical literature review and proposed next steps. Med Educ 43: 303-311.

8.  Ellaway RH, Davies D (2011) Design for learning: deconstructing virtual patient activities. Med Teach 33: 303-310.

9.   Cook DA, Erwin PJ, Triola MM (2010) Computerized virtual patients in health professions education: a systematic review and meta-analysis. Acad Med 85: 1589-1602.

10.  Eva KW (2005) What every teacher needs to know about clinical reasoning. Med Educ 39: 98-106.

11.  Posel N, Mcgee JB2, Fleiszer DM1 (2015) Twelve tips to support the development of clinical reasoning skills using virtual patient cases. Med Teach 37: 813-818.

12.  Muntean V, Calinici T, Tigan S, Fors UG (2013) Language, culture and international exchange of virtual patients. BMC Med Educ 13: 21.

13.  Ellaway R, Poulton T, Fors U, McGee JB, Albright S (2008) Building a virtual patient commons. Med Teach 30: 170-174.

14.  eViP consortium 2010.Final report.

15.  Huang G, Reynolds R, Candler C (2007) Virtual patient simulation at US and Canadian medical schools. Acad Med 82: 446-451.

16.  Garde S, Bauch M, Haag M, Heid J, Huwendiek S, et al. (2005) CAMPUS - computer-based training in medicine as part of a problem-oriented educational strategy. Stud Learn Eval Innov Dev 2: 10-19

17.  Hege I, Kononowicz A, Pfähler M, Adler M, Fischer M (2009) Implementation of the Medbiquitous standard into the learning system CASUS. BAMS 5 :51–55

18.  Zary N, Johnson G, Boberg J, Fors UG (2006) Development, implementation and pilot evaluation of a Web-based Virtual Patient Case Simulation environment--Web-SP. BMC Med Educ 6: 10.

19.  Poulton T, Conradi E, Kavia S,Round J, Hilton S (2009) The replacement of 'paper' cases by interactive online virtual patients in problem-based learning Med Teach 31:752–758

20.  Ellaway R (2010) OpenLabyrinth: An abstract pathway-based serious game engine for professional education. Digital information management (ICDIM), Fifth International Conference, 2010 July 5–8. Thunder Bay: 490–495

# 34

# The Impact of Nursing Leadership Training on Evidence-based Leadership and Practice

Tarja Kvist[1], Katja Tähkä[2], Miia Ruotsalainen[3] and Tarja Tervo-Heikkinen[4]

[1]University Researcher, PhD, RN, University of Eastern Finland, Kuopio Campus, Department of Nursing Science, Finland

[2]Nurse Manager, MNS, RN, Helsinki University Hospital, Finland

[3]Nurse Manager, MNS, RN, Kuopio University Hospital, Finland

[4]Clinical Nurse Consultant, PhD, RN, Kuopio University Hospital, Finland

*Corresponding author: Tarja Kvist, University Researcher, PhD, RN, University of Eastern Finland, Kuopio Campus, Department of Nursing Science, P.O. Box 1627, 70211 Kuopio, Finland, E-mail: tarja.kvist@uef.fi

## Abstract

**Aim:** To assess the impact of leadership training on nurse leaders' perceptions of evidence-based leadership (EBL) and practice (EBP).

**Background**: Nurse leaders are the key persons for promoting EBP. They have to use evidence skillfully both in practice and leadership.

**Methods**: 47 nurse leaders participated in EBL training (2010 – 2011) for the "At Safe" project. Data were collected from 42 leaders before the training and 34 after. The questionnaires were developed as part of the project. The data were analyzed using frequency analysis.

**Results:** Before the training most of the nurse leaders had the positive perceptions of using research knowledge to develop the practice and leadership. The training had helped nurse leaders to understand that decisions can be justified with research knowledge, which strengthened the leaders' responsibility to develop EBP, EBL and their work unit. Most of the nurse leaders seldom brought research publications for their staff to read or discussed findings with them.

**Conclusions:** Nurse leaders have a positive attitude to EBP and EBL but they need to more promote it to their staff and use it for their own leadership. The EBL courses might highlight the importance of using evidence in leadership, but changing their leadership style needs time and willingness. The nurse leaders should become aware of the importance of EBL and EBP. There is an urgent need for training and new innovations to support EBL.

**Keywords:** Evidence-Based Leadership; Evidence-Based Practice; Nurse Leaders; Web-Based survey, TrainingIntroductionEvidence-based practice (EBP) is a systematic approach to the use of the best research evidence applied to clinical expertise and patient values [1,2]. Evidence-based leadership (EBL) covers the best use of evidence to organize, guide, deliver, finance and improve the quality of care and patient safety [3]. Since the 1990s, there have been many discussions, guidelines and articles published all over the world about the importance of EBP [1,2,4-6] . The change from experience-based practice to EBP is going on and urgently needed; like the Institute of Medicine (IOM) [6] has set the goal that health care should be evidence-based in 2020.According to one American study, 53.6% (n=544) of nurses agreed or strongly agreed that EBP was implemented in their organizations [7] whilst another American study [8] found that 43% of the practicing nurses reported that 61 – 100% of their practice was evidence-based. A Norwegian study [9] showed that the nurses used more experience-based knowledge than research evidence in practice. The Finnish National Programs since 2004 have recommended developing evidence-based health care [4,5]. The Finnish Health Care Act says "The provision of health care shall be based on evidence and recognized treatment and operational practices.

The health care provided shall be of high quality, safe and appropriately organized." [10]. There are no Finnish studies showing what proportion of practice is evidence-based.Nurse leaders are central to developing evidence-based nursing practice [3,7,8,11-15] because they create a culture of evidence-based practice and have the responsibility of designing and supporting nursing environments that promote the high quality of care, based on the best available evidence [7,11,16,17]. Nurse leaders themselves need to be able to use scientific evidence and embrace continuous learning [3,8].Leadership is a key element in developing EBP in health care organizations [8,11, 18-21]. Porter-O'Grady and Malloch (2008) [22] wrote the implementation of EBP is in progress. The nurse leaders need be skillful at evidence-based leadership and practice in order to spearhead the change from experience-based to evidence-based practice. The key skills of leaders trying to advance EBP are innovative thinking, planning and implementation of the change [22]. Leaders have to be able to change continuously. The application and integration of evidence-based principles into nursing leadership is a complex process, itself part of a complex system. The process needs the passion, respect and knowledge of nursing science [14,21,22]. Support from nurse leaders is vital to the promotion of EBP. Research by Eneh et al. [23] about the transformational leadership style of Finnish nurse leaders (nurse managers, nursing directors) asked from the nursing staff (n=1497) showed that Finnish nursing directors appeared not to use evidence-based knowledge at all, whilst 50% of nursing staff had no perception if their nurse directors' used it.Many nurse leaders perceive EBP as being desirable, but they do not know how they might implement it [16]. Marshall [24] highlighted the nurse leaders' slow pace of application of EBP in their work. There are still many ineffective routines in nursing practice and leadership. There have been many different programs to develop leadership generally, or from specific views, such as empowerment of nurse leaders [19,25], effects of education on evidence-based practice courses [20], development and evaluation of a joint academic-service nursing journal club [3] and an advanced educational program promoting evidence-based practice [21]. This study introduces one Finnish evidence-based nursing leadership training program.Nurse leaders who carry out evidence-based practice appreciate the expertise of other evidence-based professionals. For example, the collaboration between nurse leaders and librarians is an important way of promoting the EBP process. Innovative nurse leaders understand this and so collaborate with the librarians, using their expertise of searching for useful research papers and articles [19,26]. Many studies underline the use of mentors implementing EBP [7,8,13,27,28].Johansson et al. [20] found that head nurses who had additional education in scientific methodology utilized more research findings than those who lacked that additional education. About half of them (n=99) searched, read and discussed research results with their colleagues. They encouraged their staff to read research findings, but their staff did not have enough time to find relevant research and read the results [20].The Finnish Health Care Act expanded the choice of public institution where someone could receive treatment [10]. The choice increases demands on organizations because people would expect to receive care based on the best available evidence. Therefore, it is most important to educate nurse leaders about EBP and EBL. Apart from the training, the willingness of nurse leaders to adopt EBP has been seen to be important in the change process [19].

## Aim

To assess the impact of leadership training on nurse leaders' perceptions of evidence-based leadership and practice.

- What are nurse leaders' perceptions of evidence-based leadership and practice before the training?
- What are nurse leaders' perceptions of evidence-based leadership and practice after the training?

## Materials and methods

### Study design

The study was a longitudinal descriptive intervention study. The intervention was the evidence-based nursing leadership (EBNL) training course (Figure 1).

### EBNL training for nurse leaders

EBNL training was carried out between September 2010 and May 2011 (Figure 1). The training was organized by Kuopio University Hospital (KUH), Department of Nursing Science, University of the Eastern Finland (UEF) and "The Attractive and Health-promoting Healthcare – At Safe" project. A total of 47 voluntary nurse leaders

from Kuopio University Hospital, Northern Savo Hospital District and Central Finland Health Care District started the course and 43 completed it and other four dropouts were mostly because of lack of time for the training.

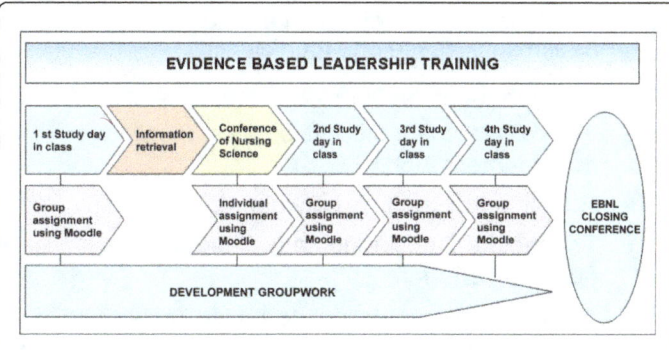

**Figure 1:** Evidence-based leadership (EBNL) training

The goals of the EBNL training were:

1. To increase nurse leaders' knowledge of EBL and EBP.

2. To help nurse leaders identify their role as a leader of EBP and as a promoter of EBP.

3. To train nurse leaders to find research information from different databases and evaluate evidence critically.

4. To increase nurse leaders' knowledge in developing and implementing effective, integrated and evidence-based best practices and procedures for their units.

The EBNL training package included four teaching days and an EBNL closing conference day. Furthermore, there was training in information retrieval by a librarian (Ovaska 2012). This course gave students information literacy skills training, necessary for the successful implementation of EBP and EBL and also for continuing professional development.

The teaching days' topics were 1) Leadership of evidence-based practice; 2) The leader as a promoter of work well-being; 3) Challenges and opportunities of leadership and 4) Patient satisfaction and patient safety. The training course included attending the national conference of nursing science in autumn 2010.

Between the teaching days, students carried out assignments on the topics taught and the group development programs, using the Moodle (Modular **Object-Oriented Dynamic Learning Environment**) e-learning environment which is a **free software e-learning** platform [29].

The students selected three of the most interesting themes suggested to them when they applied for the course. The themes were mostly drawn from the results of the At Safe Project, e.g. Eneh et al. [23] and Kvist et al. [30]. They were health promotion, rewarding and feedback, human resource planning and evaluation, patient safety, the management of expertise, change management and well-being at work. Participants carried out their development assignments (Figure 2) in groups assigned in accordance with the themes. Each group consisted of three to six nurse leaders who had similar interests. Every group had a mentor. All the mentors had a Master or Doctoral Degree and worked in KUH or in the department of Nursing Science in UEF.

Figure 2: The Development Program Topics

The Development Program Topics

- The Management of health promotion in primary health care - case one municipality
- How the nurse leaders can reward their staff?
- The development discussion as a knowledge management tool
- Handling the conflicts between nursing staff
- The factors that contribute well-bring of the nursing manager
- Implementation of evidence-based knowledge in nursing practice
- The nurse manager's role in staff com mitment to change management
- The outcome figures in the gesigning and evaluating of nurse staffing
- Use of evidence-based information to reducing medication errors and the development of management practices to promotr patient safety

## Data collection and participants

Before the EBNL training started, data were collected from 47 nurse leaders with 42 of them responding (89%) in autumn 2010. After completing the training, data were collected from 41 nurse leaders, who had given the permission to send the questionnaire at the beginning of the training, with 34 of them (83%) responding in spring 2011. Web-based surveys were used for data collection. Two weeks after requesting responses from either survey, a reminder e-mail was sent.

### Instruments and their reliability

The instruments were developed at the At Safe project and were based on literature reviews, expert panels and pilot studies.

The questionnaire used before the EBNL training covered two areas: "current own leadership work" (26 items) and "use of evidence in own leadership work and promoting EBP" (15 items). In addition, there were 14 background variables. In this article, we report the results in the area "use of evidence in own leadership work and promoting EBP". The area "current own leadership work" was omitted because the items of it were concerning general leadership issues. The items used a four point scale (totally disagree, partly disagree, partly agree and totally agree). The reliability of this area was good, having a measured Cronbach's α value of 0.82 [31].

The questionnaire used after the EBNL training had 53 items concerning EBL and EBP which covered 7 areas:

- Impact of training on the nurse leaders' perceptions of EBL and EBP (6 items)
- Responsibility of nurse leaders (9 items)

- Development of EBP (7 items)
- Motivating the staff to reach common goals and participate (7 items)
- Confirming the use of research knowledge (7 items)
- Leadership in development of staff (8 items)
- Evaluation of own development as an evidence-based leader during training (8 items)

Eight background variables described the respondents. Three open-ended questions were included in the survey.

In this article, we report the results from areas 1, 2, 5 and 7. These areas are concentrated in evidence-based practice and leadership and the others more on general leadership. The items used a four point scale (totally disagree, partly disagree, agree, totally agree). The reliability of each was considered to be good as measured by Cronbach's α values (0.88 – 0.91).

## Data analysis

The data were analyzed using descriptive statistics and SPSS version 17.0 for Windows (SPSS inc., Chicago, IL, USA).

The responses to Likert-scale items were categorized in three groups because of the exiguous size of the totally disagree group. The groups were in before survey: 1 Disagree = totally or partly disagree, 2 Partly agree = partly agree and 3 Totally agree = totally agree and after survey: 1 Disagree = totally or partly disagree, 2 Agree = Agree and 3 Totally agree = totally agree.

## Ethical considerations

Following the organization codes, the chief nursing officer of the university hospital gave permission for the surveys to be conducted. Participation was voluntary and anonymous. The web-based survey was sent to the participants of the training who had given written permission to be sent a survey before starting the course and at the end of the course.

## Results

### Demographic characteristics of nurse leaders

All respondents were women. In the survey before the training, the mean age of nurse leaders was 47 years (range 30 – 59 years); after the survey, it was 48 years (34 – 59 years). Most of them worked in specialized health care (2010: 69%; 2011: 68%) and nearly half of them at the university hospital (50%, 47%). Before and after the course, they mostly worked as nurse managers (71%, 76%). Most of them (79%, 90%) were in charge of between 0 and 49 staff. About 40% of them had a university degree. Most of the nurse leaders (78%, 88%) had under 10 years working experience in their current job but had a total work experience in health care of over 10 years (90%, 91%) (Table 1).

### Nurse leaders' perceptions of EBL and EBP before the training

The majority (62%) had the positive perceptions towards developing nursing using research knowledge. 41% of them felt that the staff in their units did not know what EBP is. 5% totally agreed and 69% partly agreed that the patient care in their units was evidence-based. Nearly half (45%) of nurse leaders appreciated the development of EBP as an important part of their leadership style. Most of the nurse leaders (88%) disagreed that their staff had sufficient time at their work to read research from their own disciplines. 29% of nurse leaders did not encourage their staff to explore the latest research in their own area. Many nurse leaders (50%) felt that they were not able to make EBP possible for their staff to perform by giving time to search for evidence. 38% disagreed that when choosing new staff, their research experience was not the first priority (Table 2).

| Demographic variable | 2010 (%) | 2011 (%) |
|---|---|---|
| Age | n=42 | n=34 |
| 30 – 39 | 19 | 12 |
| 40 – 49 | 38 | 41 |
| 50 – 59 | 43 | 47 |
| Working health care sector | n=42 | n=34 |
| Specialized health care | 69 | 68 |
| Other | 31 | 32 |
| Organization | n=42 | n=34 |
| University hospital | 50 | 47 |
| Other | 50 | 53 |
| Work position | n=42 | n=34 |
| CNO | 7 | 3 |
| Nursing director | 12 | 9 |
| Nurse manager | 71 | 76 |
| Specialist, other | 10 | 12 |
| Number of staff | n=42 | n=29 |
| 0 – 49 | 78 | 90 |
| 50 – 100 | 5 | 3 |
| Over 100 | 5 | 7 |
| None | 12 | |
| Highest educational qualification | n=42 | n=34 |
| University | 40 | 41 |
| University of applied sciences, nursing school | 60 | 59 |
| Working experience in current job | n=42 | n=33 |
| Under 10 years | 78 | 88 |
| 10 – 20 years | 17 | 9 |
| Over 20 years | 5 | 3 |
| Working experience in health care | n=42 | n=33 |
| Under 10 years | 10 | 9 |
| 10 – 20 years | 50 | 35 |
| Over 20 years | 40 | 56 |

Table 1 : Demographics of nurse leaders in 2010 (N=42) and 2011 (N=34)

## Nurse leaders' perceptions of EBL and EBP after training

Most of the nurse leaders (59%) totally agreed that the EBL training had helped them to understand that decisions can be justified with research knowledge. 15% of nurse leaders totally agreed, 76% agreed and 9% disagreed that the training had developed their own EBL. 9%

of them disagreed that the training had improved their knowledge of EBL whereas 27% totally agreed (Table 3).

| Item | Totally, partly disagree | Partly agree | Totally agree |
|---|---|---|---|
| I search for research evidence from publications in my own discipline. (n=42) | 19 | 60 | 21 |
| I use the research to develop my unit.(n=42) | 29 | 52 | 19 |
| The staff of my unit knows what evidence-based practice is.(n = 42) | 41 | 52 | 7 |
| The patient care in my unit is evidence-based. (n = 42) | 26 | 69 | 5 |
| I use research knowledge to help my leadership work (n = 42) | 17 | 69 | 14 |
| Developing evidence-based practice is an essential part of my leadership practice. (n = 42) | 19 | 62 | 19 |
| I appreciate that evidence-based practice is an important part of my leadership style. (n=42) | 7 | 48 | 45 |
| I understand about developing nursing using research knowledge (n = 42) | 0 | 38 | 62 |
| I encourage my staff to explore the latest research in my own area. (n=42) | 29 | 64 | 7 |
| The staff in my unit have opportunities to participate in evidence-based nursing training. (n = 42) | 17 | 64 | 19 |
| The staff in my unit are interested in developing nursing using evidence-based knowledge. (n = 42) | 33 | 62 | 5 |
| I make it possible for my staff to develop evidence-based practice by giving time to search for evidence. (n = 42) | 50 | 45 | 5 |
| My staff have enough time at work to read about research in own discipline. (n=42) | 88 | 12 | 0 |
| When I select new staff members, it is important they have an interest in research. (n=42) | 19 | 62 | 19 |
| When I choose new staff members, it is important that they have research experience. (n=42) | 38 | 55 | 7 |

Table 2 : Using EB knowledge in leadership and promoting EBP in their own unit (n=42) (%)

The nurse leaders recognized their responsibility to develop EBP and their working unit. Nurse leaders agreed that they had a responsibility to develop evidence-based practice and use evidence-based knowledge in their leadership. The responsibilities of planning the additional training of staff, developing professionalism and work orientation were not as clearly recognized (Table 4).

| Item | Totally, partly disagree (%) | Agree (%) | Totally agree (%) |
|---|---|---|---|

| | | | |
|---|---|---|---|
| EBNL increased my knowledge about evidence-based practice. (n=34) | 6 | 50 | 44 |
| EBNL improved my knowledge about evidence-based leadership. (n=34) | 9 | 64 | 27 |
| EBNL developed my evidence-based leadership. (n=34) | 9 | 76 | 15 |
| EBNL promoted my understanding of how nursing has to be based on research knowledge. (n=34) | 3 | 47 | 50 |
| EBNL promoted my understanding of how evidence-based practice increases the quality of care. (n=34) | 3 | 47 | 50 |
| EBNL helped me to understand that decisions can be justified with research knowledge. (n=34) | 3 | 38 | 59 |

**Table 3 :** Impact of training on the nurse leaders' perceptions of EBL and EBP (%).

| Item<br>Nurse leader<br>is responsible | Totally, partly disagree (%) | Agree (%) | Totally agree (%) |
|---|---|---|---|
| for developing evidence-based practice. (n=34) | 0 | 50 | 50 |
| for developing a working unit. (n=34) | 3 | 41 | 56 |
| for planning the additional training of staff. (n=33) | 12 | 46 | 42 |
| for developing the professionalism of staff. (n=34) | 9 | 59 | 32 |
| for work orientation. (n=33) | 9 | 42 | 49 |
| for coordinating nursing practices. (n=34) | 0 | 59 | 41 |
| for developing multi-professional collaboration. (n=33) | 3 | 61 | 36 |
| for using evidence-based knowledge in their leadership. (n=33) | 0 | 52 | 48 |
| for making the staff participate in evidence-based practice. (n=34) | 3 | 62 | 35 |

**Table 4:** The nurse leaders' responsibilities for changing the culture of EBP (%).

Most of the nurse leaders (64%) did not discuss scientific publications with their staff. One third of them did not provide the research knowledge available to staff. All (34% totally agreed and 66% agreed) of them connected their research knowledge to their previous experiences (Table 5).

| Item | Totally, partly disagree (%) | Agree (%) | Totally agree (%) |
|---|---|---|---|
| I recognize the need for research knowledge about nursing in developing my own skills. (n=34) | 6 | 68 | 26 |

| | | | |
|---|---|---|---|
| I use research knowledge to develop my own professional skills. (n=34) | 3 | 68 | 29 |
| I have made my goals in leadership clear. (n=34) | 9 | 76 | 5 |
| I link research knowledge to my previous experience. (=32) | 0 | 66 | 34 |
| I will systematically use research knowledge to support my leadership work. (n=31) | 7 | 74 | 19 |
| I regularly bring research knowledge for my staff. (n=33) | 33 | 55 | 12 |
| I regularly discuss scientific publications with my staff. (n=33) | 64 | 33 | 3 |

**Table 5 :** How nurse leaders felt about the use of research knowledge in leadership (%).

### Own development during the training

Mostly, nurse leaders assessed that they had developed their skills of supporting the staff, setting an example in their working unit and developing collaboration (24 – 27% totally agreed). 12% of nurse leaders felt that they had not developed their skills in motivation towards common goals or using research knowledge (Table 6).

| Item<br>Training has developed my work as an evidence-based leader… | Totally, partly disagree (%) | Agree (%) | Totally agree (%) |
|---|---|---|---|
| supporting my staff (n=33) | 6 | 70 | 24 |
| using research knowledge (n=33) | 12 | 61 | 27 |
| setting an example in working unit (n=33) | 9 | 64 | 27 |
| making the staff participate. (n=33) | 6 | 81 | 13 |
| motivating to reach common goals. (n=33) | 12 | 70 | 18 |
| developing the skills of the staff. (n=33) | 9 | 67 | 24 |
| developing the practice. (n=33) | 9 | 64 | 27 |
| developing collaboration. (n=33) | 9 | 67 | 24 |

**Table 6 :** How nurse leaders felt about their own development as an EB leader (%).

### Discussion

Nurse leaders are conscious of the importance of EBL and EBP. They emphasize their responsibility to develop EBP and their working unit. On the other hand, according to these results, they do not encourage their staff enough to carry out EBP. Over 60% of nurse leaders assessed the care in their units to be evidence-based; the results reflect the same kind of situation as is present in America and in Norway, as evaluated by nurses [7,9]. Nurse leaders in this study felt that the research skills of new nurses are not the main priority when they choose new staff. It should be one of the main criterions, because if the staff have good research skills, they can develop their evidence-based work with high quality care as a result. It should be one of the most important priorities of nurse leaders to start to understand the power of evidence-based practice.

Though the mean age of nurse leaders was quite high (47 years), it is possible that they have had little education in EBP: it might still be quite a new issue for them. On the other hand, nearly half of them had a university degree. It is worth asking what they have learnt about EBL and EBP at university and how they are implementing the knowledge of EBL and EBP. Melnyk et al. [7] criticized the contents of EBP teaching at universities, saying that they might be considered old-fashioned; this may be the case in Finland.

The goal of EBNL training was to increase the knowledge of EBL and EBP and to emphasize the role of nurse leaders in promoting EBL and EBP. The nurse leaders were satisfied with EBL, thus agreeing with the results from Johansson et al. [20], who reported that head nurses had a positive attitude towards EBP. Despite that assessment, there were many critical points which need to be discussed. Only a few of the nurse leaders felt that the training had improved their knowledge or developed their EBL. There might be different reasons for these evaluations. The training took place over two terms, so it was too short time to effect a change. Of course, there were critics of the training, though mostly the training was seen as being of good quality. So, was the training what they expected? Every fourth nurse leader felt that it did not cover certain areas of EBP or EBL and spent too long on others. In future, the contents of the courses need to be analyzed carefully beforehand.

The nurse leaders understood their responsibilities to change to a culture of EBP. Some of the nurse leaders did not recognize that they had responsibility to plan additional training or help develop the professionalism of their staff. If these issues are not on the agenda of the nurse leaders, EBP may end up not being implemented as soon as expected.

There were only a few nurse leaders who made research knowledge available to, or discussed scientific publications with their staff. The first step to develop evidence-based nursing is to make the most recent research knowledge available. There could be journal clubs in units, divisions and hospitals, which would be potential ways to learn about research. The results tell us that there were nurse leaders who had felt that the course had not developed them as a user of research knowledge. This is surprising since everyone on the course had the opportunity to learn about searching for research knowledge, though it is only a one part of the use of research. The librarians were involved in the training as educators and their role was highly appreciated [26].

Every group had an advanced mentor to supervise their development work. According to earlier studies [7,8,13,27,28], mentors play an important role in the implementation of EBP. However, in this study, the results of one open-ended question (not reported) suggested that their role was confusing due to the variability in the quality of the mentoring mostly because of the lack of reserved time for it.

However, the results show us that there is good progress in Finnish nursing. The nurse leaders support EBL, but they need more training and support for their work which will allow them to implement EBP in nursing.

## Reliability

The reliability of the instrument has been studied for both surveys. Both instruments had good reliability as measured by Cronbach's value. The response rates were high (89% and 83%), but the sample sizes were small, so any generalization of the results, even for research organizations, needs to be made very carefully.

## Limitations

The small sample sizes are due to the size of the training course. The small sample sizes meant that only the results of the descriptive analyses were reasonable to report here. The two surveys were carried out using two different survey questionnaires. This was an outcome of the inadequate planning of this project. Therefore, the results are not comparable, but still they give a unique overview of the stage of the study phenomenon.

## Conclusions

The nurse leaders have a positive attitude towards EBP and EBL but they have to do more to promote it in their units and through their own leadership. EBL courses might raise awareness of the importance of using evidence in leadership, but the change in leadership style needs time and passion. More work has to be done so that EBP and EBNL can be implemented in leadership practice and, through that, applied to clinical nursing practice.

## Acknowledgements

The authors gratefully acknowledge the CNO of the university hospital and the head of the Attractive and Health –promoting Healthcare –project. The Attractive and Health –promoting Healthcare- At Safe project was funded by National Development Programme for Social Welfare and Health Care (KASTE) and Northern Savo Hospital District.

## References

1. Sackett DL, Rosenberg WM, Gray JA, Haynes RB, Richardson WS (1996) Evidence based medicine: what it is and what it isn't. BMJ 312: 71-72.

2. DiCenco A, Guyatt G, Ciliska D (2005) Evidence-based nursing. A Guide to clinical practice 23: 743

3. Duffy JR, Thompson D, Hobbs T, Niemeyer-Hackett NL, Elpers S (2011) Evidence-based nursing leadership: Evaluation of a Joint Academic-Service Journal Club. J Nurs Adm 41: 422-427.

4. Ministry of Social Affairs and Health. Health and well-being by evidence based nursing. The national target and action plan 2004 - 2007(2003) Publications of the Ministry of Social Affairs and Health, Helsinki.

5. Ministry of Social Affairs and Health. Increasing the effectiveness and attraction of nursing care by means of management. An action plan for the years 2009â€"2011 (2009) Publications of Ministry of Social Affairs and Health, Helsinki.

6. Institute of Medicine (IOM) (2010) The future of nursing: leading change, advancing health. The National Academics Press, Washington DC.

7. Melnyk BM, Fineout-Overholt E, Gallagher-Ford L, Kaplan L (2012) The state of evidence-based practice in US nurses: critical implications for nurse leaders and educators. J Nurs Adm 42: 410-417.

8. Linton MJ, Prasun MA (2013) Evidence-based practice: collaboration between education and nursing management. J Nurs Manag 21: 5-16.

9. Dalheim A, Harthug S, Nilsen RM, Nortvedt MW (2012) Factors influencing the development of evidence-based practice among nurses: a self-report survey. BMC Health Serv Res 12: 367.

10. Ministry of Social Affairs and Health (2010) Health Care Act. No 1326/2010. Section 8. Quality and patient safety.

11. Everett LQ, Sitterding MC (2011) Transformational leadership required to design and sustain evidence-based practice: a system exemplar. West J Nurs Res 33: 398-426.

12. Crozier K, Moore J, Kite K (2012) Innovations and action research to develop research skills for nursing and midwifery practice: the Innovations in Nursing and Midwifery Practice Project study. J Clin Nurs 21: 1716-1725.

13. Gawlinski A, Becker E (2012) Infusing research into practice: a staff nurse evidence-based practice fellowship program. J Nurses Staff Dev 28: 69-73.

14. Hauck S, Winsett RP, Kuric J (2013) Leadership facilitation strategies to establish evidence-based practice in an acute care hospital. J Adv Nurs 69: 664-674.

15. Schaffer MA, Sandau KE, Diedrick L (2013) Evidence-based practice models for organizational change: overview and practical applications. J Adv Nurs 69: 1197-1209.

16. Sredl D (2008) Evidence-based nursing practice: what US nurse executives really think. Nurse Res 15: 51-67.

17. Staffileno BA, Carlson E (2010) Providing direct care nurses research and evidence-based practice information: an essential component of nursing leadership. J Nurs Manag 18: 84-89.

18. Newhouse RP, Dearholt S, Poe S, Pugh LC, White KM (2007) Organizational change strategies for evidence-based practice. J Nurs Adm 37: 552-557.

19. Pipe TB, Cisar NS, Caruso E, Wellik KE (2008) Leadership strategies: inspiring evidence-based practice at the individual, unit, and organizational levels. J Nurs Care Qual 23: 265-271.

20. Johansson B, Fogelberg-Dahm M, Wadensten B (2010) Evidence-based practice: the importance of education and leadership. J Nurs Manag 18: 70-77.

21. Cullen L, Titler MG, Rempel G (2011) An advanced educational program promoting evidence-based practice. West J Nurs Res 33: 345-364.

22. Porter-O'Grady T, Malloch K (2008) Beyond myth and magic: the future of evidence-based leadership. Nurs Adm Q 32: 176-187.

23. Eneh VO, Vehviläinen-Julkunen K, Kvist T (2012) Nursing leadership practices as perceived by Finnish nursing staff: high ethics, less feedback and rewards. J Nurs Manag 20: 159-169.

24. Marshall DR (2008) Evidence-based management: the path to best outcomes. J Nurs Adm 38: 205-207.

25. Macphee M, Skelton-Green J, Bouthillette F, Suryaprakash N (2012) An empowerment framework for nursing leadership development: supporting evidence. J Adv Nurs 68: 159-169.

26. Ovaska T (2012) Making evidence-based decisions when organising information retrieval training for nurses and head nurses. Health Info Libr J 29: 252-256.

27. Wallen GR, Mitchell SA, Melnyk B, et al. (2010) Implementing evidence-based practice: effectiveness of a structured multifaceted mentorship programme. J Adv Nurs 66: 2761-71.

28. Adeniran RK, Bhattacharya A, Adeniran A (2012) Professional excellence and career advancement in nursing. A conceptual framework for clinical leadership development. Nursing Administration Quarterly 36: 41-51.

29. https://moodle.org/

30. Kvist T, Mäntynen R, Turunen H, Partanen P, Miettinen M, et al. (2013) How magnetic are Finnish hospitals measured by transformational leadership and empirical quality outcomes? J Nurs Manag 21: 152-164.

31. Burns N, Grove S.K (2009) The practice of nursing research. Appraisal, synthesis, and generation of evidence. 6th ed. Elsevier, St. Louis.

# 35

# The Burden of Care: Experiences of Parents of Children with Thalassemia

Batool Pouraboli[1], Heidar Ali Abedi[2*], Abbas Abbaszadeh[3] and Majid Kazemi[4]

[1]School of Nursing and Midwifery, Department of Pediatric and Neonatal Nursing, Tehran University of Medical Sciences, Tehran, Iran

[2]Department of Nursing, School of Nursing and Midwifery, Khorasgan (Isfahan) Branch, Islamic Azad University, Isfahan, Iran

[3]School of Nursing and Midwifery, Shahid beheshti University of Medical Sciences, Tehran, Iran

[4]School of Nursing and Midwifery, Rafsanjan University of Medical Sciences, Rafsanjan, Iran

*Corresponding author: Ali Abedi H, Professor of Nursing, Department of Nursing, School of Nursing and Midwifery, Khorasgan (Isfahan) Branch, Islamic Azad University, Isfahan, Iran, E-mail: drabediedu@yahoo.com

## Abstract

**Introduction:** Parents who care for Thalassemia children tolerate a great burden. Understanding these sufferings seems necessary in order to provide appropriate care. This study was aimed to explore the experiences of parents who have children with thalassemia.

**Method:** A qualitative approach was used to obtain rich data. Twenty-two parents were recruited purposefully from one charity clinic in South East of Iran. Semi-structured interviews were used. Data were analyzed by Lundman and Granheim's content analysis method.

**Results:** Data analysis led to form one main theme including "Parents' Burden of care". Within this theme the following categories created: immersion in suffering, stigma and social death, uncertainty about future, and absence of a support network.

**Conclusion:** The findings of this study showed that Caring for children with thalassemia have a significant impact on the lives of caregivers and alleviating caregivers' burden is critical to managing parents. This research may be useful in terms of increasing information about thalassemia and raising consciousness of nurses and other health care providers.

**Keywords:** Burden of care; Parents; Thalassemia; Qualitative study; Iran

## Introduction

Major thalassemia is a genetic disease. This defect may cause an abnormal development of red blood cells and ultimately anemia [1]. Furthermore Thalassemia is a common disorder worldwide with a predominant incidence in Mediterranean countries and Southeast Asia [2]. Approximately, 240 million people are estimated as carriers for β-thalassemia throughout the world while 100,000 children with thalassemia major are born annually [2]. In Iran the prevalence of thalassemia is approximately 3-4% in general population and there are over three million β -thalassemia carriers [3]. Almost 26,000 patients with major thalassemia and 800 infants with thalassemia are born annually in Iran [4].

Children living with β-thalassemia major need a life-long treatment of regular blood transfusions and iron chelation therapy [5], which cause major social and financial burdens on patients, families, and health care system [6]. According to Pillitteri thalassemia poses a remarkable impact on children's life; patients become anemic and thus physical activities are exhausting and intolerable for them. He added that the overstimulation of bone marrow leads children to manifest changes in their craniofacial features as well as delayed growth, osteoporotic tissue, ascites and enlarged liver and finally arrhythmias as well as death resulted from heart failure [5].

Parents suffer from weakness and disability of their ill child. They feel worried, frustrated, despaired and helpless [7]. Also they have numerous physical, psychosocial and financial sufferings [6,8] which are relatively connected to the chronic nature of the disease and strenuous treatments. Recognition the nature of parent's burden is curtailed because it enables nurses to intervene effectively and reduce parental burden [9]. During recent decades, there has been a substantial increasing concern and attention given to the phenomenon of suffering in healthcare literature [10,11]. Rodger et al. used the method of concept analysis and defined the concept of suffering as an individualized, subjective and complex experience [12]. Nahalla et al. in a phenomenological study showed the impact of regular hospitalization of children with thalassemia on their parents. Ten parents were interviewed. Three themes were used to present the participant's experience: worries, medical services, and helping and being helped [13]. Also, Prasomsuk et al. [6] in a qualitative study in Thailand explored the lived experiences of mothers of children with thalassemia major by conducting semi structured interviews. Six themes were identified including: lack of knowledge about thalassemia, psychosocial problems, and concerns for the future, social support systems deficiencies, financial difficulty, and effectiveness of healthcare services. Sapountzi et al. in Greece conducted a qualitative study on the experiences of mothers caring for their children with thalassemia and interviewed with 19 mothers that had children with thalassemia. Emotional distress, fear of death and difficulties in dealing with feelings were some of the mothers' concerns [14].

Iran is one of the countries with the high rate of thalassemia [4] where the parents play the key role in caring for their sick children [15]. They have to take care their sick child and perform other responsibilities for their professional, social and familial roles simultaneously. Since they have to spend more time for a sick child, the quality of their social, professional and familial roles may be greatly influenced by this issue [15]. Although above studies have investigated some dimensions of this disease on the parents. However culture and healthcare service system can have an influential impact on this experience. As a result, regarding the particular rules and culture of Iran, in this qualitative study, we addressed the question "what are the experiences of caregiver having a child with thalassemia?"

Qualitative content analysis is one of the methods of qualitative researches and also qualitative data analysis [16]. Content analysis method contains techniques for systematic text analysis [17] because it is an unobtrusive technique of analysis that can simply accommodate a great amount of data [18]. Thus, this approach could help understand the meaning of Living with suffering as voiced by parents of children with thalassemia. Moreover, a cultural-based understanding may help healthcare policy makers establish effective context-based interventions. This study was aimed to explore the experiences of parents who have children with thalassemia.

## Materials and Methods

### Study design and setting

This study was a conventional qualitative content analysis with a descriptive-explorative approach. Content analysis is a qualitative method for analyzing written, verbal or visual communication messages. The aim at Content analysis research is to attain a condensed and broad description of the phenomenon. According to Graneheim et al., content analysis can be performed with various degrees of interpretation. They added that in each text, there are manifest messages to be described and latent meanings to be interpreted, although both manifest messages and latent meanings require interpretations which may vary in depth and level of abstraction [19].

This qualitative study was conducted from March 2012 to September 2013 in Kerman, a south-eastern city in Iran. In Kerman, Kerman Province is located in southeast of Iran; with an area of 11% of the whole country and more than 2.5 million populations [20]. This province is among ten provinces in the country where incidences of thalassemia are high due to humid tropical climate of some regions of the province, high frequency of β-thalassemia Gene as well as numerous consanguineous marriages [21]. There is one educational charity hospital with thalassemia disease centers which are affiliated to Kerman University of Medical Sciences. The majority of children suffering from thalassemia who reside in the south-east of Iran are referred to this hospital.

### Participants

The main inclusion criterion was: parents who had a child diagnosed with thalassemia that required regular blood transfusions and experienced at least 1 year of caregiving their child.

The qualitative research interview was semi structured, participants were asked to narrate their experiences of caring from their child with thalassemia and related disease. As in qualitative researches, no absolute rules determine the estimated number of participants, sampling continued and data were saturated, until no new information

was extracted. In the present study, the saturation was achieved after interviewing with 22 participants. There were 11 mothers and 11 fathers in the study. Also each of the parents in the study has 1-3 children with thalassemia. Purposive sampling was used to select participants. To reach rich and divers information, individuals with different and rich experience about the research concept were invited to do the interviews. In addition, individuals with different characteristics such as age, role, and work experience were chosen by the first researcher to provide a wide range of information. The characteristics of the participants are shown in Table 1.

| Participant | Age (year) | Level of education | Experience of caring of children with thalassemia (year) | Job/relative to parents |
|---|---|---|---|---|
| Fathers | 37-46 | Uneducated: 2 | 2-18 | Pensioner: 1 |
| | | Diploma: 8 | | Employee:9 |
| | | B.A: 1 | | Teacher: 1 |
| Mothers | 37-45 | Uneducated:3 | 9-12 | Housewife: 8 |
| | | Diploma: 8 | | Employee: 3 |

**Table 1:** Characteristics of the participants (n=22).

### Data collection

Data were collected through semi-structured, face-to-face interviews. A nurse who was trained for deep interviews performed them (the first author). First, she introduced herself as a nurse and researcher and explained the research aims and the interview process for the parents. Then, she asked them if they were willing to participate, and then they signed a consent form. . In the cases the participant did not sign the consent form, it was read loudly and his/her permission was taken orally due to the cultural structure of Iran. Sometimes, the participant did not trust on giving an informed written consent. Afterwards, the suitable time and place for interview was determined for each participant based on her comfort. The interview was done in a room in thalassemia clinic. At the beginning of conversation, the interviewer explained the study aims and the benefits of the study and reminded the interviewee that they can withdraw the interview Session whenever they did not want to continue. Then, the primary questions were asked. For Example, "What is your perception of caring for your child?" And please describe your experience of one day of caring about your child." The interview was conducted using follow up questions such as: "Please tell me more about it", "How do you feel about them", "Please give me an example". Every interview lasted at least 20 and at most 60 min. All interviews were recorded with previous permission of participants. Also, the key points were written during the interview.

### Data analysis

The first author recorded, transcribed, and analyzed the audio responses verbatim, read the transcripts interviews repeatedly and allocated codes to recurrent themes. The MAXQDA 2007 software (VERBI GmbH, Berlin, and Germany) was used to manage and sort the coding. The analytical process was guided by qualitative content analysis, as described by Granheim and Lundman. Content analysis is initially interpretative; the narratives were read several times to obtain a comprehensive view of the attributes associated with a meaningful encounter. After that, words and sentences that applied to the attributes which were related by content and context were broken into meaning units without losing the content of the text, meaning units were condensed and labeled with codes at a low level of abstraction. After rereading and understanding the coded, they were sorted into preliminary categories representing similarities and differences. Finally, the preliminary categories were formulated as categories and subcategories according to the manifest content at a higher level of abstraction. During the analysis process, focus moved between the whole and parts of the text to ensure that interpretations were made at a high level of abstraction [19].

## Ethical considerations

The study was approved by the ethical center committee, in Medical Research at the Faculty of Nursing and Midwifery supervised by Kerman University of Medical Sciences (ethical code 91/93). All participants provided informed consent and some oral information was given to them including the goals and objectives of the study. They were assured of anonymity and confidentiality of the data. Also they were informed about their rights to withdraw from participation in the study at any time. Furthermore, they could refuse to answer any unfavorable question.

## Rigor

Trustworthiness is a criterion which constitutes rigor in qualitative researches. Usually four issues use to describe various aspect of trustworthiness: credibility, conformability, dependability, and transferability [19,22]. Several techniques were used to enhance trustworthiness of the following study. Peer checking has done by researcher's supervisors through frequent sessions between the first researcher and the supervisors, the study's progress and process was reported and discussed. Member-checking was completed with some of participants for validation of interpreted findings (codes and categories). Some of the faculty members checked the encoding process and access to categories (external checks). In addition, a clear and detailed description of culture, context, selection and characteristics of participants, data collection and process of analysis were provided. Interviews lasted between 35-60 min. The interviews were audio taped and then the transcripts were written out verbatim by the first author (B.P).

## Results

In total, 22 parents were interviewed: 11 mothers and 11 fathers. The age of the participants ranged from 37 to 46 years. Their level of education ranged from illiterate to bachelor and had different jobs. 8 mothers were housewives and 3 were full-time employees. 10 fathers were full-time employees and 1 was retired (Table 1).

According to data analysis, the main theme was "Parents Burden of care" was emerged. Through this theme, we created the following categories: 1- immersion in suffering, 2- stigma and social death, 3- uncertainty about future 4- absence of a support network.

## Immersion in suffering

The mothers faced multiple problems in care process. They endured a lot of sufferings. This category was extracted from the following subcategories: exhaustion with the past, tensions of caring, new-age sufferings, and concerns about transplant, psychological tension.

## Exhaustion with the past

Suffering of these parents has been started since the past; however, this suffering has continued and reformed. Parents complained about lack of pre-marital tests, preventive methods for birth of thalassemia children, and lack of diagnostic tests of thalassemia in the past. Some families blamed this factor for having three or four children with thalassemia. They complained about some difficulties including: spending extended periods of time due to lack of diagnostic facilities in the past, the untimely diagnosis of their child's disease and endured suffering of purchasing blood for required frequent transfusions as well as lack of desferal pump and medications. Due to these shortages, some patients received ineffective treatment because they forced to share one desferal pump with other siblings with thalassemia.

A father with two children with thalassemia said: *"I was always searching for someone to donate blood. I donated my own blood several times. Some soldiers were ready to sell their blood. I had to find them to pay for and purchase their blood. I myself had to take them to the blood transfusion center to receive their blood."*

Some patients who lived in remote districts had to commute frequently to receive treatments. In order to be close to an equipped center, they moved to another city and their problem was unfamiliarity with their residential place.

The father of two thalassemia boys (one of whom was dead) stated:

*"We forced to move in this city (Kerman). I remembered the terrible night when we arrived Kerman. We were chased by some stray dogs. I carried two of my children on my shoulders to get rid of those animals."*

## Caring tensions

Parents suffered from uncooperative of their thalassemia children for self-care for example non-cooperation of children with Deferoxamine injections. Some parents living in remote area lost their spouses in road accidents due to frequent commuting to an equipped center to provide treatment for their sick child. These participants stated that they had to follow-up treatments for their ill child lonely. They tolerated insomnia and fatigue due to the fortnightly journey to charity center for blood transfusions. Also parents stated that the child's treatment program interfered with their routine life and severely restricted parents' activities.

A father said: *"One of the most annoying days of the week is the day I come here. I miss a lot of my plan and have to take a day off to come here."*

Children's high iron levels (Hemosidrosis ), Defroxamine injections, insertion of IV lines and withdrawing blood, in addition to the potential complications of hepatitis C left parents distraught and exhausted during caring for these children.

A mother who cared for her two daughters and a son with hepatitis C stated:

*"I was hurting more than my ill children. Their disease stressed me a lot. Once they had fever I stayed awake all the night to care for them."*

In addition, the comparison of the child's growth with other children and having no answer to their childish questions about these differences was a heavy burden of parents.

A father stated: *"My child asks me why Mr. X's son is taller than me. Why has he grown more than me? Why do I have to receive frequent injections and my sister not? These questions really hurt me."*

Also parents were worrying about their children being called by 'offensive names' and teased by their peers for their shorter height.

A mother stated: *"Children at school bother my daughter and they call her MRS.PEPPERPOT."*

## New-age sufferings

The history of having a thalassemia child imposed pregnant mothers to great stress of amniocentesis and possible mandatory abortion. A positive result of a thalassemia test in a pregnant mother reminded them bitter memories of the operating room, abortion and surgical complications. In some cases, the false answer led to the birth of a child with thalassemia. Also lack of technology required patients to travel to Tehran to receive services such as T2 star Magnetic resonance Imagine that is a new device for assessment Iron in heart and liver and a fully equipped laboratory with polymerase chain reaction (PCR) tests that is a laboratory test for detecting hepatitis in thalassemia patients in their province.

The mother of two daughters and one son with thalassemia and hepatitis C (they should do a test for hepatitis C due to effective treatment) stated:*"Their treatment will be finished here but I have to carry them to Tehran for Echo and laboratory tests. It is very difficult for me, I always think about it and I cannot sleep at night."*

## Concerns about transplant

Parents sought for certain treatment of their children's diseases that is transplant of stem cells. At first, the donor of stem cells should be searched for. In addition, it is not possible in small cities and patients should refer to an equipped center. Therefore, lack of a bone marrow transplantation center in their province, lack of a suitable donor and unaffordable expenses concerned parents.

A father said: *"The most important challenge is that I only think about my child's health and I try my best to treat him/her even if I die in direction of my goals. I will sell all my properties and spend them for his/her treatment (even for transplant)."*

A parent stated:*"The biggest suffering is that, since foundation of this charity clinic in 1998, a transplantation center has not been established in the province."*

## Psychological tension

Parents suffered psychological tensions due to the difficulties of caring for the thalassemic child. They stated that they were distressed and grieved to see their upset child. Also, they expressed concern about birth of next children with thalassemia too. Furthermore, parents narrate their experiences of receiving abrupt diagnosis of thalassemia, which caused despair, sadness and they did not believe their child disease. A father of two children with thalassemia stated: *"When we were informed about our children disease, we were distraught and disheartened. Our life became bitter."*

The next reaction of parents was denial; disbelief in the diagnosis which led them to change medical team or hospital. One father living in a village near to Jiroft (a city in Southern Kerman) said: *"After receiving the thalassemia test result, Dr. F informed us about our child diagnosis. We went to Jiroft to confirm the result by another doctor. We could not trust him too; therefore, we went to Kerman."*

Parents believed that the diagnosis of thalassemia for their child impacted their mental and emotional status, family relationship as well as love and affection between couples. Fearing from birth of a thalassemia child, some of the mothers underwent tubal ligations surgery which led to separation and divorce in a number of families.

One of the fathers stated: *"We liked to have at least four children. With this happening, we do not want any more children. This matter bothered us and family problems appeared. This was not the woman I used to love. My love for this child is gone."*

## Stigma and social death

This category was extracted from three subcategories: 1- poverty of the society, 2- concealment, 3- censure.

## Cultural poverty of society

Parents suffered from cultural poverty, misconception and lack of knowledge and insufficient information about the disease in the society. A father said:

*"People treat unwisely. They talk about my child disease unfairly when they speak together.*

*The false beliefs and superstitions about thalassemia also troubled parents."* A parent stated that:

*"People stigmatize us. Unfortunately, that is how they perceive thalassemia and blame this disease.*

## Concealment

In order to escape from other people's reproach, a number of parents followed their child treatments and care secretly which annoyed them. One of the interviewed mothers who concealed her child's disease expressed:

*"I swear to God, that we annoy of secret living. We are scared of our own shadow. We cannot tell anyone; therefore, we have to do everything alone". On the other hand, more parents worried about their child's marriage which causes them to reveal their child disease. A mother said: "some men proposed marriage to my daughter but I had to refuse. I'm worried and this bothers me."*

## Censure

Censure was another reaction experienced by participants, in verbal or non-verbal forms (a blaming look). Despite some parents were bothered by their relatives' reproach, they had to ignore their behavior, suffer or terminate the relationship with these relatives. A mother of two daughters with thalassemia said:

*"Everybody reproaches us, including relatives and strangers. They allow themselves to talk about our child disease in an unfair and unreasonable manner. Well, it's a small town and the news spreads quickly. Thus it is not wondering if a mother is hurt by these behaviors."* Another father described people's reproach:

*"I married to a non-relative woman and my relatives blamed me for it. They believe that my child disease is a consequence of my marriage and my suffering is a punishment and torture from God".*

## Uncertainty about future

Uncertainty about their children future, job prospects of children, education of children, marriage of children, and definite treatment of their children caused another stress. A father of two children with thalassemia whose daughter was attending the university this year expressed his concerns: *"We worry about their future and their work prospects. "Can they get a job? Will they be able to manage themselves? I have butterfly in my stomach"*

## Absence of a support system

Participants complained about lack of effective management of thalassemia. High expenses of treatments transportation and hospitalization, besides the living costs imposed a heavy burden for families. They mentioned some deficiencies in health care system such as lack of expertise among the medical team, absence of an equipped team and lack of experienced nurses in IV (intra venous) lines administration. A father said:

*"There is effective management for all diseases except this disease; there is no stable management. It is annoying when you realize no one cares about this disease".*

In spite of free medical treatments for thalassemia, most interviewees complained of the financial treatment costs of thalassemia. Financial burden of expensive costs of the disease caused economic consequences on families which they could no longer afford it. Most parents considered these as the most important suffering. This includes the cost of transportation, accommodation, and child's hospitalization. A father stated:

*"Our main problem is financial costs and that's all.' One of the fathers whose child took iron chelating pills said: "I like to buy "Exjade" pill manufactured in foreign countries for my child to stop more nausea and vomiting caused by Iranian pills, but I can't afford it. This is really bothering."*

Parents complained about medication shortage and lack of insurance support. Due to recent sanctions in Iran, providing Deferoxamine and Exjade is difficult and this torments parents.

A father said:

*"To provide pills we have to search everywhere. But they are not easily available and this is so distressing."*

## Discussion

In this study, the parents considered their care experiences of children with thalassemia. The

Burden of the child care by parents was found as the main theme of this study.

According to the findings, four categories for the main theme were found: immersion in suffering, - stigma and social death, uncertainty about future, absence of a support network.

All categories existed in their experiences of parents. In this part, the scientific documentations on the significance of codes are explained. Although there were few qualitative studies, it was tried to use both quantitative and qualitative literature.

## Immersion in suffering

One of significant results of this study was difficulties that participants buckled with and did not forget their unpleasant memories during the years. These difficulties profoundly impact their mental and physical conditions. This finding is agreed with the study of Pouraboli et al. that revealed lack of social support and health insurance, lack of a regular program for thalassemia treatment and lack of fixed custodians were the most burdens of participants [3]. However, in a study conducted in Italy, the authors reported extremely lower difficulties faced by parents of thalassemia children [23]. These differences could be associated to the lower incidence rate of this disease in such countries resulting in a better well-being and effective management of the disease. Also, this discrepancy may be related to cultural differences and different social attitudes toward this disease in western countries compared to Iranian context. Fortunately, recent requirements of thalassemia patients and their families have taken more concentration than before with cooperation of non-governmental organizations and charities.

In the current study, participants reported suffering when comparing their child's physical features with healthy children; furthermore they were tormented by questions asked by their ill child. This result is in agreement with findings of a study conducted by Wahab et al., which stated that not attaining the average height compared to their peers was perceived as a major problem by both parents and patients. Also, patients were being called by 'nick names' and teased by their peers for their shorter stature. Participants in their study reported that these children were compared to other siblings at home regarding their height and thus they were not respected by younger siblings [24].

According to the findings of the following study, interviewees experienced great psychological tensions and emotional distress caused by thalassemia and its treatment. In a similar study conducted by Åstedt-Kurki et al., they reported various emotional symptoms and feelings of shock induced by illness of a family member in 50% of cases; negative psychological symptoms such as depression and grief were reported in 71% of families [25]. Widayanti stated that parents of children with thalassemia suffer tremendously from provision of daily life-long care for their child [26]. Also Mashayekhi et al. reported that psychological problems annoyed families more than other problems [27]. Also Liem et al. reported feelings of concern and despair experienced by these parents [28]. Despite numerous psychological problem experienced by parents unfortunately effective psychosocial consulting services which lead to a healthy mind and sense of well-being, are not available properly for these parents in the context. Furthermore, the important role of psychologists and assistance of psychiatric nurses has not been considered in identifying and resolving such problems.

In this study, parents also reported that they were angry and shocked when being informed about their child diagnosis. They felt guilty. This finding is in congruent with the other studies which reported that parents described the shock of being informed about their child's disease and reluctantly accepted the diagnosis of disease and sought the possibility of misdiagnosis [15,29].

Insomnia and fatigue reported by parents as caregivers also are confirmed by other studies. Mashayekhi et al. reported that families had experienced Insomnia and fatigue more than other problems [27].

## Stigma and social death

Concealment and censure reported by interviewees were other significant findings of the present study which both are rooted in cultural beliefs, stigma and inadequate knowledge about thalassemia in the society. In a similar research, Furness et al. reported people's comments and verbal taunts as one of the parents suffering [30]. According to Pouraboli et al., in Iran patients with thalassemia conceal their illness as a result of stigma [3]. Also In the study by Shum et al., participants also considered thalassemia as a reason for shame and stigma leading to social isolation and reduction of their communications [31]. In study of Else et al breast cancer patients had experienced shame and stigma [32] however, in a study conducted in Greece acceptance of these patients by the society was reported [23]. The reason for this difference may be related to lack of knowledge and favorable attitude toward this illness which result in lack of a social position and poor acceptance of these patients by the society.

Also according to the results, interviewees experienced stigma. This finding is disagreed with the finding of Wahab et al.'s study in which stigma is not mentioned by participants [33]. Chenard stated that Stigma is a socially constructed concept that identifies a person or social group that has aberrance from some norms, ideals, or expectations. He goes on that Stigmatized persons are viewed negatively for having violated certain rules or for possessing traits that are negative or socially devalued [34]. According to Chenard, stigmatized persons to preserve themselves from the shame, embarrassment, blame, and social rejection, consistently struggle with the decision of whether to conceal or disclose their stigmatizing attributes [35].

In the following study all mothers wished their children to be accepted and treated normally by others. This will not cause stigmatization and social isolation associated with a chronic disease like thalassemia. False beliefs in Iranian Culture are main reason of related problems. This challenge may be overcome through educating people in order to change the society misconception.

Based on the results, parents suffered from uncooperative children under medical care which was in congruent with the study conducted by Wahab et al. The authors reported that parents complained about non-cooperative children with deferoxamine injections, which was attributed to the presence of rashes at the injection site [33]. Patients with thalassemia major must receive at least 150-350 mL of packed red cells every two or four weeks. Although blood transfusion is lifesaving, it causes painful IV line insertion and loads body with excess iron. Iron accumulation eventually may result in hemosiderosis and its associated complications [36]. Prognosis for survival will be greatly improved if the serum ferritin level is kept below 2,000 m g/L by regular chelation by deferoxamine (DFO) [37]. However to achieve a satisfactory result, DFO has to be administered via painful subcutaneous infusions, for 8-10 hours each day and five to seven days a week [36].

## Uncertainty about future

Participants also revealed their uncertainty about the future of their children. Marriage and employment were major concerns reported by participants. All participants hoped for their children to get married, continue education, find a job and become independent in future. Parents in Previous studies have similar concerns about their children [27,33] Concern about children's marriages was not reported in some studies conducted in other countries [10] . This concern reflects the importance of marriage in the Iranian/Islamic culture. In this respect,

people's perspective toward thalassemia patients' marriage should be changed through educating and informing via mass media. However, in recent years more attention has paid to marriage of these patients. The health care system accompanied by some charities support them by paying the cost of their wedding celebration, housing and furniture. Therefore marriage of two thalassemia patients or even marriage of a patient with a non-thalassemia person has increased.

## Absence of a support system

Absence of a support system was among the most important concerns stated by interviewees which are in disagreement with mothers' statements reported in Shosha's research. They appreciated the support given by their neighbors, friends, and teachers. Moreover, Shosha reported psychosocial support provided by physicians and nurses which was vital to alleviate the suffering of mothers and their children [10]. This supportive behavior was not reported by parents in the following research. Despite available psychosocial support and services for patients with thalassemia in recent years in the Iranian context, some parents' needs are ignored to a large extent. Some services have offered by health care system, non-governmental organizations and charities, but mostly are focused on patients welfare including: providing these patients with some pilgrimage and recreational trips, performing some celebrations in some special days such as thalassemia day in May 8, dedicating some foods, clothes, stationery and toys. Lack of supportive behaviors in health care and lack of a holistic care system for families may reflect many challenges that require effective strategies to be overcome in the Iranian context

Finally, financial issues were another major concern that participants expressed. High expenses of treatments, transportation and hospitalization, besides the living costs imposed a heavy burden for families. Previous studies found similar findings [6,33,38]. According to Sattari et al., the cost of therapy in thalassemia as well as any other disease does not only include medication cost. They stated that these extra costs include the cost of medical consultation, laboratory tests, diagnostic tests, cost of treatments, side effects of therapies and many other indirect costs. They added that indirect costs include travel expenses, the impairment of well-being. Concerning high costs of this disease as well as poor economic condition of most thalassemia patients in this region of the country, effective strategies are required to reduce the financial burden [39]. More financial support and favorable insurance should be considered by national health care policy makers and administrators. Additionally, The Iranian Ministry of Health should continue supporting free treatment for thalassemia patients. Sattari et al. stated that almost all medications in Iran are subsidized by the government and a small fraction of the total cost of treatment/care is paid by the patients such as iron chelating therapies in thalassemia treatment. Also they added there is insurance coverage for these patients. Despite coverage of most costs of therapy, parts of the cost are not paid by the government or the insurance companies and are paid by the patients themselves [39]. Also overcoming this challenge is required charity and non-governmental organizations support because the numerous expenses of this disease burden significant financial load to the health care system annually. According to Habibzadeh et al., about 350,000 blood bags are needed annually for thalassemia patients costing about US $3 apiece. This is equal to US $1,000,000 per year. Also DFO is an expensive drug, and US $40,000,000 should be spent annually to provide the adequate amount for thalassemics in Iran [21].

## Limitations of the Study

Despite the strategies we applied to enhance the rigor of this study, some limitations may be inherent. The sample size was small and the context confined to a particular geographic location. However, the study provides some valuable insights for the parents suffering from children with Thalassemia. But we believe that these findings would support further research of wider scope. The findings of this study can be generalized to other mothers, families and special professional in health services.

## Conclusion

According to the findings of this study, parents of children with thalassemia face many problems when caring their child. Results of this study showed that some parents manage their problems alone. Also, deep cognition of parents' needs was obtained considering the experiences of parents. Thus, it is necessary that health provider provides support and education by appropriate planning. Nurses are recommended to help these parents by appropriate interventions. Training life skills to them can be very helpful in reducing the severe difficulties imposed on these parents in Iran. Furthermore, it is helpful to determine the parents' burden of care to improve the family function.

## Acknowledgement

Special thanks to all parents who took part in this study. This study was undertaken in part fulfillment of the degree of nursing doctoral by the first author.

## References

1. Mazzone L, Battaglia L, Andreozzi F, Romeo MA, Mazzone D (2009) Emotional impact in ß-thalassaemia major children following cognitive-behavioural family therapy and quality of life of caregiving mothers. Clin Pract Epidemiol Ment Health 5: 5.

2. Bala J, Sarin J (2014) Empowering parents of children with thalassemia. Int J Nurs Care 2: 22-25.

3. Pouraboli B, Abedi HA, Abbaszadeh A, Kazemi M (2015) Living in a misty marsh: A qualitative study on the experiences of self-care suffering of patients with thalassemia. Iran J Nurs Midwifery Res 19: 77-82.

4. Moridi GVS, Khaled's, Khiladi S, Fathi M, Shafiian M (2012) Quality of life compared to healthy children and thalassemic. Journal of Pajoohesh Parastari 1: 675-684.

5. Pillitteri A (2010) Maternal and child health nursing: Care of the childbearing and childrearing family: Lippincott Williams and Wilkins.

6. Prasomsuk S, Jetsrisuparp A, Ratanasiri T, Ratanasiri A (2007) Lived experiences of mothers caring for children with thalassemia major in Thailand. J Spec Pediatr Nurs 12: 13-23.

7. Ammad SA, Mubeen SM, Shah S, Mansoor S (2011) Parents' opinion of quality of life (QOL) in Pakistani thalassaemic children. J Pak Med Assoc 61: 470.

8. Ali S, Sabih F, Jehan S, Anwar M, Javed S (2012) Psychological distress and coping strategies among parents of beta-thalassemia major patients. Int Proc Chem Biol Environ Eng 27: 124-128.

9. Mg (2009) Significant effect of group therapy on life expectancy, education and public health in female patients with thalassemia. J Appl Psychol 42:25-45.

10. Shosha GMA (2014) Needs and concerns of Jordanian mothers with thalassemic children: A qualitative study. J Am Sci 10.

11. Barton-Burke M, Barreto Jr RC, Archibald LI (2008) Suffering as a multicultural cancer experience. Semin Oncol Nurs 24:229-236.

12. Rodgers BL, Cowles KV (1997) A conceptual foundation for human suffering in nursing care and research. J Adv Nurs 25: 1048-1053.

13. Nahalla CK, FitzGerald M (2003) The impact of regular hospitalization of children living with thalassaemia on their parents in Sri Lanka: A phenomenological study. Int J Nurs Pract 9: 131-139.

14. Sapountzi-Krepia D, Roupa Z, Gourni M, Mastorakou F, Vojiatzi E, et al. (2006) A qualitative study on the experiences of mothers caring for their children with thalassemia in Athens, Greece. J Pediatr Nurs 21: 142-152.

15. Sabzevari S, Nematollahi M, Mirzaei T, Ravari A (2016) The burden of care: Mothers' experiences of children with congenital heart disease. Int J Commun Based Nurs Midwifery 4: 374-385.

16. Thyme KE, Wiberg B, Lundman B, Graneheim UH (2013) Qualitative content analysis in art psychotherapy research: Concepts, procedures, and measures to reveal the latent meaning in pictures and the words attached to the pictures. Arts Psychother 40: 101-107.

17. Vaismoradi M, Turunen H, Bondas T (2013) Content analysis and thematic analysis: Implications for conducting a qualitative descriptive study. Nurs Health Sci 15: 398-405.

18. Molavi Vardanjani H, Baneshi MR, Haghdoost A (2015) Cancer visibility among Iranian familial networks: To what extent can we Rely on family history reports? PloS ONE 10: e0136038.

19. Graneheim UH, Lundman B (2004) Qualitative content analysis in nursing research: Concepts, procedures and measures to achieve trustworthiness. Nurse Educ Today 24: 105-112.

20. Nayeri ND, Dehghan M, Iranmanesh S (2015) Being as an iceberg: Hypertensive treatment adherence experiences in southeast of Iran. Global Health Action 8: 28814.

21. Habibzadeh F, Yadollahie M, Merat A, Haghshenas M (1998) Thalassemia in Iran; an overview. Arch Irn Med 1: 27-33.

22. Lam KK, Hung SYM (2013) Perceptions of emergency nurses during the human swine influenza outbreak: A qualitative study. Int Emerg Nurs 21: 240-246.

23. Shum Sk (2002) Living with thalassemia major: The process of adjustment: The University of Hong Kong (Pokfulam, Hong Kong).

24. Melzack R, Bentley KC (1983) Relief of dental pain by ice massage of either hand or the contralateral arm. Journal (Canadian Dental Association) 49: 257-260.

25. Åstedt-Kurki P, Paunonen M, Lehti K (1997) Family members' experiences of their role in a hospital: a pilot study. J Adv Nurs 25: 908-914.

26. Widayanti CG (2011) The perceived role of god in health and illness: The experience of Javanese mothers caring for a child with thalassemia. Jurnal Psikologi Undip 9:50-56.

27. Mashayekhi F, Rafati S, Rafati F, Pilehvarzadeh M, Mohammadi-Sardo M (2014) A study of caregiver burden in mothers with thalassemia children in Jiroft, 2013. Modern Care Journal 11: 229-235.

28. Liem RI, Gilgour B, Pelligra SA, Mason M, Thompson AA (2011) The impact of thalassemia on southeast Asian and Asian Indian families in the United States: A qualitative study. Childhood 11:12.

29. Yeh CH (2003) Dynamic coping behaviors and process of parental response to child's cancer. Appl Nurs Res 16: 245-255.

30. Furness P, Garrud P, Faulder A, Swift J (2006) Coming to terms a grounded theory of adaptation to facial surgery in adulthood. J Health Psychol 11: 453-66.

31. Melzack R, Guité S, Gonshor A (1980) Relief of dental pain by ice massage of the hand. Can Med Assoc J 122: 189-191.

32. Else-Quest NM, LoConte NK, Schiller JH, Hyde JS (2009) Perceived stigma, self-blame and adjustment among lung, breast and prostate cancer patients. Psychol Health 24: 949-964.

33. Wahab IA, Naznin M, Nora MZ, Suzanah AR, Zulaiho M, et al. (2011) Thalassaemia: A study on the perception of patients and family members. Med J Malaysia 66: 326-334.

34. Robinson TE, Berridge KC (2000) The psychology and neurobiology of addiction: An incentive-sensitization view. Addiction 95: S91-117.

35. Chenard C (2007) The impact of stigma on the self-care behaviors of HIV-positive gay men striving for normalcy. J Assoc Nurses AIDS Care 18: 23-32.

36. Moradi G, Ghaderi E (2013) Chronic disease program in Iran: Thalassemia control program. Chronic Dis J 1: 98-106.

37. Pouraboli B, Abedi HA, Abbaszadeh A, Kazemi M (2014) Living in a misty marsh: A qualitative study on the experiences of self-care suffering of patients with thalassemia. Iran J Nurs Midwifery Res 19: S77-82.

38. Medway M, Tong A, Craig JC, Kim S, Mackie F, et al. Parental perspectives on the financial impact of caring for a child with CKD. Am J Kidney Dis 65: 384-393.

39. Sattari M, Sheykhi D, Nikanfar A, Pourfeiz A, Nazari M, et al. (2012) The financial and social impact of thalassemia and its treatment in Iran. Pharmaceutical Sciences 18: 171-176.

# 36

# Experiences of Healing Yoga among Breast Cancer Women with Adjuvant Chemotherapy

**Hsiao-Yun Chang\*, Shu-Ming Chen and Wen-Li Lin**

*Department of Nursing, Fooyin University, Taiwan*

\***Corresponding author:** Chang HY, Department of Nursing, Fooyin University, Taiwan. E-mail: FT045@fy.edu.tw

## Abstract

**Objective:** To illustrate the experiences and perceived benefits of healing yoga as described by patients with breast cancer participating in a healing yoga program.

**Methods:** The qualitative research with naturalistic design was conducted after the completion of an 8 weeks healing yoga program. A total of 11 breast cancer women with adjuvant chemotherapy were interviewed using the semi-structured interview guidelines.

**Findings:** Participants expressed their experiences of healing yoga, including transforming concern to confidence, regaining a sense of belonging, gaining experience and satisfaction, and leading the way for life, were critical in developing these benefits. The perceived benefits of participating in this program was described as positive mental support, promoted a mind-body interaction and provided benefits ascribed to social activities, leading to a reported increase in active participation in life.

**Conclusion:** This study gives support for the positive experiences of healing yoga among patients with a breast cancer. The objective effect of the healing yoga must be examined further to guide nurses in implementing suitable health promotional strategies for breast cancer patients.

**Keywords:** Healing yoga; Breast cancer; Qualitative research; Adjuvant chemotherapy

## Introduction

Breast cancer is the most common cancer worldwide in women. Nearly 1.7 million women were diagnosed with breast cancer in 2015, and this number is expected to increase rapidly because of more than 25% the incidence rate which can become a major concern in health care systems [1]. Patients with breast cancer are typically treated using surgery followed by chemotherapy which is the most popular method used to treat breast cancer. The types of chemotherapy for breast cancer include CMF (cyclophosphamide, methotrexate, fluorouracil), FAC (fluorouracil, doxorubicin, cyclophosphamide), FEC (fluorouracil, epirubicin, cyclophosphamide) and TAC (docetaxel, doxorubicin, cyclophosphamide) [2]. However, the side effects of chemotherapy often cause psychosocial distress and physical discomfort [3]. Conditions induced by chemotherapy include nausea, vomiting, diarrhoea, loss of appetite, and bone marrow inhibition, which substantially affect the quality of life of patients if not alleviated [4]. In addition, previous studies have indicated that 40%–100% of breast cancer patients experienced psychological distress such as anxiety, general unhappiness negative thoughts, physical problems, fatigue and depression when undergoing chemotherapy [5-7]. Intervention targeting psychological distress is of great importance for patient with breast cancer who undergoing chemotherapy.

Multiple studies provided mechanisms on the vast on the vast mental health and physical benefits associated with yoga among healthy population8-10. The mechanisms behind this improvement are often a result of changes in the electrical activity of neurons within the brain which stimulating the activation of alpha, beta, and theta brainwave. Alpha ($\alpha$) waves in associated with calmness can be increased after breathing, meditation, and asana-based yoga practice, beta waves in associated with task performance to be improved in frequency and amplitude during and after mainly breathing based yoga and theta ($\theta$) wave in associated with repetitive tasks and autonomy to be increased in asana and breathing based yoga practice [8-10]. Healing yoga can also generate controlled high-frequency gamma waves which is associated with intelligence, compassion, self-control and feelings of happiness in result of decrease psychosocial distress [9,11]. In addition to brain activation, healing yoga can lower morning and 5 p.m. salivary cortisol and improved emotional well-being and fatigue in breast cancer survivors [12].

Understanding the mechanisms behind the healing yoga within the brain can lead to better knowledge of a constructive effect on the anatomy of the brain from healing yoga. Using a randomized controlled trial to examine the effect of healing yoga on improving depression, anxiety and fatigue of breast cancer women have been undertaken [13]; however, qualitative research to explore the benefits of healing yoga among patients with breast cancer remains unclear. What can elicit changes in individual that are occurring psychological benefits, can give insight into the development of interventions in patients with breast cancer as well as both healthy and clinical populations. Therefore, the purpose of this qualitative study is to illustrate participants' perceived benefits and experiences of healing yoga following the completion of participating the experimental study.

## Methods

### Design

This study reported exploratory findings from one substantial section of the experimental study [13] examining the perceptions and experience of patients participating in healing yoga. The qualitative research approach undertaken in this study was a form of naturalistic inquiry. The aim of this approach is to understand how people make meaning of naturally occurring situation or phenomena within a real-world setting [14]. This study involved interview guide with participants who were interested in contributing their perceived benefits and experiences of healing yoga.

### Study sample and recruitment

Researchers used a purposive sampling technique to recruit participants from the first phase study (n=30) of a randomized controlled trial on the efficacy of healing yoga for women with breast cancer at the hospital in the Southern of Taiwan. The authors targeted participants who would be able to offer valuable descriptions of the phenomena being studied. The participants were required to (a) be breast cancer patients who completed an 8 weeks healing yoga

program; (b) be able to provide informed consent. All of the participants received medical clearance before joining the group. At the end of the follow-up questionnaire, participants from the intervention group were asking if the she was willing to participate in a qualitative interview regarding their experiences and signed the consent form. All 30 participants in the healing yoga intervention been asked to enter into the qualitative study and 11 gave a consent to participate. The Institutional Review Board of Chi Mei Medical Center approved this study (No. 09912-L01).

### Intervention-healing yoga

All participants were from the experimental group who not only received the standard care, but also participated 60 min healing yoga, twice a week for 8 weeks. A team of yoga instructors and rehabilitation teachers designed a healing yoga followed the principle of healing yoga for people living with cancer written by Holtby [15]. The exercise cycled through three segments including (a) 10 min of meditation and breathing exercises that focused participant attention on breathing and on internal body sensations; (b) 40 min of healing yoga with a series of 10 modified *Asana* yoga composed of gentle stretching and strengthening exercises targeting specific groups of muscle, tendons, and ligaments; and (c) 10 min of cool-down exercises (Table 1).

| Segments | Activities |
|---|---|
| Meditation for 10 min | Accomplished Pose (Siddhasana) |
| | 1. Meditation (Dhyana) for determination of a part of the body and internalization of being-for-self. |
| | 2. Yoga breathing (Pranayama) for controlling the breath and internalize body sensations. |
| yoga exercises for 40 min | Legs Up the Wall Pose (Viparita Karani) |
| | A series of modified yoga asana : |
| | 1. Mountain Pose (Tadasana) |
| | 2. Tree Pose (Vrksasana) |
| | 3. Pelvic Tilts Pose (Setu Bandha Sarvangasana) |
| | 4. Cobra Pose (Bhujangasana) |
| | 5. Yawning Dog Pose (Adho Mukha Svanasana) |
| | 6. Resting Child Pose (Balasana) |
| | 7. Pigeon Pose (Eka Pada Rajakapotasana) |
| | 8. Fire Log Pose (Agnistambhasana) |
| | 9. Supported Forward Fold (Uttanasana) |
| | 10. Repose Pose (Pranayama) |
| Relaxation for 10 min | Resting Pose (Shavasana) for relaxation |
| | Restorative yoga pose for ending |

**Table 1:** The Segments and activities of intervention for breast cancer patients.

### Interviews

Those who agreed to participate in the study were conducted in a private room at the medical teaching hospital following the final activity session of program and were asked about their experiences of

participating in the healing yoga. Each focus group interviews usually last about 90 min. All interviews were done by one of the study coordinators not involved with the group intervention. Participants were asked the following questions: *"How was your previous experience with a healing yoga or similar practiced during the program?"; "What were your expectations from this exercise and what extent were they met?"; "What have you learned from this program?"; "What have you experienced any adverse reaction to this program?"; "How did this program affect your life now and in the future?"* The interviews were terminated when thematic saturation was achieved – new interviews producing no new significant themes resulting in 11 participants.

## Data analysis

All of the audio records were transcribed into written documentation. Two researchers independently transcribed recordings verbatim and thematically analyzed the recordings inductively. The content analysis methods were used by first coding each individual interview and then by comparing the interviews. This involved coding at the sentence level, developing categories and overarching themes. Discrepancies between the two researchers were discussed and a consensus was attained. The final themes were compared with those of the participants and the confirmed notes taken during the interview, and these themes were discussed with the members of the research team to identify implicit assumptions, plus an outsider invited as an independent reviewer, verified the validity and reliability of the analysis. We discussed the meanings of emerging themes until agreement was reached.

## Results

### Demographic information

This article is based on data from the participants in the intervention group who agreed to participate in a qualitative interview after the intervention. All of the participants were receiving chemotherapy (n=11) (Table 2). Of these patients, mean age was 46.55 years (range: 26-70 years). Most of the participants were married (n=9, 82%), had a college education (n=8, 73%), were Buddhist (n=6, 55%) and were employed (n=6, 55%) at the beginning of the study. Most of the participants were in stages II (n=4, 36%) and III (n=4, 36%) of breast cancer; only 3 participants were in stage I (n=3, 28%). The types of chemotherapy received by participants were: 4 in CMF (37%), 3 in CAF (27%), 2 in CMF (18%) and 2 in FEC (18%). The chemotherapy is usually given in cycles following by a period of rest and each course of chemotherapy generally consists of six cycles lasting for half year.

| characteristics | n=11 | % |
|---|---|---|
| **Age** | | |
| 20-40 | 3 | 27 |
| 41-60 | 7 | 64 |
| 61-70 | 1 | 9 |
| **Educational levels** | | |
| Junior school | 1 | 9 |
| High school | 2 | 18 |
| College | 8 | 73 |
| **Religious** | | |
| Buddhism | 6 | 55 |
| Christian | 2 | 18 |
| Not religious | 3 | 27 |
| **Marital status** | | |
| Single | 2 | 18 |
| Married | 9 | 82 |
| **Occupational status** | | |
| Employed | 6 | 55 |
| Unemployed | 5 | 45 |
| **Cancer status** | | |
| Stage I | 3 | 28 |
| Stage II | 4 | 36 |
| Stage III | 4 | 36 |
| **Chemotherapy regimen** | | |
| TAC | 4 | 37 |
| FAC | 3 | 27 |
| CMF | 2 | 18 |
| FEC | 2 | 18 |
| **The adherence rate of yoga exercise among participants with a month post-surgery** | | |
| Yes | 10 | 90 |
| No | 1 | 10 |

**Table 2:** Demography characteristics of patients with breast cancer, TAC: Docetaxel/Doxorubicin/Cyclophosphamide; FAC: Fluorouracil, Doxorubicin, Cyclophosphamide; CMF: Cyclophosphamide, Methotrexate, Fluorouracil; FEC: Fluorouracil, Epirubicin, Cyclophosphamide.

### Themes

After the creation of a codebook based on the research questions, researchers identified relevant paraphrase, reduced and summarized of the data and four main themes with 13 subthemes were developed in the following sections which were substantiated among the participants through member checks (Figure 1).

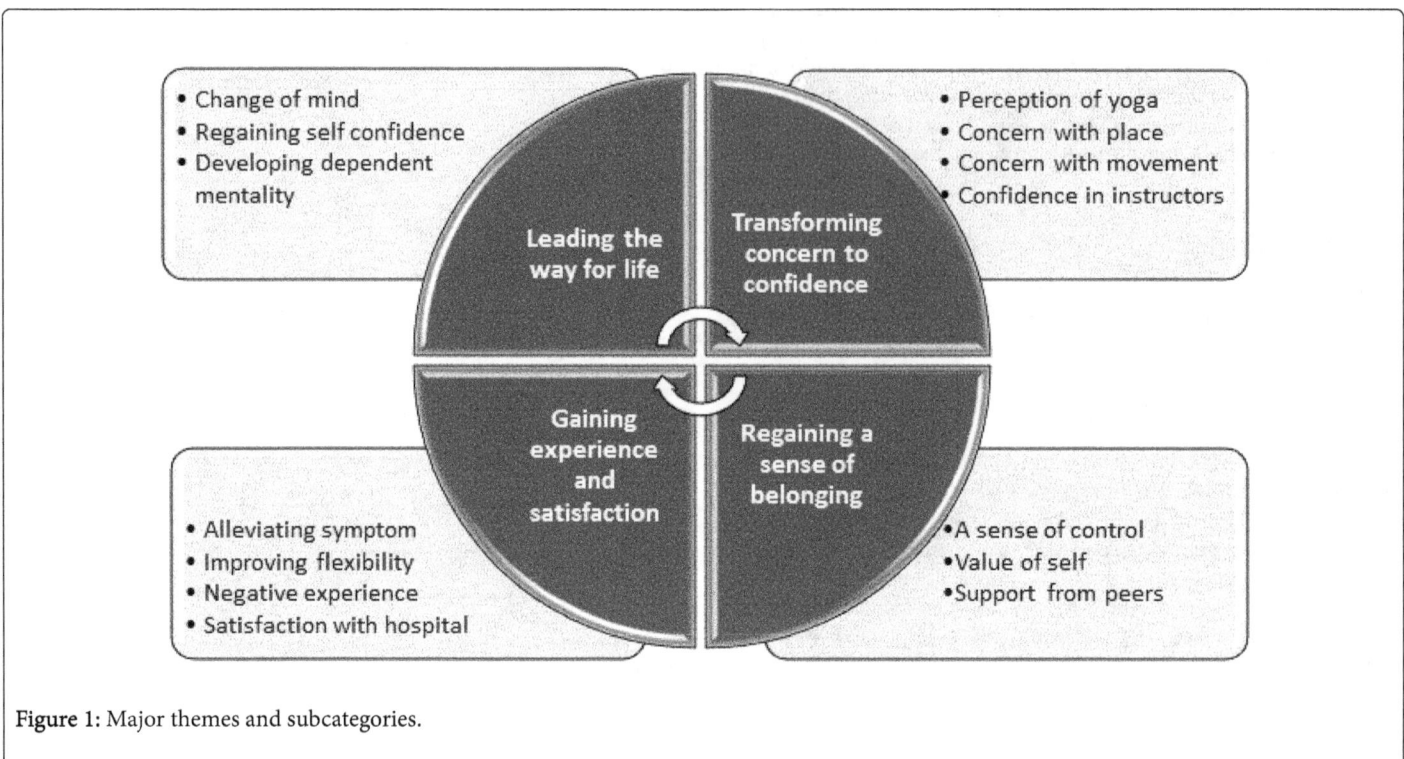

**Figure 1:** Major themes and subcategories.

### Transforming concern to confidence

Before the participants participated in the healing yoga, their perception of yoga was ambivalent and they were concerned that healing yoga would result in postsurgical injuries to the limbs on the side on which they were operated or other uncertain effects. These concerns included fears of training sites, yoga movements and instructors. Several participants who had no yoga experience expressed stereotypical perceptions of healing yoga and stated, *"I always thought yoga was for older people because I felt that the exercise is not strenuous enough"* (Participant H). They believed that healing yoga does not yield substantial health benefits. Another concern was the safety and appropriateness of the learning sites. Participant D said, *"To be honest, I'm afraid that the place (learning site) I find will be inappropriate, and that I might injure myself during yoga practice."* Most of the participants wanted to locate a healing yoga learning site specifically for patients with breast cancer because they were afraid that the instructor may not be aware of suitable types of healing yoga for them.

The other participants were concerned about whether the movements during healing yoga would cause injuries and whether the healing yoga was specifically designed for patients with breast cancer. For example, one participant stated, *"You can never be sure if body-mind yoga class is suitable for patients like us"* (Participant I) and another participant asked, *"Are they (instructors) aware of the types of movement that breast cancer patients are capable of?"* (Participant B). Therefore, several participants were afraid that yoga movements might injure the limbs on the side on which they were operated, causing them to refrain from performing some movements and preventing them from relaxing their bodies completely during the section of Shavasana yoga. After several classes, numerous participants reported that the healing yoga movements are safe to perform and thus gained trust in the instructor, enabling them to open their bodies and minds and

follow the instructor's tempo in performing deep meditation, relaxation, symptom relief, and stretching. One participant reported, *"I can achieve the movement based on instructions from the instructor"* (Participant C) and *"another participant stated, "The instructor does a wonderful job in guiding us in breathing and moving"* (Participant G). During yoga practice, the participants gradually acquired a sense of comfort in the learning site and yoga movements through the guidance of professional yoga instructors.

### Regaining a sense of belonging

Healing yoga can promote a calm awareness of the body, feelings, and mind by enabling participants to focus on the moment with openness, reducing their anxiety, fatigue and promoting a sense of calmness and relaxation. Factors that emerged from this category included a sense of control, recognizing self-value and support from others. Several participants indicated that the breathing exercises helped them increase their cognition and awareness. Participant J indicated that *"breathing control and relaxation enables me to consciously control my spine (for relaxing)."* Yoga meditation enabled the participants to obtain a sense of control over their bodies, release thoughts of unease, and develop their inner energy. Once the participants acquired control of their bodies, they began learning to focus on and value themselves. Participant G reported, *"I've started focusing on myself and valuing myself more. I did not care for myself so much in the past, but now I do."* The improved sense of control enabled participants to cope effectively with breast cancer, facilitating optimal psychosocial adjustment.

Two of the participants stated that, because all of the members had the same disease, they did not feel socially isolated, enabling them to share disease-related experiences with each other. *"It feels like everyone's heart is closely tied together"* (Participant F). Healing yoga provided the participants with a sense of belonging and the ability to inspire and encourage other people, enhancing the self-esteem of the participants and enabling them to overcome their personal problems and progress toward recovery.

*When I come here and see a lot of people, I do not feel lonely at all...We are all breast cancer patients...I think the support, the power of support becomes very strong. At least you do not feel as if you are fighting this (disease) alone and you know that there are a bunch of people just like you, trying to become better (Participant F).*

The release of emotions and feelings of care and attention may result not only from healing yoga but also from instructor support and companionship among members. Healing yoga alleviates stiffness. Numerous participants reported that healing yoga helped them relax.

### Gaining experience and satisfaction

Several of the participants experienced that healing yoga provides extensive benefits, including improved flexibility, strength, and concentration. The subcategories of this theme are alleviating symptoms, improving flexibility, negative experience and satisfaction with the hospital. The health benefits associated with healing yoga reported by the participants included improved flexibility, increased strength, improved sleep, reduced depression, and a healthy appetite. Participant K said, *"It helped reduce my tiredness and relieve feelings of depression!"* Participant G said, *"I used to have trouble sleeping and now I use meditation to concentrate and relax, which, in turn, helps me get truly restful sleep. I am so thankful for it. "*

Numerous participants reported that healing yoga helped them relax tension, tension, improve flexibility, and ease stiff muscles in the back, hips, and legs. Participant F stated, "it loosened my neck, entire spine, and head. *I felt tense (before the class), but my entire body felt relaxed and very comfortable (after healing yoga)." "I used to feel stiff in my tendons, but I have not experienced this problem since participating in these 8 weeks haling healing yoga classes,"* stated Participant J. Participant G happily announced *"after sweating, the arm that was operated on is less swollen."* Participant D stated, *"I do not feel as tight as usual."* Several participants felt bodily changes of tension to relaxation, decreased swelling of the limbs, and alleviation of pain.

The participants also described negative experiences, including muscle ache, nausea, and concern about their ability to maintain progress in healing yoga. Participant B reported, *"My back pain may be caused by doing too much yoga."* Participant A stated, *"At the beginning, I had muscle pain...the pain was pretty severe."* Some participants expressed a fear of being late and that it may cause difficulty in following the instructor. *"When I was driving to yoga class, I was afraid that I would be late and would miss some moves,"* reported Participant I.

Several participants expressed appreciation to the hospital for providing this service to them and gave a high rating of overall satisfaction with healing yoga. Participant E stated, *"I feel so thankful and my heart is full of gratitude. I thank the hospital for taking care of our bodies and health after surgery and this has made the hospital become such a warm place."*

Ten of the participants reported a decrease in symptom distress, increase in flexibility, and relaxation of the mind and body attributable to the healing yoga. Although some of them experienced negative symptoms caused by healing yoga at the beginning, they continually participated in the 8 weeks healing yoga program until the end. In addition, the hospital not only attracted the participants but also attracted the employees because of the participants' support and satisfaction.

### Leading the way for life

Healing yoga helped nine participants change their perspectives on life. They learned to disregard all trivial matters, treat themselves well and re-evaluate their self-value. The participants recalled that they rarely slowed down to relax and that the pace of everyday life was fast. Participant G reported, *"I used to think about nothing but making money...every day. Now I know that I should live for myself...all my confidence has come from yoga!"* Healing yoga enabled them to learn to increase their awareness and value themselves, causing them to feel happy and carefree. Participant J reported, "When you exercise, your thoughts tend to be more positive and cheerful." "I feel very happy and confident, and it (yoga) makes me realize that this is just what I want," explained Participant F. After experiencing relief from the pain and suffering of illness, the participants gradually regained confidence in the process of exercising. This was indicated by Participant G:

*My emotions have changed so much, and now I have begun thinking in a positive way. I do yoga every day now because I have started to focus on myself and value myself more. I did not take care of myself enough in the past, but now I do.*

Through exercise, the participants learned to manage situations with a calm and positive mind, enabling them to regain confidence, identify goals in life, and live their own lives in a meaningful manner. Six participants stated that they did not have regular exercise habits before they participated in the healing yoga program. After 8 weeks of haling healing yoga, it became part of their lives. Participant C proudly stated, *"I do yoga regularly on my own now and I feel more relaxed after yoga; it is like I depend on it."* This was supported by Participant G: *"It (yoga) becomes a thing I must do now...like I am dependent on it."* Throughout the 8 weeks healing yoga practice, a habit of regular exercise was gradually established, and healing yoga became an interesting and essential event in the lives of the participants.

## Discussion

The 8 weeks healing yoga combined postures, breathing techniques, and meditation to help participants make a difference in their lives through apprehension, camaraderie, involvement, and transformation. Patients with breast cancer often have little information on physical activities suitable for post-surgery exercise and are concerned that exercise may cause them harm, reinjures, and side effects. Therefore, they are hesitant to perform physical exercise. Another reason may be concern that health care professionals do not actively provide patients with post-surgery exercise plans. This explains why the participants in this study avoided physical activity before they participated in the healing yoga. However, the participants felt comfortable with the yoga postures and gradually began to trust the yoga instructor, express their approval and provide positive feedback. The results indicate that most participants seen to find the program beneficial and expressed feelings of reduced distress symptoms both during and after the completion of the program.

The techniques of breathing control and meditation in healing yoga are based on the mindfulness theory [16,17]. The techniques stimulate the arousal systems in the brain, including the brain-stem reticular activating system, which is a core sleep-energy center and part of the subcortical-cortical arousal axis controlling energy distribution in the brain and body [8-10]. The benefits of the techniques are a decrease in fatigue and increase in sleep latency and well-being. Mindfulness affects a person's self-consciousness, integrative awareness and attention [16,17]. The participants experienced greater control over their bodies after performing the breathing exercise because they focused on their bodies and minds, enabling them to gain a clear awareness of their inner and outer worlds and to relax completely both physically and spiritually. This finding is consistent with Mackenzie et al. [18] studies.

The participants shared a supportive and positive environment because of the benefits of exercises and felt cared for and valued because of both cancer survivorship and therapeutic relationships. Receiving support from other trial participants heavily influenced the participants' experience with healing yoga because it enabled them to share useful information, encourage one another and provide emotional catharsis. This created a sense of connection among the participants, enabling them to express thoughts and feelings about how to cope with a stressful life and live with breast cancer [19].

Numerous participants practiced healing yoga independently and frequently because they experienced increased flexibility, alleviation of physical symptoms, and improved body function. The participants reported that previous problems, such as amnesia, headaches, tightness, pain in the limbs, swollen limbs, and fatigue were alleviated. This is consistent with the results of other yoga studies that reported reduced pain, anxiety and swelling; increased energy, flexibility, and physical function; a sense of control; feelings of comfort and relaxation; and the ability to maintain self-control [20-22]. In particularly, a previous study reported that the participants who provided positive feedback on healing yoga stated that it enabled them to enjoy the exercise process [20]. However, three participants reported negative experiences caused by healing yoga, such as muscle ache, pain, nausea, and concern about missing sessions or not being punctual. Similar results were obtained by Kvillemo and Branstrom [20], who indicated that two patients reported problems with stiffness and back pain. Nevertheless, most of the participants were grateful that the hospital provided this yoga program, which increased their satisfaction with the overall treatment.

Healing yoga helped the participants transform feelings of passivity into activity to cope with their illness. Previous studies have indicated that participants learned to focus on positive thinking, learned how to forgive, and found meaning in their lives [6,22]. Our study revealed that most participants learned to slow the pace of everyday life, redirect their thoughts to positive aspects, and value themselves as a first priority. Through this program, the participants gradually regained confidence and perceived a new sense of control over their well-being. As the results, the healing yoga seemed to help patients with breast cancer focus their attention on their bodies and renew awareness to their inner and outer well-being. Further qualitative research should focus on understanding the perceived differences between group yoga and individual yoga or should compare yoga with other exercises.

## Limitations

A weakness in this study was that only 11 of 30 possible interviewees (these randomized into the intervention group). This could be a result of the fact that the interview was a voluntary additional part of the experimental study. It is possible that those who decided to participate in the interviews were more positive to the healing yoga than those who declined. A difficulty with interview study

is that the questions can be biasing the answers and influence the responses collected. The participants' knowledge about the expected effect of the healing yoga can also influence both the experience of the interview and the interview responses.

## Implications for Practice

Based on the positive experiences of the patients with breast cancer who participated in the healing yoga, health care professionals should consider implementing healing yoga in clinical practice and nursing education. Although individuals may suffer different conditions and symptoms from chemotherapy, the improvements in the neurobiological changes due to healing yoga can have implications in mood, anxiety, fatigue and an over-all sense of well-being among clinical populations. Especially, these improvements in a sense of well-being remain a universal demand. We suggest that healing yoga be a complementary therapy for clinical practice in oncology. Future studies should investigate the importance of following elements on the influence of the healing yoga, such as reflections on patients' education level, religion, treatment how these factors influence on the patients' own perceptions; reflections on the intensity, frequency and duration of yoga program how it can the patients' perception of fatigue. The findings of this study provide as a reference for nursing education, research design, and clinical practice that can be applied in healing yoga schemes for cancer patients. The format and the amount of time required by the participants make this intervention most suitable for highly motivated participants with interest in the use of mind-body-spiritual relaxation techniques.

## Conclusion

This study gained insight into patients with breast cancer through process of healing yoga. Four themes emerged from the data: transforming from concern to confidence; regaining a sense of belonging; receiving experience and satisfaction; and leading the way for life. Participants expressed positive experiences both of participating in the healing yoga and of the perceived effect of the healing yoga. Moreover, the participants perceived the healing yoga approach to exert a crucial influence on fatigued breast cancer patients. This includes a suitable support level of personal challenge. The study findings strengthen the experience of healing yoga to support the long-term needs of breast cancer patients. However, this study provides insight into the remarkable changes in the bodies and mind of breast cancer patients, as well as the perspectives, beliefs, values and life lessons that they gained through healing yoga.

## References

1.  Health Organization (2011) The World Health Report 2011. Media centre, World Health Organization.

2.  Denduluri N, Somerfield MR, Wolff AC (2016) Selection of optimal adjuvant chemotherapy regimens for early breast cancer and adjuvant targeted therapy for her2-positive breast cancers: an American society of clinical oncology guideline adaptation of the cancer care Ontario clinical practice guideline summary. J Oncol Pract 12: 485-488.

3.  Lorusso D, Bria E, Costantini A, Di Maio M, Rosti G, et al. (2017) Patients' perception of chemotherapy side effects: Expectations, doctor-patient communication and impact on quality of life - An Italian survey. Eur J Cancer Care. 26.

4.  Mortimer JE, Waliany S, Dieli-Conwright CM et al. (2017) Objective physical and mental markers of self-reported fatigue in women undergoing (neo)adjuvant chemotherapy for early-stage breast cancer. Cancer.

5.  Thompson P1 (2007) The relationship of fatigue and meaning in life in breast cancer survivors. Oncol Nurs Forum 34: 653-660.

6.  Leigh M, Roth E, Galvin D, Mary FB, Ellen H, et al. (2012) The impact of resistive exercise and psychosocial support on quality of life and fatigue in cancer survivors via utilization of a community-based program: A case series. Rehabil Oncol 30: 12-17.

7.  Noelia GC, Angelica AG, Irene CV, Carolina FL, Lourdes DR, et al. (2014) Depressed mood in breast cancer survivors: Associations with physical activity, cancer-related fatigue, quality of life and fitness level. Eur J Oncol Nurs 18: 206-210.

8.  Desai R, Tailor A, Bhatt T (2015) Effects of yoga on brain waves and structural activation: A review. Complement Ther Clin Pract 21: 112-118.

9.  Vialatte FB, Bakardjian H, Prasad R, Cichocki A (2009) EEG paroxysmal gamma waves during Bhramari Pranayama: A yoga breathing technique. Conscious Cogn 18: 977-988.

10. Field T, Diego M, Hernandez-Reif M (2010) Tai chi/yoga effects on anxiety, heart rate, EEG and math computations. Complement Ther Clin Pract 16: 235-238.

11. Chen SM, Lin WL, Lin SH, Chang HY (2011) Cancer nursing care: A systematic review of yoga intervention. J Nurs Healthc Res 7: 151-160.

12. Jacquelyn B, Holly W, Mel H, Sally B, Robert B (2011) Effect of Iyengar yoga practice on fatigue and diurnal salivary cortisol concentration in breast cancer survivors. J Am Acad Nurse Pract 23: 135-142.

13. Taso CJ, Lin HS, Lin WL, Chen SM, Huang WT, et al. (2014) The effect of healing yoga on improving depression, anxiety and fatigue in women with breast cancer: A randomized controlled trial. J Nurs Res 22: 155-164.

14. Erlandson DA (1993) Doing naturalistic inquiry: A guide to methods. Newbury Park, Sage, California.

15. Holtby L (2004) Healing yoga for people living with cancer, Taylor Trade Publishing, USA.

16. Brown KW, Ryan RM, Creswell JD (2007) Mindfulness: Theoretical foundations and evidence for its salutary effects. Psychol Inq 18: 211-237.

17. Lindsay EK, Creswell JD (2017) Mechanisms of mindfulness training: Monitor and acceptance theory (MAT). Clin Psychol Rev 51: 48-59.

18. Mackenzie MJ, Wurz AJ, Yamauchi Y, Pires LA, Culos-Reed SN (2016) Yoga helps put the pieces back together: a qualitative exploration of a community-based yoga program for cancer survivors. Evid Based Complement Alternat Med 2016: 1832515.

19. Fiori F, Aglioti SM, David N (2017) Interactions between body and social awareness in yoga. J Altern Complement Med 23: 227-233.

20. Kvillemo P, Bränström R (2011) Experiences of a mindfulness-based stress-reduction intervention among patients with cancer. Cancer Nurs 34: 24-31.

21. Pan Y, Yang K, Wang Y, Zhang L, Liang H (2017) Could yoga practice improve treatment-related side effects and quality of life for women with breast cancer? A systematic review and meta-analysis. Asia Pac J Clin Oncol 13: e79-e95.

22. Greysen HM, Greysen SR, Lee KA, Hong OS, Katz P, et al. (2017) A qualitative study exploring community yoga practice in adults with rheumatoid arthritis. J Altern Complement Med.

# Permissions

# List of Contributors

**John J Power, Johanna McMullan and Tony O'Connor**
School of Nursing and Midwifery, Queen's University Belfast, Ireland

**Dessalegn Haile, Tenaw Gualu and Haymanot Zeleke**
Department of Nursing, College of Health Sciences, Debre Markos University, Debre Markos, Ethiopia

**Berhanu Dessalegn**
Department of Nursing and Midwifery, College of Health Sciences, School of Allied Health Sciences, Addis Ababa University, Addis Ababa, Ethiopia

**Poonam Sheoran, Manisha Rani, Yogesh Kumar and Navjyot Singh**
M.M. Institute of Nursing, Mullana, Ambala, India

**Sukhpal Kaur, Anoop Kumar K.P, Baljeet Kaur, Bhawana Rani, Sandhya Ghai and Monaliza Singla**
National Institute of Nursing Education, Post Graduate Institute of Medical Education and Research, Chandigarh, India

**Hussen SH**
Department of Reproductive Health, Arba Minch University, Arba Minch, Ethiopia

**Estifanos WM and Moga FE**
Department of Nursing, Arba Minch University, Arba Minch, Ethiopia

**Melese ES**
Department of Statistics, Arba Minch University, Arba Minch, Ethiopia

**Philip Onuoha, Denis Isreal-richardson, Lu-Ann Caesar and Chidum Ezenwaka**
The Diabetes & Metabolism Research Group (DMRG), Faculty of Medical Sciences, The University of the West Indies, St Augustine Campus, Trinidad and Tobago

**Michiko Moriyama**
Institute of Biomedical & Health Sciences, Hiroshima University, Japan

**Cris Renata Grou Volpe, Diana Lucia Moura Pinho, Marina Morato Stival Lima, Walterlânia Silva Santos, Tania Cristina Santa Barbara Rehen and Silvana S Funghetto**
Universidade de Brasilia, Brazil

**Reena Thakur**
Kol Vally Institute of Nursing, India

**Rajesh Kumar Sharma, Laxmi Kumar and Sanchita Pugazhendi**
Swami Rama Himalayan University, India

**Maan Hameed Ibrahim Al-Ameri**
Psychiatric Mental Health Nursing Department, College of Nursing/ University of Baghdad, Iraq

**Nadia Mohamed Taha, Howida Kameel Zatton and Hala Ibrahem Zatton**
Department of Medical Surgical Nursing, Faculty of Nursing Zagazig University, Zagazig, Egypt

**Louise Tourigny**
University of Wisconsin-Whitewater, Whitewater, USA

**Vishwanath V Baba**
McMaster University, Hamilton, ON, Canada

**Terri Lituchy**
CETYS Universidad, Mexico

**Dorah Ursula Ramathuba**
Department of Nursing, University of Venda, South Africa
Tshilidzini Hospital, Department of Health, South Africa

**Ramutumbu Neo Jacqueline and Ndou ND**
Department of Nursing, University of Venda, South Africa

**Vitoria H Maciel Coelho**
Federal University of Triângulo Mineiro, Department of Physiotherapy, Uberaba-MG, Brazil

**Luiza D Alvares**
UNICEP, Physiotherapy Faculty, Miguel Petroni, Sao Carlos-SP, Brazil

**Fernanda M Carbinatto, Antonio E de Aquino Junior, Dora Patricia Ramirez Angarita and Vanderlei S Bagnato**
Sao Carlos Institute of Physics, University of São Paulo, Sao Carlos-SP, Brazil

**Bisrat Hailemeskel, Imbi Drame, Min Choi and Pawvana Pansiri**
College of Pharmacy, Howard University, Silver Spring, USA

**Ayanos Taye**
Department of Nursing, College of Health Sciences, Jimma University, Ethiopia

**Iyobe Asmare**
Department of Nursing, College of Health Sciences, Debreberhan University, Ethiopia

**Jan Johansson Hanse**
Nordic School of Public Health NHV, Sweden
Department of Psychology, University of Gothenburg, Sweden

**Ulrika Harlin**
Swerea IVF, Mölndal, Sweden

**Caroline Jarebrant**
Swerea IVF, Mölndal, Sweden
Department of Sociology and Work Science, University of Gothenburg, Sweden

**Kerstin Ulin**
Institute of Health and Care Science, Sahlgrenska Academy, University of Gothenburg, Sweden
Sahlgrenska University Hospital, Gothenburg, Sweden

**Jörgen Winkel**
Department of Management Engineering, Technical University of Denmark, Denmark
Department of Sociology and Work Science, University of Gothenburg, Sweden

**Shu-Ming Chen and Huey-Shyan Lin**
Fooyin University, Kaohsiung city, Taiwan

**Mary Beth Maguire, Marie N Bremner and Daniel J. Yanosky**
Kennesaw State University, Kennesaw, United States

**Phyllis Montgomery, Denise Newton-Mathur, Sarah Benbow and Sharolyn Mossey**
School of Nursing, Ramsey Lake Road, Laurentian University, Sudbury, Ontario, Canada

**Laura Hall**
York University, 4700 Keele St., Toronto, Ontario, Canada

**Cheryl Forchuk**
Arthur Labatt Family School of Nursing, Lawson Health Research Institute, 1151, Richmond Street, Western University, London, Ontario, Canada

**Fase Badriah**
Syarif Hidayatullah Islamic State University, Faculty of Medicine and Health Sciences, Department of Public Health, Indonesia

**Takeru Abe**
Waseda University, Faculty of Human Sciences, Department of Health Sciences and Social Welfare, Saitama, Japan

**Baequni**
Syarif Hidayatullah Islamic State University, Faculty of Medicine and Health Sciences, Department of Public Health, Indonesia
Osaka University, School of Human Science, Department of International Collaboration, Osaka, Japan

**Akihito Hagihara**
Osaka University, School of Human Science, Department of International Collaboration, Osaka, Japan

**Fukuoka, Japan Zeljko Vlaisavljević and Ivan Rankovic**
University of Mississippi Clinical Centre of Serbia, Clinic for Gastroenterolgy and Hepatology, Street of Dr Koste Todorovica 2, 11 000 Belgrade, Serbia

**Annette Burgess**
Education Office, Sydney Medical School, The University of Sydney, Sydney, NSW, Australia

**Heather Jeffery**
School of Public Health, Sydney Medical School, The University of Sydney, Sydney, NSW, Australia

**Shinetugs Bayanbileg**
United Nations Population Fund, Mongolia

**Erdenekhuu Nansalmaa**
Education, Policy and Management, Mongolian National University of Medical Sciences, Mongolia

**Kirsten Black**
Sydney Medical School – Central, The University of Sydney, Sydney, NSW, Australia

**Kathleen Bradshaw LaSala**
University Of South Carolina, USA

**Karen Gorton**
University of Colorado Anschutz Medical Campus, USA

**Frilund Marianne**
Faculty of Medicine and Health Sciences, NTNU University, Aalesund, Norway

**Lisbeth Maria Fagerstrom**
Department of Nursing Science, Drammen, Norway

**Ali Hamzah and Sugiyanto**
Bandung Nursing Department, Bandung Health Politechnic, Indonesia

**Li-Li Xiang**
Physical examination center, Taihe Hospital, Hubei University of Medicine, Shiyan, Hubei, China

**Duo-Shuang Xie**
Department of Infection Control, Taihe Hospital, Hubei University of Medicine, Shiyan, Hubei, China Center of Health Administration and Development studies, Hubei University of Medicine, Shiyan, Hubei, China

**Rui Li, Xiang-Yun Fu, Hui-Fang Wang, Qiao Hu, Qin-Qing Luo, Rui-Ping Lai and Han-Lin Liao**
Department of Infection Control, Taihe Hospital, Hubei University of Medicine, Shiyan, Hubei, China

**Lei Wang**
Hospital Administration Office, Taihe Hospital, Hubei University of Medicine, Shiyan, Hubei, China

**Soon Min, Yun-Ju Ha, Jung-Hwa Kang and Hee-Young Kang**
Chosun University, Gwangju, Korea, Republic of Korea

**Anna E Van den Heever**
University of the Witwatersrand, South Africa

**Judith Kutzleb, Nancy Elmann, Andrew Fruhschien, Stephen Angeli, Angel Mulkay, Jarrett Bauer, Rohan Udeshi and Dan Priece**
Advanced Practice Professionals at Holy Name Medical Center, 718 Teaneck Road, Teaneck, New Jersey, USA

**Erdaw Tachbele**
Department of Nursing and Midwifery, College of Health Sciences, Addis Ababa University, Ethiopia

**Biruhalem Taye**
Aklilu Lemma Institute of Pathobiology, Addis Ababa University, Addis Ababa, Ethiopia

**Begna Tulu and Gobena Ameni**
Microbiology, Immunology and Parasitology Department, Bahir Dar University, Ethiopia

**Anne Kuusisto**
Satakunta Hospital District, 28500 Pori, Finland

**Pirkko Nykänen**
University of Tampere, School of Information Sciences, 33014 Tampere, Finland

**Johanna Kaipio**
Aalto University, School of Science, 00076 Aalto, Finland

**Daren Anderson, Khushbu Khatri and Mary Blankson**
Weitzman Institute, Community Health Center, Inc. Middletown, CT, USA

**Tudor Calinici**
Iuliu Hatieganu" University of Medicine and Pharmacy Cluj-Napoca, Romania

**Tarja Kvist**
University of Eastern Finland, Kuopio Campus, Department of Nursing Science, Finland

**Katja Tähkä**
Helsinki University Hospital, Finland

**Miia Ruotsalainen and Tarja Tervo-Heikkinen**
Kuopio University Hospital, Finland

**Batool Pouraboli**
School of Nursing and Midwifery, Department of Pediatric and Neonatal Nursing, Tehran University of Medical Sciences, Tehran, Iran

**Heidar Ali Abedi**
Department of Nursing, School of Nursing and Midwifery, Khorasgan (Isfahan) Branch, Islamic Azad University, Isfahan, Iran

**Abbas Abbaszadeh**
School of Nursing and Midwifery, Shahid beheshti University of Medical Sciences, Tehran, Iran

**Majid Kazemi**
School of Nursing and Midwifery, Rafsanjan University of Medical Sciences, Rafsanjan, Iran

**Hsiao-Yun Chang, Shu-Ming Chen and Wen-Li Lin**
Department of Nursing, Fooyin University, Taiwan

# Index

* 9 7 8 1 6 3 2 4 1 5 4 1 7 *